**NINTH EDITION**

# LANGE Q&A™

# OBSTETRICS & GYNECOLOGY

**Vern L. Katz, MD**
Clinical Professor
Department of Obstetrics and Gynecology
Oregon Health Science University
Medical Director, Perinatal Services
Sacred Heart Medical Center
Eugene, Oregon

**Sharon Phelan, MD**
Professor of Obstetrics & Gynecology
School of Medicine
Department of Obstetrics and Gynecology
University of New Mexico
Albuquerque, New Mexico

**Vicki Mendiratta, MD**
Associate Professor
Department of Obstetrics and Gynecology
University of Washington School of Medicine
Seattle, Washington

**Roger P. Smith, MD**
The Robert A. Munsick Professor of Clinical
Obstetrics & Gynecology
Director, Medical Student Education
Director, Division of General Obstetrics &
Gynecology
Department of Obstetrics and Gynecology
Indiana University School of Medicine
Indianapolis, Indiana

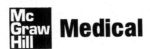
**Medical**

New York   Chicago   San Francisco   Lisbon   London   Madrid   Mexico City
Milan   New Delhi   San Juan   Seoul   Singapore   Sydney   Toronto

**Lange Q&A™: Obstetrics & Gynecology, Ninth Edition**

1 2 3 4 5 6 7 8 9 0 QDB/QDB 15 14 13 12 11

ISBN 978-0-07-171213-2
MHID 0-07-171213-5

---

## Notice

Medicine is an ever-changing science. As new research and clinical experience broaden our knowledge, changes in treatment and drug therapy are required. The authors and the publisher of this work have checked with sources believed to be reliable in their efforts to provide information that is complete and generally in accord with the standards accepted at the time of publication. However, in view of the possibility of human error or changes in medical sciences, neither the authors nor the publisher nor any other party who has been involved in the preparation or publication of this work warrants that the information contained herein is in every respect accurate or complete, and they disclaim all responsibility for any errors or omissions or for the results obtained from use of the information contained in this work. Readers are encouraged to confirm the information contained herein with other sources. For example and in particular, readers are advised to check the product information sheet included in the package of each drug they plan to administer to be certain that the information contained in this work is accurate and that changes have not been made in the recommended dose or in the contraindications for administration. This recommendation is of particular importance in connection with new or infrequently used drugs.

---

This book was set in Palatino by Aptara, Inc.
The editors were Kirsten Funk and Christine Diedrich.
The production supervisor was Catherine Saggese.
Project management was provided by Shikha Sharma, Aptara, Inc.
Quad/Graphics was printer and binder.

This book is printed on acid-free paper.

**Library of Congress Cataloging-in-Publication Data**

Lange Q & A. Obstetrics & gynecology / Sharon Phelan . . . [et al.]. – 9th ed.
     p. ; cm.
   Lange Q and A. Obstetrics & gynecology
   Obstetrics & gynecology
   Includes bibliographical references and index.
   Summary: More than 1400 exam-style Q&A deliver an unbeatable review of obstetrics and gynecology for the USMLE Step 2 CK and shelf exam Covers the clerkship's core competencies LANGE Q&A Obstetrics & Gynecology, 9th ed. features more than 1400 USMLE-style questions and answers with concise but comprehensive explanations of correct and incorrect answer choices. This trusted review simulates the USMLE Step 2 CK test-taking experience by including 100% clinical vignette questions and updates on the latest in obstetric and gynecologic treatment, therapies, diseases and disorders. Questions are carefully selected to match the style and difficulty level of what students will see on the actual exams. The ninth edition features more than 35 images and is student tested and reviewed to assure the most relevant, up-to-date content possible. The content you need to ace the exam"–Provided by publisher.
   ISBN-13: 978-0-07-171213-2 (pbk. : alk. paper)
   ISBN-10: 0-07-171213-5 (pbk. : alk. paper)
   1. Gynecology—Examinations, questions, etc.   2. Obstetrics—Examinations, questions, etc.   I. Phelan, Sharon T.
II. Title: Lange Q and A. Obstetrics & gynecology.   III. Title: Obstetrics & gynecology.
   [DNLM: 1. Genital Diseases, Female–Examination Questions.   2. Obstetrics–Examination Questions. WS 18.2]
   RG111.V66 2011
   618.076–dc22                                                                 2011005064

McGraw-Hill books are available at special quantity discounts to use as premiums and sales promotions, or for use in corporate training programs. To contact a representative, please e-mail us at bulksales@mcgraw-hill.com.

# Contents

# Student Reviewers

**Adam Darnobid, MD**
Resident Physician
UMass Memorial Medical Center
Worcester, Massachusetts
Class of 2009

**Barrett Little**
Temple University
School of Medicine
Philadelphia, Pennsylvania
Class of 2010

**Radhika Lu Sundararajan**
New York University
School of Medicine
New York, New York
Class of 2010

# Preface

*Education is the kindling of a flame, not the filling of a vessel.*
*—Socrates*

The ninth edition of *Lange Q&A: Obstetrics and Gynecology* book has been written, as were the prior editions, to be a study aid for self-examination and review in the field of obstetrics and gynecology. Each chapter has been updated with new questions written to cover new information. These encompass new areas in the field, updates in other areas, and some of the new clinical guidelines from national organizations.

The questions are designed to review many topics commonly covered in tests such as the clerkship examination and United States Medical Licensing Examination (USMLE) Step 2 CK. The style and presentation of the questions have been fully revised to conform with the USMLE. This will enable readers to familiarize themselves with the types of questions to be expected and practice answering questions in each board format used in the actual examination. The majority of questions are multiple-choice one best answer–single-item questions. For these questions, you will choose the **one best** response to the question. Some questions are matching sets consisting of a group of questions preceded by a list of lettered options. For these questions you will select **one** lettered option that is **most** closely associated with the question. In some cases, a group of two or three questions may be related to one patient situation. These questions—often called second- or third-order questions—will require you to think through the entire set of questions to reach the correct answers in the patient scenario. Since the USMLE seems to prefer questions requiring judgment and critical thinking, we have attempted to emphasize these questions. In addition, some questions have images that require understanding and interpretation to reach the correct answer.

Each chapter of this book presents questions covering important topics in the obstetrics and gynecology specialty. The question sections are followed by a section containing the answers and explanations. These answer sections provide background information on the subject matter and discuss the various issues raised by the question and its answer. After answering a question, we encourage you to review the explanations further—even if you have answered the question correctly—to enhance your study and understanding. These explanations will often discuss not only why one answer is correct, but also why the other choices are incorrect. This reinforces your knowledge and provides feedback to guide further study.

At the end of the book we have included a practice test that contains randomly ordered questions of all styles covering all the topics. This test is designed to more closely approximate the form of the USMLE Step 2 CK examination. An answer and comment section follows the practice test and relates to the questions contained in it.

We hope that using this review will help you consolidate your knowledge, evaluate your capabilities, and motivate you to continually expand your horizons to levels far beyond this study aid.

# Abbreviations

| | | | |
|---|---|---|---|
| **ABH:** | A and B are blood antigens; H is the substrate from which they are formed. | **G6 PD:** | glucose-6-dehydrogenase deficiency |
| **ACTH:** | adrenocorticotropic hormone | **GH:** | growth hormone |
| **ADH:** | antidiuretic hormone | **GI:** | gastrointestinal |
| **AFP:** | alpha$_1$ fetoprotein | **GU:** | genitourinary |
| **AP:** | anteroposterior | **Hb A:** | adult hemoglobin |
| **ATN:** | acute tubular necrosis | **Hb F:** | fetal hemoglobin |
| **B:** | basophils | **HCG:** | human chorionic gonadotropin |
| **BMR:** | basal metabolic rate | **HCS:** | human chorionic somatomammotropin |
| **BP:** | blood pressure | **Hct:** | hematocrit |
| **BSO:** | bilateral salpingo-oophorectomy | **H&E:** | hematoxylin and eosin (stain) |
| **BSU:** | Bartholin, Skene's, and urethral glands | **HLA:** | histocompatibility locus antigen |
| **CAH:** | congenital adrenal hyperplasia | **HPF:** | hepatic plasma flow |
| **CHD:** | congenital heart disease | **HPV:** | human papilloma virus |
| **CHF:** | congestive heart failure | **ICSH:** | interstitial-cell stimulating hormone |
| **CIN:** | cervical intraepithelial neoplasia | **INH:** | isonicotinoylhydrazine |
| **CNS:** | central nervous system | **IRDS:** | infant respiratory distress syndrome |
| **CP:** | cerebral palsy | **IVP:** | intravenous pyelogram |
| **CPD:** | cephalic disproportion | **KUB:** | kidneys, ureters, & bladder |
| **CSF:** | cerebrospinal fluid | **L:** | lymphocytes |
| **CST:** | contraction stress test | **LE:** | lupus erythematosus |
| **D&C:** | dilation and curettage | **LH:** | luteinizing hormone |
| **DES:** | diethylstilbestrol | **LHRH:** | luteinizing hormone–releasing hormone |
| **DHEA:** | dehydroepiandrosterone | **LMP:** | last menstrual period |
| **DHEAS:** | dehydroepiandrosterone sulfate | **LMT:** | left mentotransverse |
| **DIC:** | disseminated intravascular coagulation | **LOA:** | left occipito-anterior |
| **E:** | eosinophils | **LOP:** | left occiput posterior |
| **E$^3$:** | estriol | **LOT:** | left occiput transverse |
| **EDC:** | estimated date of confinement | **L/S:** | lecithin/sphingomyelin |
| **ESR:** | erythrocyte sedimentation rate | **LSB:** | left sternal border |
| **EUA:** | examination under anesthesia | **LST:** | left sacrotransverse |
| **5-FU:** | 5-fluorouracil | **M:** | monocytes |
| **FHTs:** | fetal heart tones | **MCH:** | mean corpuscular hemoglobin |
| **FIGLU:** | formiminoglutamic acid | **MCHC:** | mean corpuscular hemoglobin concentration |
| **FIGO:** | International Federation of Gynecology and Obstetrics | **MCV:** | mean corpuscular volume |
| | | **MeV:** | mega electron volt |
| **FSH:** | follicle-stimulating hormone | **MF:** | menstrual formula |
| **FTA:** | fluorescent treponemal antibody (test) | **MI:** | maturation index |

| | | | | |
|---|---|---|---|---|
| **MIF:** | müllerian-inhibiting factor | | **ROP:** | right occipitoposterior |
| **mm:** | muscles | | **SGOT:** | serum glutamic-oxaloacetic transaminase |
| **MMK:** | Marshall–Marchetti–Krantz procedure | | **SLE:** | systemic lupus erythematosus |
| **NST:** | nonstress test | | **SRT:** | sacrum right transverse |
| **OA:** | occipito-anterior | | **SS:** | sickle cell anemia |
| **OCT:** | oxytocin challenge test | | **TAH:** | total abdominal hysterectomy |
| **OD:** | optical density | | **TB:** | tuberculosis |
| **OP:** | occiput posterior | | **TNM:** | tumor, node, metastasis |
| **OR:** | operating room | | **TRH:** | thyrotropin-releasing hormone |
| **P:** | plasma cells | | **TSH:** | thyroid-stimulating hormone |
| **PAS:** | para-aminosalicylic acid | | **UA:** | urinalysis |
| **PBI:** | protein-bound iodine | | **UPD:** | urinary production (rate) |
| **PG:** | prostaglandin | | **UTI:** | urinary tract infection |
| **PID:** | pelvic inflammatory disease | | **WBC:** | white blood cell count |
| **PIF:** | prolactin-inhibiting factor | | | |
| **PKU:** | phenylketonuria | | | |

# USMLE Step 2 CK Laboratory Values

| | REFERENCE RANGE | SI REFERENCE INTERVALS |
|---|---|---|
| **BLOOD, PLASMA, SERUM** | | |
| *Alanine aminotransferase (ALT), serum | 8–20 U/L | 8–20 U/L |
| Amylase, serum | 25–125 U/L | 25–125 U/L |
| *Aspartate aminotransferase (AST), serum | 8–20 U/L | 8–20 U/L |
| Bilirubin, serum (adult) Total // Direct | 0.1–1.0 mg/dL // 0.0–0.3 mg/dL | 2–17 $\mu$mol/L // 0–5 $\mu$mol/L |
| *Calcium, serum ($Ca^{2+}$) | 8.4–10.2 mg/dL | 2.1–2.8 mmol/L |
| *Cholesterol, serum | Rec: <200 mg/dL | <5.2 mmol/L |
| Cortisol, serum | 0800 h: 5–23 $\mu$g/dL // 1600 h: 3–15 $\mu$g/dL | 138–635 nmol/L // 82–413 nmol/L |
| | 2000 h: ≤50% of 0800 h | Fraction of 0800 h: ≤0.50 |
| Creatine kinase, serum | Male: 25–90 U/L | 25–90 U/L |
| | Female: 10–70 U/L | 10–70 U/L |
| *Creatinine, serum | 0.6–1.2 mg/dL | 53–106 $\mu$mol/L |
| Electrolytes, serum | | |
|   Sodium ($Na^+$) | 136–145 mEq/L | 136–145 mmol/L |
|   *Potassium ($K^+$) | 3.5–5.0 mEq/L | 3.5–5.0 mmol/L |
|   Chloride ($Cl^-$) | 95–105 mEq/L | 95–105 mmol/L |
|   Bicarbonate ($HCO_3$) | 22–28 mEq/L | 22–28 mmol/L |
|   Magnesium ($Mg^{2+}$) | 1.5–2.0 mEq/L | 0.75–1.0 mmol/L |
| Estriol, total, serum (in pregnancy) | | |
|   24–28 wks // 32–36 wks | 30–170 ng/mL // 60–280 ng/mL | 104–590 nmol/L // 208–970 nmol/L |
|   28–32 wks // 36–40 wks | 40–220 ng/mL // 80–350 ng/mL | 140–760 nmol/L // 280–1210 nmol/L |
| Ferritin, serum | Male: 15–200 ng/mL | 15–200 $\mu$g/L |
| | Female: 12–150 ng/mL | 12–150 $\mu$g/L |
| Follicle-stimulating hormone, serum/plasma | Male: 4–25 mIU/mL | 4–25 U/L |
| | Female: premenopause 4–30 mIU/mL | 4–30 U/L |
| |        midcycle peak 10–90 mIU/mL | 10–90 U/L |
| |        postmenopause 40–250 mIU/mL | 40–250 U/L |
| Gases, arterial blood (room air) | | |
|   pH | 7.35–7.45 | [$H^+$] 36–44 nmol/L |
|   $Pco_2$ | 33–45 mm Hg | 4.4–5.9 kPa |
|   $Po_2$ | 75–105 mm Hg | 10.0–14.0 kPa |
| *Glucose, serum | Fasting: 70–110 mg/dL | 3.8–6.1 mmol/L |
| | 2-h postprandial: <120 mg/dL | <6.6 mmol/L |
| Growth hormone—arginine stimulation | Fasting: <5 ng/mL | <5 $\mu$g/L |
| | provocative stimuli: >7 ng/mL | >7 $\mu$g/L |
| Immunoglobulins, serum | | |
|   IgA | 76–390 mg/dL | 0.76–3.90 g/L |
|   IgE | 0–380 IU/mL | 0–380 kIU/L |
|   IgG | 650–1,500 mg/dL | 6.5–15 g/L |
|   IgM | 40–345 mg/dL | 0.4–3.45 g/L |
| Iron | 50–170 $\mu$g/dL | 9–30 $\mu$mol/L |
| Lactate dehydrogenase, serum | 45–90 U/L | 45–90 U/L |
| Luteinizing hormone, serum/plasma | Male: 6–23 mIU/mL | 6–23 U/L |
| | Female: follicular phase 5–30 mIU/mL | 5–30 U/L |
| |        midcycle 75–150 mIU/mL | 75–150 U/L |
| |        postmenopause 30–200 mIU/mL | 30–200 U/L |
| Osmolality, serum | 275–295 mOsmol/kg $H_2O$ | 275–295 mOsmol/kg $H_2O$ |
| Parathyroid hormone, serum, N-terminal | 230–630 pg/mL | 230–630 ng/L |
| *Phosphatase (alkaline), serum (p-NPP at 30°C) | 20–70 U/L | 20–70 U/L |
| *Phosphorus (inorganic), serum | 3.0–4.5 mg/dL | 1.0–1.5 mmol/L |
| Prolactin, serum (hPRL) | <20 ng/mL | <20 $\mu$g/L |

(*continued*)

| | REFERENCE RANGE | SI REFERENCE INTERVALS |
|---|---|---|
| *Proteins, serum | | |
| Total (recumbent) | 6.0–7.8 g/dL | 60–78 g/L |
| Albumin | 3.5–5.5 g/dL | 35–55 g/L |
| Globulin | 2.3–3.5 g/dL | 23–35 g/L |
| Thyroid-stimulating hormone, serum or plasma | 0.5–5.0 μU/mL | 0.5–5.0 mU/L |
| Thyroidal iodine ($^{123}$I) uptake | 8%–30% of administered dose/24 h | 0.08–0.30/24 h |
| Thyroxine ($T_4$), serum | 5–12 μg/dL | 64–155 nmol/L |
| Triglycerides, serum | 35–160 mg/dL | 0.4–1.81 mmol/L |
| Triiodothyronine ($T_3$), serum (RIA) | 115–190 ng/dL | 1.8–2.9 nmol/L |
| Triiodothyronine ($T_3$) resin uptake | 25%–35% | 0.25–0.35 |
| *Urea nitrogen, serum | 7–18 mg/dL | 1.2–3.0 mmol/L |
| *Uric acid, serum | 3.0–8.2 mg/dL | 0.18–0.48 mmol/L |

### BODY MASS INDEX (BMI)

| | | |
|---|---|---|
| Body mass index | Adult: 19–25 kg/m$^2$ | |

### CEREBROSPINAL FLUID

| | | |
|---|---|---|
| Cell count | 0–5/mm$^3$ | 0–5 × 10$^6$/L |
| Chloride | 118–132 mEq/L | 118–132 mmol/L |
| Gamma globulin | 3%–12% total proteins | 0.03–0.12 |
| Glucose | 40–70 mg/dL | 2.2–3.9 mmol/L |
| Pressure | 70–180 mm $H_2O$ | 70–180 mm $H_2O$ |
| Proteins, total | <40 mg/dL | <0.40 g/L |

### HEMATOLOGIC

| | | |
|---|---|---|
| Bleeding time (template) | 2–7 minutes | 2–7 minutes |
| Erythrocyte count | Male: 4.3–5.9 million/mm$^3$ | 4.3–5.9 × 10$^{12}$/L |
| | Female: 3.5–5.5 million/mm$^3$ | 3.5–5.5 × 10$^{12}$/L |
| Erythrocyte sedimentation rate (Westergren) | Male: 0–15 mm/h | 0–15 mm/h |
| | Female: 0–20 mm/h | 0–20 mm/h |
| Hematocrit | Male: 41%–53% | 0.41–0.53 |
| | Female: 36%–46% | 0.36–0.46 |
| Hemoglobin $A_{1c}$ | ≤6% | ≤0.06 |
| Hemoglobin, blood | Male: 13.5–17.5 g/dL | 2.09–2.71 mmol/L |
| | Female: 12.0–16.0 g/dL | 1.86–2.48 mmol/L |
| Hemoglobin, plasma | 1–4 mg/dL | 0.16–0.62 mmol/L |
| Leukocyte count and differential | | |
| Leukocyte count | 4,500–11,000/mm$^3$ | 4.5–11.0 × 10$^9$/L |
| Segmented neutrophils | 54%–62% | 0.54–0.62 |
| Bands | 3%–5% | 0.03–0.05 |
| Eosinophils | 1%–3% | 0.01–0.03 |
| Basophils | 0%–0.75% | 0–0.0075 |
| Lymphocytes | 25%–33% | 0.25–0.33 |
| Monocytes | 3%–7% | 0.03–0.07 |
| Mean corpuscular hemoglobin | 25.4–34.6 pg/cell | 0.39–0.54 fmol/cell |
| Mean corpuscular hemoglobin concentration | 31%–36% Hb/cell | 4.81–5.58 mmol Hb/L |
| Mean corpuscular volume | 80–100 μm$^3$ | 80–100 fL |
| Partial thromboplastin time (activated) | 25–40 seconds | 25–40 seconds |
| Platelet count | 150,000–400,000/mm$^3$ | 150–400 × 10$^9$/L |
| Prothrombin time | 11–15 seconds | 11–15 seconds |
| Reticulocyte count | 0.5%–1.5% | 0.005–0.015 |
| Thrombin time | <2 seconds deviation from control | <2 seconds deviation from control |
| Volume | | |
| Plasma | Male: 25–43 mL/kg | 0.025–0.043 L/kg |
| | Female: 28–45 mL/kg | 0.028–0.045 L/kg |
| Red cell | Male: 20–36 mL/kg | 0.020–0.036 L/kg |
| | Female: 19–31 mL/kg | 0.019–0.031 L/kg |

### SWEAT

| | | |
|---|---|---|
| Chloride | 0–35 mmol/L | 0–35 mmol/L |

### URINE

| | | |
|---|---|---|
| Calcium | 100–300 mg/24 h | 2.5–7.5 mmol/24 h |
| Chloride | Varies with intake | Varies with intake |
| Creatinine clearance | Male: 97–137 mL/min | |
| | Female: 88–128 mL/min | |

*(continued)*

| | REFERENCE RANGE | SI REFERENCE INTERVALS |
|---|---|---|
| Estriol, total (in pregnancy) | | |
|   30 wks | 6–18 mg/24 h | 21–62 μmol/24 h |
|   35 wks | 9–28 mg/24 h | 31–97 μmol/24 h |
|   40 wks | 13–42 mg/24 h | 45–146 μmol/24 h |
| 17-Hydroxycorticosteroids | Male: 3.0–10.0 mg/24 h | 8.2–27.6 μmol/24 h |
| | Female: 2.0–8.0 mg/24 h | 5.5–22.0 μmol/24 h |
| 17-Ketosteroids, total | Male: 8–20 mg/24 h | 28–70 μmol/24 h |
| | Female: 6–15 mg/24 h | 21–52 μmol/24 h |
| Osmolality | 50–1400 mOsmol/kg $H_2O$ | |
| Oxalate | 8–40 μg/mL | 90–445 μmol/L |
| Potassium | Varies with diet | Varies with diet |
| Proteins, total | <150 mg/24 h | <0.15 g/24 h |
| Sodium | Varies with diet | Varies with diet |
| Uric acid | Varies with diet | Varies with diet |

*Included in the Biochemical Profile (SMA-12).

# CHAPTER 1

# Anatomy

## Questions

**DIRECTIONS (Questions 1 through 35): For each of the multiple choice questions in this section, select the lettered answer that is the one *best* response in each case.**

1. A healthy 5 ft 6 in. tall, adult female is most likely to have a pelvic inlet that would be classified as which of the following Caldwell–Moloy types?

   (A) android
   (B) platypelloid
   (C) anthropoid
   (D) gynecoid
   (E) triangular

2. Hernias occur more commonly in men than in women beneath the thickened lower margin of a fascial aponeurosis extending from the pubic tubercle to the anterior superior iliac spine. This thickened fascia is called which of the following?

   (A) inguinal ligament
   (B) Cooper's ligament
   (C) linea alba
   (D) posterior rectus sheath
   (E) round ligament

3. The inguinal canal in an adult female was opened surgically. Which of the following structures would normally be found?

   (A) a cyst of the canal of Nuck
   (B) Gartner's duct cyst
   (C) Cooper's ligament
   (D) the round ligament and the ilioinguinal nerve
   (E) the pyramidalis muscle

4. The human pelvis is a complex structure that permits upright posture and being capable with childbirth despite the relatively large fetal head. Which option includes all of the bones that make up the pelivs?

   (A) trochanter, hip socket, ischium, sacrum, and pubis
   (B) ilium, ischium, pubis, sacrum, and coccyx
   (C) ilium, ischium, and pubis
   (D) sacrum, ischium, ilium, and pubis
   (E) trochanter, sacrum, coccyx, ilium, and pubis

5. During normal delivery, an infant must pass through the maternal true pelvis. Which of the following most accurately describes the characteristics of the true pelvis?

   (A) It has an oval outlet.
   (B) It has three defining planes: an inlet, a midplane, and an outlet.
   (C) It has an inlet made up of a double triangle.
   (D) It is completely formed by two fused bones.
   (E) It lies between the wings of the paired ileum.

6. The part of the pelvis lying above the linea terminalis has little effect on a woman's ability to deliver a baby vaginally. What is the name of this portion of the pelvis?

   (A) true pelvis
   (B) midplane
   (C) outlet
   (D) false pelvis
   (E) sacrum

7. The plane from the sacral promontory to the inner posterior surface of the pubic symphysis is an important dimension of the pelvis for normal delivery. What is the name of this plane?

   (A) true conjugate
   (B) obstetric conjugate
   (C) diagonal conjugate
   (D) bi-ischial diameter
   (E) oblique diameter

8. During an operation, a midline incision was made at an anatomic location 2 cm below the umbilicus. Which of the following lists (in order) the layers of the anterior abdominal wall as they would be incised or separated?

   (A) skin, subcutaneous fat, superficial fascia (Camper's), deep fascia (Scarpa's), fascial muscle cover (anterior rectus sheath), rectus muscle, a deep fascial muscle cover (posterior rectus sheath), preperitoneal fat, and peritoneum
   (B) skin, subcutaneous fat, superficial fascia (Scarpa's), deep fascia (Camper's), fascial muscle covering (anterior abdominal sheath), transverse abdominal muscle, a deep fascial muscle cover (posterior rectus sheath), preperitoneal fat, and peritoneum
   (C) skin, subcutaneous fat, superficial fascia (Camper's), deep fascia (Scarpa's), fascial muscle cover (anterior rectus sheath), rectus muscle, a deep fascial muscle cover (posterior rectus sheath), peritoneum, and preperitoneal fat

   (D) skin, subcutaneous fat, superficial fascia (Scarpa's), deep fascia (Camper's), fascial muscle cover (anterior rectus sheath), rectus muscle, a deep fascial muscle cover (posterior rectus sheath), preperitoneal fat, and peritoneum
   (E) skin, subcutaneous fat, superficial fascia (Camper's), deep fascia (Scarpa's), fascial muscle cover (anterior rectus sheath), transverse abdominal muscle, a deep fascial muscle covering (posterior rectus sheath), preperitoneal fat, and peritoneum

9. Under the influence of relaxin and the pressure of pregnancy the junction between the two pubic bones may become unstable near the time of delivery. This will result in a waddling gait in the woman to minimize discomfort. What is this junction called?

   (A) sacroiliac joint
   (B) symphysis
   (C) sacrococcygeal joint
   (D) piriformis
   (E) intervertebral joint

10. The shape of the escutcheon may change with masculinization. The presence of a male escutcheon in a female is one of the clinical signs of hirsutism or increased testosterone. What is the usual shape of the escutcheon in the normal female?

    (A) diamond shaped
    (B) triangular
    (C) oval
    (D) circular
    (E) heart shaped

11. During the performance of a pelvic examination, the area of the Bartholin's ducts should be inspected. Where do the Bartholin's glands' ducts open?

    (A) into the midline of the posterior fourchette
    (B) bilaterally, beneath the urethra
    (C) bilaterally, on the inner surface of the labia majora

(D) bilaterally, into the posterior vaginal vestibule

(E) bilaterally, approximately 1 cm lateral to the clitoris

12. During a physical examination myrtiform caruncles may be noted. What are they?

(A) circumferential nodules in the areola of the breast

(B) healing Bartholin's cysts

(C) remnants of the Wolffian duct

(D) remnants of the hymen

(E) remnants of the Müllerian duct

13. The clitoris is a major sensory sexual organ. Where does it get its major nerve supply from?

(A) lumbar spinal nerve

(B) pudendal nerve

(C) femoral nerve

(D) ilioinguinal nerve

(E) anterior gluteal nerve

14. In the uterus of a normal female infant, what is the size relationship of the cervix, isthmus, and fundus?

(A) The cervix is larger than the fundus.

(B) The isthmus is longer than either the cervix or the fundus.

(C) They are of equal size.

(D) The fundus is the largest portion.

(E) The cervix is smaller than either the isthmus or the fundus.

15. How do nabothian cysts occur?

(A) Wolffian duct remnants

(B) blockage of crypts in the uterine cervix

(C) squamous cell debris that causes cervical irritation

(D) carcinoma

(E) paramesonephric remnants

16. What is the uterine corpus mainly composed of?

(A) fibrous tissue

(B) estrogen receptors

(C) smooth muscle

(D) elastic tissue

(E) endometrium

17. The uterus and adnexa have some relatively fixed anatomic characteristics that can be noted on pelvic examination or laparoscopic observation. Which of the following characteristics would you most likely find in a normal patient?

(A) retroflexion of the uterus

(B) ovaries caudad to the cervix

(C) round ligaments attached to the uterus posterior to the insertion of the fallopian tubes

(D) immobility of the uterus

(E) cervix not palpable on rectal examination

18. A patient presents approximately 10 years postmenopausal with complaints of pressure vaginally and the sensation that something is falling out. When told she has a fallen uterus, she wonders if it is due to the damage from her round ligaments since she had a great deal of round ligament pain during her pregnancies. Which of the following ligaments provide the most support to the uterus in terms of preventing prolapse?

(A) broad ligaments

(B) round ligaments

(C) utero-ovarian ligaments

(D) cardinal ligaments

(E) arcuate ligament

19. Pelvic inflammatory disease (PID) occurs in women because of which of the following characteristics of the fallopian tube?

(A) It is a conduit from the peritoneal space to the uterine cavity.

(B) It is found in the utero-ovarian ligament.

(C) It has five separate parts.

(D) It is attached to the ipsilateral ovary by the mesosalpinx.

(E) It is entirely extraperitoneal.

20. In a female, which of the following best describes the urogenital diaphragm?

    (A) includes the fascial covering of the deep transverse perineal muscle
    (B) encloses the ischiorectal fossa
    (C) is synonymous with the pelvic diaphragm
    (D) is located in the anal triangle
    (E) envelops the Bartholin's gland

21. The levator ani is the major component of the pelvic diaphragm, which is commonly compromised during pregnancy and delivery with resulting prolapse of uterus, bladder/urethra, and/or rectum. This is especially true if obstetric lacerations are not repaired keeping the normal anatomical relationships in mind. Which of the following is the best description of the levator ani?

    (A) a superficial muscular sling of the pelvis
    (B) a tripartite muscle of the pelvic floor penetrated by the urethra, vagina, and rectum
    (C) is made up of the bulbocavernosus, the ischiocavernosus, and the superficial transverse perineal muscle
    (D) a muscle that abducts the thighs
    (E) is part of the deep transverse perineal muscle

22. Which of the following is the best description of the pelvic diaphragm?

    (A) made up mainly by the coccygeus
    (B) covered on one side by fascia and on the other by peritoneum
    (C) a muscle innervated by L2, L3, and L4
    (D) an extension of the sacrococcygeal ligament
    (E) synonymous with the pelvic floor

23. When performing a hysterectomy, the surgeon should be aware that at its closest position to the cervix, the ureter is normally separated from the cervix by which of the following distances?

    (A) 0.5 mm
    (B) 1.2 mm

    (C) 12 mm
    (D) 3 cm
    (E) 5 cm

24. When performing surgery, the position of important structures should be well known to avoid injury. What is the ureter's relationship to the arteries in its course through the pelvis?

    (A) anterior to the internal iliac and uterine arteries
    (B) posterior to the iliac artery and anterior to the uterine artery
    (C) anterior to the uterine artery and posterior to the iliac artery
    (D) posterior to the uterine artery and medial to the iliac artery
    (E) posterior to the uterine artery and posterior to the hypogastric artery

25. Urinary incontinence is a major problem for some women. Which of the following characteristics of the female urethra helps prevent incontinence?

    (A) its 15- to 20-cm length
    (B) its junction with the bladder at the level of the midtrigone
    (C) its true anatomic sphincter
    (D) its upper two-thirds integration with the anterior vaginal wall
    (E) its intrinsic resting tone

26. The anatomy of the spinal cord and dural space is important when giving regional spinal anesthesia. At what approximate spinal level do the dural space and the spinal cord, respectively, end?

    (A) T10, T8
    (B) L2, T10
    (C) L5, T12
    (D) S2, L2
    (E) S5, S2

27. During a hysterectomy, vaginal bleeding may be a significant complication even after removal of the uterus. Such bleeding would most likely originate from which of the following arteries?

   (A) internal pudendal
   (B) superior hemorrhoidal
   (C) inferior mesenteric
   (D) superior vesical
   (E) ovarian

28. Anterior vulvar cancer is most likely to spread primarily to which of the following lymph nodes?

   (A) inguinal
   (B) para-aortic
   (C) obturator
   (D) femoral
   (E) ovarian

29. Which artery provides the main blood supply to the vulva?

   (A) pudendal
   (B) inferior hemorrhoidal
   (C) ilioinguinal
   (D) femoral
   (E) inferior hypogastric

30. During delivery, which of the following muscles is most likely to be obviously torn?

   (A) ischiocavernosus muscle
   (B) bulbocavernosus muscle
   (C) superficial transverse perineal muscle
   (D) levator ani muscle
   (E) coccygeus

31. A patient develops a neurologic disease that destroys components of S2, S3, S4 bilaterally. What clinical manifestation would you expect the patient to have as a result?

   (A) inability to abduct her thigh
   (B) rectal incontinence
   (C) painless menses
   (D) labor without pain
   (E) inability to extend her knees

32. A 56-year-old woman comes to your office for a yearly examination. During physical examination, you notice that her left breast has a 2-cm area of retraction in the upper-outer quadrant that can be seen by simple inspection. What is the most likely diagnosis?

   (A) Mondor's disease
   (B) benign fibroadenoma
   (C) fibrocystic change
   (D) breast cancer
   (E) intraductal polyp

33. A woman who is 32 weeks pregnant comes in complaining of lumps in her breasts. These lumps are multiple in number and on inspection are within the areola. By palpation they seem to be small, superficial, uniform in size, nontender, and soft. What is the most likely diagnosis?

   (A) Mondor's disease
   (B) Montgomery's follicles
   (C) inflammatory breast carcinoma
   (D) fibrocystic breast changes
   (E) lactiferous ducts

34. A woman has a radical hysterectomy and pelvic lymphadenectomy for Stage I carcinoma of the cervix. After surgery she complains that she cannot adduct her left leg and there is an absence of sensation on the medial aspect of her left thigh. What is the most likely explanation?

   (A) injury to the obturator nerve
   (B) femoral nerve injury
   (C) hematoma in the pouch of Douglas
   (D) injury to the uterosacral nerve
   (E) injury to the pudendal nerve

35. During delivery of a first twin, a very tight nuchal cord is reduced from the baby's neck by clamping and dividing it. After this, the second twin (as yet unborn) develops severe fetal distress. Of the following, what is the most likely mechanism for the distress in the second twin?

   (A) a twin-to-twin transfusion before birth
   (B) the second twin may no longer be connected to its placenta
   (C) placenta previa in the second twin
   (D) amniotic fluid embolism
   (E) uterine rupture

**DIRECTIONS (Questions 36 through 59): The following groups of questions are preceded by a list of lettered options. For each question, select the one lettered option that is most closely associated with it. Each lettered option may be used once, multiple times, or not at all.**

**Questions 36 through 39**

   (A) a thick band of fibers filling the angle created by the pubic rami
   (B) passes from the anterior superior iliac spine to the pubic tubercle
   (C) triangular and extends from the lateral border of the sacrum to the ischial spine
   (D) attaches to the crest of the ilium and the posterior iliac spines superiorly with an inferior attachment to the ischial tuberosity
   (E) passes over the anterior surface of the sacrum

36. Sacrospinous ligament

37. Sacrotuberous ligament

38. Ilioinguinal ligament

39. Arcuate ligament

**Questions 40 through 43**

   (A) obturator foramen
   (B) greater sciatic foramen
   (C) lesser sciatic foramen
   (D) sacrospinous ligament
   (E) pudendal (Alcock's) canal
   (F) sacral foramina

40. Formed by the superior and inferior pubic rami and covered by a central membrane through which a nerve, artery, and vein pass

41. The internal pudendal vessels and pudendal nerve exit the pelvis but then reenter through this structure

42. Divides and demarcates the greater and lesser sciatic foramen

43. A sheath of fascia on the lateral wall of the ischiorectal fossa containing vessels and nerve

**Questions 44 through 49**

   (A) anterior hypogastric nerve (T12)
   (B) posterior iliac nerve (T12–L1)
   (C) ilioinguinal nerve (L1)
   (D) genitofemoral nerve (L1–L2)
   (E) the pudendal nerve (S2, S3, S4)
   (F) terminal branch of the pudendal nerve

44. Mons veneris and anterior labia majora

45. Gluteal area

46. Anterior and medial labia majora

47. Deep labial structures

48. Main innervation of the labia

49. Clitoris

**Questions 50 through 56**

   (A) Battledore placenta
   (B) bipartite placenta
   (C) circumvallate placenta
   (D) multiple-pregnancy placenta
   (E) placenta accreta
   (F) placenta previa
   (G) succenturiate lobe

50. A small central chorionic plate surrounded by a thick whitish ring, associated with increased rates of perinatal bleeding and fetal death

51. An accessory cotyledon that is possible not to remove with the placenta at birth and cause postpartum atony and hemorrhage

52. Divided into two lobes

53. Umbilical cord inserted at the placental margin

54. Placenta abnormally adherent to the myometrium

55. Placenta covers the cervical os

56. May be distinct entities or fused

**Questions 57 through 59: For each of the following postoperative patients with areas of skin anesthesia, pain, and/or muscle weakness, select the most likely cause.**

- (A) electrolyte imbalance
- (B) obturator nerve injury
- (C) pudendal nerve injury
- (D) femoral nerve injury
- (E) disruption of peripheral (skin) nerves
- (F) ilioinguinal nerve injury
- (G) spinal cord injury
- (H) sciatic nerve injury
- (I) diabetes

57. A 56-year-old white woman who had paravaginal suspension and Burch procedure 2 days ago complains of pain over the right mons pubis, right labia, and right medial thigh.

58. A 36-year-old patient who underwent a total abdominal hysterectomy for uterine fibroids complains of weakness of her left leg and numbness of her left anterior medial thigh.

59. A patient, following a pelvic lymphadenectomy for cervical cancer, complains of some numbness in the medial thigh. On examination, she is found to have full range of motion of her leg, but weakness to adduction.

# Answers and Explanations

1. **(D)** Pelvises in most U.S. women are gynecoid, but they may be of a mixed type (for instance, having a gynecoid forepelvis and an anthropoid posterior pelvis). The obstetrician has to judge the capacity of the pelvis on the basis of its total configuration, including midplane and outlet capacities, and always in relation to the size and position of the fetus.

2. **(A)** From the pubic tubercle to the anterior superior iliac spine, the thickened lower margin of the fascial aponeurosis forms the inguinal ligament. This aponeurosis of the external oblique muscle fuses with its counterpart from the opposite side and with the underlying internal oblique fascia. Cooper's ligament is a thickening of fascia along the pubic bone. The linea alba is in the midline and the round ligament attaches to the uterus.

3. **(D)** The superficial inguinal ring is just cephalad to the pubic tubercle and just lateral to it, the deep inguinal ring passes through the transversalis fascia. The connection of these rings forms the inguinal canal. The round ligament, the ilioinguinal nerve, and the processus vaginalis pass out of the abdomen through this canal (as does the spermatic cord in the male). Gartner's ducts are found in the lateral walls of the vagina. One would not normally find a cyst of the processus vaginalis (cyst of the canal of Nuck).

4. **(B)** The pelvis surrounds the birth passage, provides attachment for muscles and fascia, and includes the ilium, ischium, pubis, sacrum, and coccyx. The ilium, ischium, and pubic bone compose the innominate bone.

5. **(B)** The true pelvis has three planes: inlet, midplane, and outlet. It is made up of the paired ileum, ischium, and pubic bones, and the single sacrum and coccyx. The true pelvis is caudad to the false pelvis, which lies between the paired ileum wings. Its inlet is usually gynecoid.

6. **(D)** The false pelvis or pelvis major lies above the linea terminalis. It seldom affects obstetric management, and measurements of the iliac crest flare do not usually aid in determining the size of the true pelvis. An important measurable indicator of the size of the true pelvis is the interspinous diameter.

7. **(B)** The obstetric conjugate is the shortest line from the inside of the symphysis to the most prominent point on the front two segments of the sacrum. It defines what is often the smallest diameter of the pelvic inlet. It should be estimated during clinical examination (pelvimetry) and considered whenever evaluating a pelvis for possible cephalopelvic disproportion, especially during abnormalities of labor. It differs from the true conjugate, which is measured from the top of the symphysis, and also from the diagonal conjugate, which is measured clinically from the bottom of the symphysis to the sacral promontory. The bi-ischial diameter is on the pelvic outlet.

8. **(A)** Layers at the midline of the abdominal wall, 2 cm below the umbilicus that would be incised or separated are skin, subcutaneous fat, superficial fascia (Camper's), deep fascia (Scarpa's), and the fascial muscle coverings (anterior rectus

sheath). The rectus muscles would be separated and the deep fascial layer (posterior rectus sheath), preperitoneal fat, and peritoneum would be incised. The posterior rectus sheath is only present cephalad to the arcuate line. Camper's is the most superficial fascia and transversus abdominal muscle would not be found in the midline (see Figure 1–1).

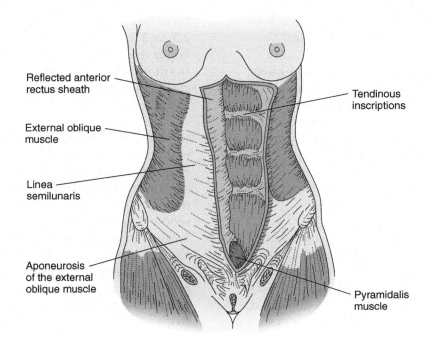

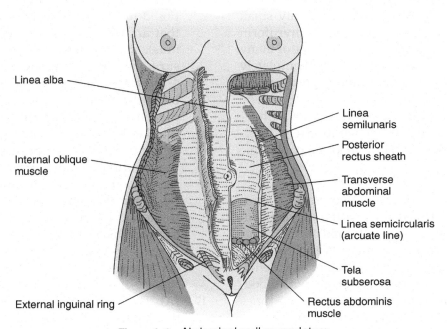

**Figure 1–1.** Abdominal wall musculature.
(Reproduced, with permission, from DeCherney AH, Nathan L. *Current Obstetric and Gynecologic Diagnosis and Treatment*, 9th ed. New York: McGraw-Hill, 2003.)

9. **(B)** The joint between the two pubic bones is the pubic symphysis. It is not a stable joint. Joints between the bones of the pelvis, such as the sacroiliac and sacrococcygeal, are called synarthroses. They have limited motion but do become more mobile and even separate a bit during pregnancy. The relaxation is attributed to the hormone relaxin. The piriformis is a muscle.

10. **(B)** The escutcheon, or configuration of the pubic hair on the mons veneris and lower abdomen, is generally an inverted triangle in the female. It is considered a secondary sex characteristic. The male pattern (a diamond shape extending upward toward the umbilicus) may exist in 25% of women. Sometimes a male-pattern escutcheon in the female may be associated with increased levels of androgens.

11. **(D)** The vestibule is an area enclosed by the labia minora. Bartholin's glands, sometimes called the major vestibular glands, open into the posterior vestibule. These glands are prone to infection with resulting occlusion of the ducts and the formation of grossly enlarged tender cysts.

12. **(D)** The hymen is a membrane that may cover all or part of the vaginal opening just above the vestibule. It may vary from being only small integumental remnants (known as myrtiform caruncles) to being perforated with one or many openings of various sizes, to being completely closed (imperforate hymen) and require surgical intervention to allow menstruum to drain. The presence of myrtiform caruncles is not pathognomonic of prior vaginal penetration (e.g., intercourse or childbirth). They are of no pathologic significance.

13. **(B)** The clitoris consists of two crura, a short body, and the glans clitoris with overlying skin called the prepuce. It is attached to the pubic bone by a suspensory ligament. Within the shaft are corpora cavernosa consisting of erectile tissue (loose in structure) that engorges with blood, causing erection and enlargement (two times usual size) during sexual excitement. The clitoris and prepuce are the primary areas of erotic stimulation in most women. The prepuce has the most innervation, which usually comes from a terminal branch of the pudendal nerve in most women. Some women, however, have alternate innervations and, in a few, innervation is sparse.

14. **(A)** The size of the cervix and corpus changes with age and hormonal status; so does the ratio of cervix to corpus. The infant uterus is only 2.5 to 3 cm in total length, and the cervix is larger than the corpus. With aging, the size of the uterus changes, as does the ratio of cervix to corpus length. The normal adult uterus is 7 to 10 cm long.

15. **(B)** Nabothian cysts are also called retention cysts because they are full of mucus from the blocked crypts. They are benign and need no specific therapy. Their appearance is characteristic both grossly and through the colposcope. Seldom is there any need for biopsy. Wolffian duct remnants cause cystic structures along the broad ligament under the fallopian tube (paraovarian cysts) or on the lateral aspect of the vagina (Gartner's duct cysts). The parmesonephron becomes the female reproductive system.

16. **(C)** The uterus has a body (corpus) composed mainly of smooth muscle, and a cervix composed mainly of connective and elastic tissues that are joined by a transitional portion (isthmus). It is an estrogen-dependent organ measuring about 7.5 cm long × 5 cm wide, with a 4-cm anterior-to-posterior diameter. After puberty, the uterus weighs about 50 g in the nullipara and 70 g in the multipara. It lies between the bladder anteriorly and the pouch of Douglas in front of the rectum posteriorly, with the cervical portion extending from the intraperitoneal area into the vagina. The opening at the distal tip of the cervix is called the external os. It is connected by the cervical canal to the internal os, which is located just below the endometrial cavity. This cavity is lined by an epithelium, the endometrium.

17. **(A)** The cervix protrudes into the fornix of the vagina, and the ovaries are intraperitoneal; therefore, they are found cephalad to the cervix. The round ligaments are attached to the uterus anterior to the attachment of the fallopian tubes.

Retroflexion implies a sharp angle between the cervix and the fundus of the uterus, which is bent posteriorly. This is a less common position of the uterus, which can also, more commonly, be midposition or anteflexed. These are all normal positions of the uterus. It is important to recognize which way the uterine body is flexed so that you do not perforate the lower uterine segment while sounding the uterus or dilating the cervix. The uterus is normally mobile and if it is not, adhesions or tumor may be present. The cervix is normally palpated anterior to the rectum on rectal examination.

18. **(D)** The cardinal ligaments are also called the transverse cervical ligaments, or Mackenrodt's ligaments, and are considered part of the uterosacral ligament complex. These ligaments serve as the major support for the apex of the vagina and are severed at the time of hysterectomy. Once divided at hysterectomy, vaginal vault prolapse becomes more likely. The broad ligaments are mainly peritoneum and the round ligaments mainly muscle. Neither provides much support. The arcuate ligament is not attached to the uterus.

19. **(A)** Fallopian tubes are a conduit from the peritoneal to the uterine cavity, which can also allow sperm or bacteria from the vagina through the uterus to the peritoneal cavity. Each tube is covered by peritoneum and consists of three layers: serosa, muscularis, and mucosa. They traverse the superior portion of the broad ligament attached by a mesentery (mesosalpinx). It has four distinct areas in its 8- to 12-cm length: the portion that runs through the uterine wall (interstitial or cornual portion), the portion immediately adjacent to the uterus (isthmic portion), the midportion of the tube (ampulla), and the distal portion containing the finger-like fimbriae that sweep the ovum into the infundibulum of the tube. The fimbriae are intraperitoneal. The tubal lumen becomes increasingly more complex as it approaches the ovary. In tubal reanastomoses, the greatest success is attained when isthmic–isthmic or isthmic–ampullary regions can be reapproximated. The longest of the fimbriae (the fimbriae ovarica) is attached to the ovary.

20. **(A)** The urogenital diaphragm is immediately cephalad to the muscles of the external genitalia. It consists of a tough fibrous fascial membrane inferiorly covering the triangular area under the pubic arch and extending posteriorly to the ischial tuberosities. It is penetrated by the urethra and vagina in the female. Just cephalad to this fascia are the deep transverse perineal muscle and the urethral sphincter mechanism. The superior fascia of the urogenital diaphragm is attached tightly to these muscles and is just caudad to the levator ani muscle. The urogenital diaphragm supplies support for the anterior vagina, urethra, and trigone of the bladder. The area encompassing the urogenital diaphragm and the superficial and deep perineal spaces is referred to as the urogenital triangle.

21. **(B)** The levator ani muscle has three portions: iliococcygeous, pubococcygeus, and puborectalis.

22. **(E)** The pelvic diaphragm (also called the pelvic floor) is made up of the levator ani muscle and the coccygeus. It is connected to the pelvic sidewall by its attachment to the obturator internus muscle at the arcus tendineus. The pelvic diaphragm provides support and closure for the intraperitoneal cavity caudally just as the thoracic diaphragm provides closure in the cephalad direction. It is covered by fascia on both sides and innervated from S2, S3, S4. The potential spaces through which the vagina, urethra, and rectum pass are the possible sites of pelvic prolapse (see Figure 1–2).

23. **(C)** A surgeon has a little more than a 1-cm space between the cervix and the ureter when performing a hysterectomy. Just lateral to the cervix is a high-risk area for injury to the ureter during gynecologic surgery. The importance of dissecting away the bladder, staying close to the cervix, and not placing clamps too far laterally or inserting wide sutures is apparent. At times, it is necessary to dissect enough to allow visualization of both ureters prior to ligation of the uterine arteries.

24. **(D)** One can remember the ureter's distal course posterior to the uterine artery by recalling that

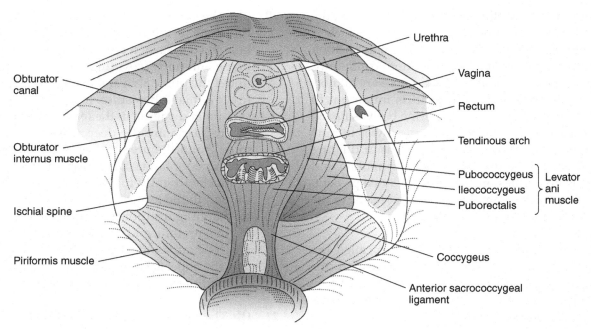

Obturator canal

Obturator internus muscle

Ischial spine

Piriformis muscle

Urethra

Vagina

Rectum

Tendinous arch

Pubococcygeus ⎫
Ileococcygeus ⎬ Levator ani muscle
Puborectalis ⎭

Coccygeus

Anterior sacrococcygeal ligament

**Figure 1–2.**

"water runs under the bridge." Do not confuse the uterine artery–ureteral relationship with the iliac artery–ureteral relationship. In the pelvis, the ureter is always anterior and medial to the iliac arteries. The position of the ureter in relation to the uterine artery makes it particularly vulnerable at the time of hysterectomy.

25. **(E)** The urethra has a higher intrinsic resting pressure than the bladder in normal women, thus helping to maintain continence. It is a hollow, multilayered tube, 2.5 to 5 cm long in the female, as opposed to being about 20 cm long in the male. It connects the bladder with the outside world. The proximal portion begins at the junction of the bladder base at the lowest portion of the trigone. It contains a functional sphincter mechanism but not a true anatomic sphincter. The distal two-thirds of the urethra is just anterior to the anterior vaginal wall.

26. **(D)** The spinal cord ends within the dura at about L2. The dural space ends at about S2. The filum terminal and cauda equina extend within the dura for some distance after the spinal cord ends. Caudal anesthesia intercepts the spinal nerves after they emerge from the dural space. When giving spinal anesthesia, one should recognize that one usually enters the subarachnoid

space at or below the termination of the spinal cord. The cauda equina extends for some distance within the dura. This relationship allows for effective anesthesia and analgesia with minimal risk of injury to the spinal cord.

27. **(A)** The arterial supply of the vagina comes from the cervicovaginal branch of the uterine artery internal pudendal, inferior vesical, and middle hemorrhoidal arteries. If the uterus is removed, neither the uterine nor ovarian arteries could be the source. Venous drainage of the vagina is accomplished through an extensive plexus rather than through well-defined channels. The same is true of the surrounding venous drainage of the bladder. The lymphatic drainage is such that the superior portion of the vagina (along with the cervix) drains into the external iliac nodes, the middle portion into the internal iliac nodes, and the lower third mainly into the superficial inguinal nodes and internal iliac nodes (like the vulva). The vagina is richly supplied with blood and lymphatics.

28. **(A)** The lymphatic drainage of the vulva has a superficial component (draining the anterior two-thirds of the vulva) and a deep drainage system (draining the posterior one-third of the vulva). The superficial drainage is to the

superficial inguinal lymph nodes, and the deep drainage is to the deep inguinal nodes, external iliac, and femoral nodes. The posterior aspects of the labia may drain to the lymphatic plexus surrounding the rectum. These anatomic relationships for lymphatic drainage are of great significance in the treatment of vulvar cancers.

29. **(A)** The major blood supply to the vulva is from the internal pudendal or its branches, the inferior hemorrhoidal and perineal. Some is provided by the external pudendal artery, which is from the femoral. There is good collateral circulation to the vulva, and either the hypogastric or pudendal artery can be occluded on either side without compromise to the vulva. The pelvic circulation provides communication so that right- and left-sided vessels may provide accessory flow to the contralateral side.

30. **(C)** The superficial transverse perineal muscle is most likely to have an obvious tear. The bulbocavernosus and ischiocavernosus are lateral. The levators and coccygeus are deep in the pelvis and not seen, though they may suffer tears (see Figure 1–3).

31. **(B)** The S2, S3, S4 innervation, if damaged at the level of the spinal cord, is most likely to produce incontinence of bladder or bowel. The patient may also have decreased vulvar sensation. Uterine pain with labor or menses is mediated by the sympathetic and parasympathetic system. Movement of the leg is mediated by L2–L4.

32. **(D)** The deep surface of the breast lies on the fascia covering the chest muscles. The fascia of the chest is condensed into many bands (Cooper's ligaments) that support the breast in its normal position on the chest wall. It is the distortion of these ligaments caused by infiltrative tumors that results in the "dimpling" appearance of the breast associated with malignancy. At age 56, the most likely cause of this is cancer. Fibroadenomas are usually found in younger women, and neither fibrocystic change nor fibroadenomas usually cause significant dimpling (see Figure 1–4). Mondor's disease is a residual of venous thrombophlebitis of the breast; it is rare. An intraductal polyp may cause a nipple discharge, but is unlikely to result in dimpling especially at a distance from the areola.

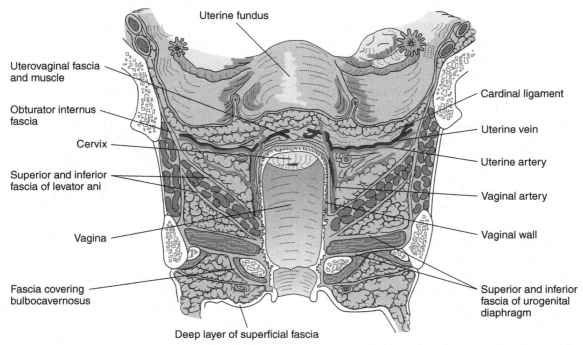

**Figure 1–3.** Fascial support of the pelvis.
(Reproduced, with permission, from DeCherney AH, Nathan L. *Current Obstetric and Gynecologic Diagnosis and Treatment*, 9th ed. New York: McGraw-Hill, 2003.)

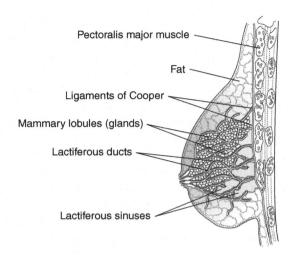

**Figure 1–4.** Sagittal section of the female breast. (Reproduced, with permission, from DeCherney AH, Nathan L. *Current Obstetric and Gynecologic Diagnosis and Treatment*, 9th ed. New York: McGraw-Hill, 2003.)

33. **(B)** These multiple, small, elevated nodules, beneath which lie the sebaceous glands, are called Montgomery's follicles. The glands are responsible for lubrication of the areola. They may hypertrophy markedly in pregnancy. The small openings of the lactiferous ducts are situated on the nipple.

34. **(A)** The injury is to the obturator nerve, which has both a sensory component on the medial thigh and a motor component to adduct the leg. At the time of the lymphadenectomy, the obturator nerve is often exposed. Just below it in the obturator space are many venous plexuses. If bleeding becomes active in this area, efforts to control it could damage the obturator nerve. This same type of nerve injury can also happen in pregnancy secondary to its compression by the fetus against the pelvic floor. Problems in the other areas would not produce this set of symptoms.

35. **(B)** In this case placenta previa can be ruled out because the first twin has already been delivered through the cervix. If there had been a severe twin–twin transfusion, it would be unlikely to manifest itself at this time in the pregnancy. An amniotic fluid embolism does not affect the fetus but rather the mother. Uterine rupture with no other signs and occurring at that precise time would be unlikely. That leaves us with a cord

accident. Using our knowledge of the placenta, we know that there may be one placenta or two, but we know that both babies have their own umbilical cord. The cord wrapped around the neck of the first twin might belong to the second twin!

36–39. **(36-C, 37-D, 38-B, 39-A)** Ligaments of the pelvis are important for their attachment and support. They are often used in the surgical repair of pelvic relaxation. The sacrospinous ligament is triangular and extends from the lateral border of the sacrum to the ischial spine. It is a common landmark in gynecologic (vaginal-suspension operations) and obstetric operations (as a marker both for the midpelvis and for the administration of regional anesthesia). The sacrotuberous ligament attaches superiorly to the posterior crest of the ilium, the posterior iliac spines, and the lateral posterior aspect of the lower sacrum. The inferior attachment is the ischial tuberosity. The ilioinguinal ligament passes from the anterior superior iliac spine to the pubic tubercle. These ligaments are very firm in the nonpregnant patient but in the pregnant patient will soften in response to the hormone relaxin, as will the symphysis and sacroiliac joints. The arcuate ligament is connective tissue that fills the space below the pubic arch (see Figure 1–5).

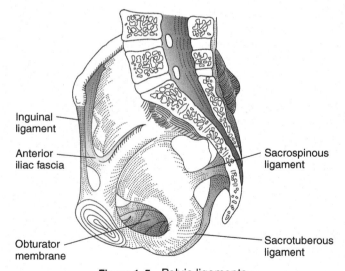

**Figure 1–5.** Pelvic ligaments. (Reproduced, with permission, from DeCherney AH, Nathan L. *Current Obstetric and Gynecologic Diagnosis and Treatment*, 9th ed. New York: McGraw-Hill, 2003.)

**40–43. (40-A, 41-C, 42-D, 43-E)** The superior and inferior pubic rami form the obturator foramen, covered by the obturator membrane with an opening (obturator canal) through which the obturator nerve, artery, and vein pass. The sacrospinous ligament divides and demarcates the greater and lesser sciatic foramina. The piriformis muscle and gluteal vessels pass out of the pelvis into the thigh through the greater sciatic foramen. The sciatic nerve and posterior femoral cutaneous nerve also pass through it. The internal pudendal vessels and pudendal nerve leave the pelvis through the greater sciatic foramen and then enter the perineal region by passing through the lesser sciatic foramen. The obturator internus muscle and its corresponding nerve also pass out of the pelvis through the lesser sciatic foramen. The pudendal canal (Alcock's canal) is a sheath of fascia on the lateral wall of the ischiorectal fossa containing the pudendal vessels and nerve.

**44–49. (44-A, 45-B, 46-C, 47-D, 48-E, 49-F)** The anterior hypogastric nerve (T12) supplies the mons veneris and the anterior labia majora, often with branches of the ilioinguinal and genitofemoral nerves. The posterior iliac nerve supplies the gluteal area. The ilioinguinal nerve supplies the anterior and medial labia majora. The genitofemoral nerve supplies the deep labial structures. The sacral plexus (S2, S3, S4), largely via the pudendal nerve, supplies the middle and posterior labia. The clitoris is supplied by the terminal branch of the pudendal nerve (see Figure 1–6). There is significant overlap in the perineal nerve distribution.

**50–56. (50-C, 51-G, 52-B, 53-A, 54-E, 55-F, 56-D)** The placenta can have many configurations. It may be small and constricted by an amniotic ring (circumvallate placenta), which predisposes to prematurity, bleeding, and early delivery. Older multiparas seem to have this predisposition. The succenturiate lobe is an accessory cotyledon. It may not deliver with the rest of the placenta and in such a case can cause significant postpartum hemorrhage. Whoever delivers a baby should therefore carefully inspect for

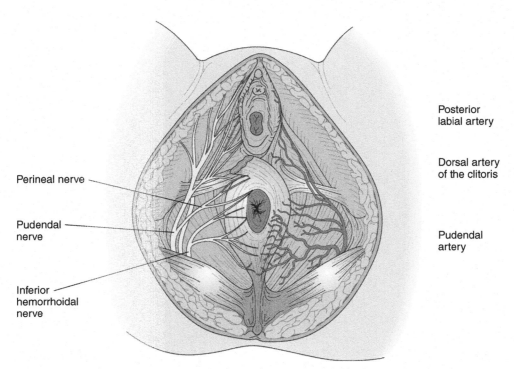

**Figure 1–6.** Arteries and nerves of the perineum.
(Reproduced, with permission, from DeCherney AH, Nathan L. *Current Obstetric and Gynecologic Diagnosis and Treatment*, 9th ed. New York: McGraw-Hill, 2003.)

large vessels that seem to run off the edge of the placenta, which suggests the possibility of an accessory lobe. The bipartite placenta, on the other hand, has two more or less equal portions connected by membranes and large vessels: retention of either half can cause major hemorrhage. The Battledore placenta (or marginal insertion of the cord) has a cord that inserts on the edge of the placenta. Placenta accreta (meaning firmly attached) forms when the decidual layer is incompletely developed and firm attachment occurs to the underlying myometrium. Percreta is even more firmly implanted, and increta means the placenta has grown completely through the myometrium. Previous surgery, grand multiparity, prior cesarean section, and placenta previa all predispose to abnormally firm placental adherence. Sometimes hysterectomy is necessary to stop the bleeding from these placental abnormalities. Multiple-pregnancy placentas can be single, connected, or even separate.

57. **(F)** The ilioinguinal nerve passes medially to the inguinal ligament and supplies the mons pubis, labia, and medial thigh. Entrapment of the nerve during surgical procedures for incontinence may result in pain over these areas. The pain may occur immediately or within a few days.

58. **(D)** The femoral nerve rises from L2 to L4 and supplies motor fibers to the quadriceps and sensation to the anterior and medial thigh. The nerve may be compressed by abdominal retractor blades that have impinged on the psoas muscle where the nerve perforates. The nerve can also undergo stretch injury from hip flexion or abduction during vaginal procedures. Either of these can result in pain or numbness or paresthesias over the anterior and medial thigh, as well as weakness of the quadriceps, causing inability to raise the knee and therefore affecting gait.

59. **(B)** Iatrogenic injury to the obturator nerve can cause sensory defects over the medial thigh. As it supplies the medial muscles of the thigh, injury may cause a decrease in ability to adduct. Fortunately, the injury is often transitory or easily compensated.

# Histology and Pathology

## Questions

1. A 65-year-old patient presents with a vulvar lesion. The pathology report of the vulvar biopsy is returned with the following description: There is hyperplasia of keratinocytes in the prickle cell layer (stratum spinosum) thickening the epidermis. This is descriptive of which of the following?

   (A) Atrophic vulvitis
   (B) Syphilitic ulceration
   (C) Acanthosis
   (D) Lichen sclerosus
   (E) Parakeratosis

2. At an annual examination of a 33-year-old woman, a 3 × 4 mm mass is noted on the lateral aspect of her vagina approximately 3 cm internally from the introitus and at the 3 o'clock position. Which of the following biopsy findings would be most abnormal?

   (A) bacteria
   (B) a small (3-mm) cyst lined by simple cuboidal epithelium
   (C) a thin keratin layer
   (D) a 3-mm-thick epithelial layer
   (E) a thin fibromuscular coat beneath the epithelium

3. Near the external os of the cervix, what is found as a normal transition from columnar epithelium?

   (A) keratinized epithelium
   (B) squamous epithelium
   (C) transitional epithelium
   (D) cuboidal epithelium
   (E) cervical erosion

4. During routine examination, an asymptomatic multiparous patient is found to have a raised 1-cm cyst on her cervix. The area is biopsied and clear mucus is extruded. Histologic examination of the specimen shows a lining of flattened columnar or cuboidal-type cells. With what would this clinical picture be most compatible?

   (A) herpes cervicitis
   (B) varicella infection
   (C) cervical intraepithelial neoplasia (CIN)
   (D) nabothian cyst
   (E) cervical adenosis

5. On a cytologic specimen, which of the following findings would be most suspicious of herpes virus infection?

   (A) intranuclear inclusion bodies
   (B) intracytoplasmic inclusions
   (C) copious glassy cytoplasm
   (D) Donovan bodies
   (E) multiple round nucleoli

6. During the menstrual cycle, the histologic appearance of the endometrium will change significantly. During the first half of the menstrual cycle, the endometrium becomes thicker and rebuilds largely in response to which of the following?

   (A) progesterone
   (B) follicle-stimulating hormone (FSH)
   (C) estrogen
   (D) luteinizing hormone (LH)
   (E) gonadotropin-releasing hormone (GnRH)

7. During repeat c-section excretances are seen on the ovary and uterine surface. These are biopsied and the report states this as decidualization. What does the term *decidualization* mean?

   (A) derived from cytotrophoblast
   (B) derived from syncytiotrophoblast
   (C) small, dark-staining cells found in the endometrium during pregnancy
   (D) endometrial cells that are proliferating
   (E) a response of cells to progesterone

8. A 44-year-old G5P5005 patient who is currently using oral contraceptive pills to control menorrhagia had a hysterectomy for uterine enlargement. You suspect adenomyosis by history. Which histological description supports the diagnosis of adenomyosis?

   (A) the metaplastic change of glandular epithelium to muscle fibers in the uterus
   (B) the same pattern and location as endometriosis
   (C) the presence of endometrial glands and stroma deep within uterine muscle
   (D) a premalignant change of the endometrium
   (E) a premalignant change of the uterine muscle

9. A 38-year-old African American woman presents with heavy menses and an enlarged uterus. After an examination the clinical diagnosis is leiomyoma of the uterus. Which of the following best describes this finding?

   (A) a soft, interdigitating mass of the uterine wall
   (B) a premalignant papule of the uterine wall
   (C) a rapidly dividing necrotic malignancy
   (D) a rounded, smooth, firm, well-circumscribed mass
   (E) erythematous, tender, and hereditary

10. A 47-year-old G0P0 patient presents with history of irregular menses, infertility, and currently increasingly heavy bleeding when it occurs. Her examination is remarkable for obesity, mild hypertension, and a clinical finding consistent with polycystic ovarian syndrome (PCOS). An endometrial biopsy is done and shows endometrial hyperplasia. Which of the following is its best histological description?

    (A) endometrial glands scattered throughout an atrophic-appearing uterine muscle
    (B) increased number of glands with a piling up of their cells and decreased intervening stroma
    (C) tightly spiraled endometrial glands with eosinophilic cytoplasm surrounding the arterioles
    (D) tortuous glands with a loose, edematous stroma
    (E) endometrial glands surrounding a fibrovascular stroma, often with a characteristic central blood vessel

11. Although thought to be primarily a conduit between the ovaries and the uterus, the fallopian tubes have been found to have a more prominent role in conception. The same cellular lining that helps in fertility also makes the patient more vulnerable for chronic infection from many of the sexual infectious diseases. Which of the following best describes the normal lining of the fallopian tube?

    (A) squamous epithelium
    (B) transitional epithelium
    (C) cuboidal epithelium
    (D) columnar epithelium with cilia
    (E) fibrous connective tissue

12. The ovaries are covered by a thin layer of epithelium called germinal epithelium. Why is it called germinal epithelium?

    (A) The germ cells arise from it during fetal life.
    (B) It produces germ cells throughout menstrual life.
    (C) It protects the ova from bacteria.
    (D) It was thought to produce germ cells.
    (E) It is made up of germ cells.

13. The cells in the layers surrounding each oocyte produce ovarian hormones. Which of the following is the correct order of cell layers surrounding an ovarian follicle from the oocyte outward?

    (A) zona pellucida, granulosa, theca interna
    (B) granulosa, theca interna, zona pellucida
    (C) theca interna, zona pellucida, granulosa
    (D) theca interna, granulosa, zona pellucida
    (E) zona pellucida, theca interna, granulosa

14. What is the fate of most of the ovarian follicles that begin to develop at each cycle?

    (A) They develop and ovulate at some time during the person's life.
    (B) They continue to grow, forming follicle cysts.
    (C) They undergo atresia.
    (D) They remain to continue their development in the next cycle.
    (E) They regress to primordial follicles.

15. Luteinization occurs normally in the ovary during each menstrual cycle. Which of the following best describes this process?

    (A) The granulosa cells turn red.
    (B) Mature granulosa and the theca interna cells become epithelioid and form a corpus luteum.
    (C) The ovarian stroma undergoes adipose degeneration prior to ovulation.

    (D) The nonovulated follicles undergo fatty degeneration.
    (E) Cysts form in the theca.

16. An ovary is removed for frozen section pathologic examination. The ovary is enlarged, with small surface excrescences. Pathologic examination reveals numerous cysts lined by serous epithelium with six to eight cell layers piled on top of one another to form the cyst walls. The cells show marked cytologic atypia, and nests of similar cells are present in the ovarian stroma. Round laminated calcium bodies are also seen. What diagnosis does this histologic description indicate?

    (A) normal proliferative phase follicle
    (B) corpus luteum cyst
    (C) ovarian endometriosis
    (D) borderline ovarian carcinoma
    (E) cystadenocarcinoma

17. Histologically, the presence of which of the following would determine that an ovarian teratoma is malignant?

    (A) squamous cells
    (B) all three germ cell lines
    (C) immature fetal-like cells
    (D) neural ectoderm
    (E) an ovarian capsule

18. A 52-year-old patient presents for her annual examination. She denies any problems other than that she has not had an "annual" examination in over 5 years due to cost. During the breast examination she is noted to have dimpling of the skin of the right breast with raising of the arms. What possibility should this sign signify?

    (A) pregnancy
    (B) weight gain
    (C) aging
    (D) fibrocystic disease
    (E) carcinoma

19. Histologic examination of the normal breast from a postmenopausal woman as compared to the breast from a premenopausal woman would show which of the following?

    (A) a decrease in the number and size of acinar glands and ductal elements, with decreased density of the breast parenchyma

    (B) an increase in breast size and turgidity because of an increase in the density of the parenchyma

    (C) increase in number and size of acinar cells and a widening of the ductal lumens

    (D) significant atrophy of the adipose tissue of the breast with little change in the actual breast parenchyma

    (E) no significant change in histology

20. A patient has a screening mammograph that shows a lesion that is high risk for carcinoma. While waiting for her biopsy to be scheduled she has done some reading on the web regarding breast cancer. She is confused by the number of different types of breast cancer and asks which is the most common pathologic type of breast cancer?

    (A) ductal
    (B) lobular
    (C) Paget's
    (D) inflammatory
    (E) adenoid cystic

21. A breast biopsy on a 35-year-old woman shows "atypical epithelial hyperplasia confined within the biopsy site." Which of the following best explains this biopsy finding?

    (A) Her biopsy is benign, and she is at no risk for cancer of the breast in the future.

    (B) Her biopsy is benign, but she is at increased risk for developing breast cancer in the future.

    (C) Her biopsy is definitely premalignant, and bilateral prophylactic subcutaneous mastectomy is indicated.

    (D) Her biopsy is malignant, and she will need to undergo radiation therapy but no further surgery since the lump has been removed.

    (E) Her biopsy is malignant, and she should undergo radical mastectomy and sampling of the axillary lymph nodes.

22. A 37-year-old woman complains of a painful lump in her breast. The lump is removed, and microscopic examination of the mass shows "microscopic cysts, papillomatosis, fibrosis, and ductal hyperplasia." Which of the following is the most likely diagnosis?

    (A) benign intraductal papilloma
    (B) endometriosis of the breast
    (C) fibrocystic changes
    (D) lobular carcinoma in situ
    (E) infiltrating ductal carcinoma

23. An asymptomatic 24-year-old college student is found to have a 4-cm, very firm mass in her breast that she has not previously noticed. The mass is mobile, smooth, and nontender in the upper, outer quadrant of her breast. An excision biopsy is performed and shows "a well-circumscribed, fibrous lesion with glands interspersed throughout the body of the tumor." Which of the following is the most likely diagnosis?

    (A) cystosarcoma phyllodes
    (B) macromastia
    (C) mastitis
    (D) fat necrosis
    (E) fibroadenoma

24. Which of the following pathologic features is most helpful in distinguishing complete hydatidiform mole from normal placenta?

    (A) trophoblastic proliferation
    (B) absence of blood vessels
    (C) hydropic degeneration of villi
    (D) cellular atypia
    (E) sex chromatin positivity

DIRECTIONS (Questions 25 through 31): The following groups of questions are preceded by a list of lettered options. For each question, select the one lettered option that is most closely associated with it. Each lettered option may be used once, multiple times, or not at all.

**Questions 25 through 28**

(A) molluscum contagiosum
(B) vulvar intraepithelial neoplasia
(C) lichen sclerosis
(D) condyloma acuminata
(E) hidradenoma

25. Grossly, a raised lesion of the vulva with an irregular appearance. Histologic section shows a papilliform shape to the epithelium. The section is acanthotic, with increased keratin and parakeratosis. The surface is irregular and spiked in appearance.

26. Found in an intertriginous area. Appears as a waxy, raised papule with an umbilicated center. Microscopically, there are eosinophilic inclusions in a central cistern within a raised lesion.

27. A thin, white epithelium. Microscopically, it has a thin epidermis, with flattened rete pegs and a dense hyaline appearance in the dermis. The dermis has a distinct lack of cellularity.

28. A discrete lesion that is slightly raised and can be white or pigmented. The microscopic appearance shows cellular disorganization, with a loss of epithelial cell stratification. There is increased cellular density and variation in cell size with numerous mitotic figures.

**Questions 29 through 31**

(A) metaplasia
(B) CIN
(C) acanthosis
(D) hyperkeratosis
(E) dyskaryosis

29. A large nuclear/cytoplasmic (N/C) ratio.

30. Transformation of areas of columnar cells to squamous cells.

31. A term that describes cellular maturation defects of the cervical epithelium.

# Answers and Explanations

1. **(C)** Acanthosis is found with syphilis, lichen planus, venereal warts, and cancer, as well as other conditions. Clinically, it refers to a hyperplasia of keratinocytes, causing a thickening of the prickle layer of the epidermis, which clinically appears as a diffusely thickened or localized plaque. Thickening of the superficial horny layer of the skin is called hyperkeratosis. The presence of nucleated surface cells is called parakeratosis. Thinning or atrophy means fewer cells and cell layers present. Ulceration means there is absence of epithelium.

2. **(C)** Keratin is not normally present in the vagina. It can occur in response to chronic irritation or infection. Many kinds of bacteria are present in the vagina as normal vaginal flora and may be seen on a biopsy. As long as they are confined to the surface, they are probably a normal variant. A 3-mm cyst lined by cuboidal epithelium is likely to be a remnant of the Wolffian duct (Gartner's duct cyst). They are common. Endocervical-type mucus-secreting glands may also be found in the vagina. If present, they are called vaginal adenosis. They are more common in women whose mothers were exposed to DES (diethylstilbestrol) during their pregnancy. The stratified squamous epithelium lining in the vagina is usually no more than 3 mm in thickness and a thin fibromuscular coat is found beneath it. For various lesions that may be found in the vagina, see Figure 2–1.

3. **(B)** The cervix is covered with glandular epithelium in childhood. The cervical epithelium will undergo change (metaplasia) as it is exposed to estrogen. The columnar epithelium is replaced by squamous epithelium. The area that changes is called the transformation zone, and the leading edge of the area of change is the squamocolumnar junction. Squamous changes are thought to begin at the squamocolumnar junction where active metaplasia is occurring. This area must be sampled by a Pap smear, and it must be completely seen with a colposcope, or biopsied during diagnostic procedures to evaluate abnormal Pap smears.

4. **(D)** Nabothian cysts occur when a cleft of columnar endocervical cells becomes walled off by epidermidization, entrapping mucous secretions. They are common and benign and are usually recognized visually. Rarely, it may be necessary to biopsy them for identification. This cyst is found on the surface of the cervix, in contrast to the histologically similar Gartner's duct cyst (Wolffian duct remnant) found deep within the stroma of the cervix. CIN is not cystic. Herpes may cause vesicles but they are thin, last a short time before rupture, and contain serous fluid. Cervical adenosis is made up of columnar glandular epithelium but is not a cyst.

5. **(A)** Intranuclear inclusion bodies, irregular nucleoli, and multinuclei are characteristic of herpes simplex virus. These findings are sometimes detected by biopsy or Tzanck staining of a cytologic smear, or sometimes with routine Pap smear (50% sensitivity). Donovan bodies are found with granuloma inguinale and sulfur granules with actinomyces.

6. **(C)** In the first half of the menstrual cycle, the endometrium is influenced by estrogen.

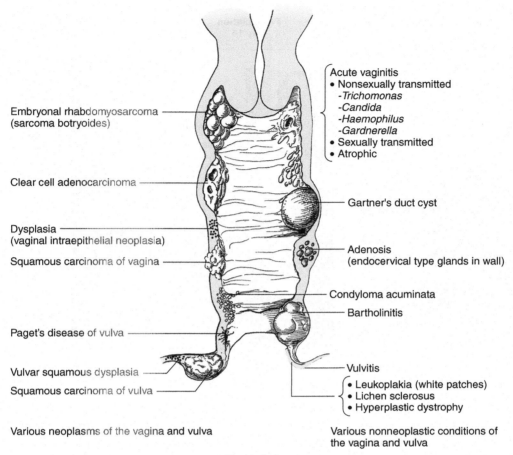

Embryonal rhabdomyosarcoma
(sarcoma botryoides)

Clear cell adenocarcinoma

Dysplasia
(vaginal intraepithelial neoplasia)

Squamous carcinoma of vagina

Paget's disease of vulva

Vulvar squamous dysplasia

Squamous carcinoma of vulva

Acute vaginitis
• Nonsexually transmitted
  - *Trichomonas*
  - *Candida*
  - *Haemophilus*
  - *Gardnerella*
• Sexually transmitted
• Atrophic

Gartner's duct cyst

Adenosis
(endocervical type glands in wall)

Condyloma acuminata

Bartholinitis

Vulvitis
  • Leukoplakia (white patches)
  • Lichen sclerosus
  • Hyperplastic dystrophy

Various neoplasms of the vagina and vulva

Various nonneoplastic conditions of
the vagina and vulva

**Figure 2–1.**

The endometrium develops from its basal layer (basalis). Estrogen makes the lining proliferate (hence, the proliferative phase). At midcycle, estrogen production continues, but with ovulation, progesterone is also produced, which causes coiling of the endometrial arteries and compaction of the endometrium. Progesterone also causes endometrial glands to secrete (hence, secretory phase). Although it is true that gonadotropins (GnRH, FSH, and LH) serve as signals for this process, they have little direct effect on endometrium. In the normal postmenopausal woman, gonadotropins are elevated, but the endometrium does not change because no estrogen or progesterone is produced (see Figure 2–2).

7. **(E)** Decidualization is a characteristic of the endometrium of the pregnant uterus. It is a response of maternal cells to progesterone.

However, decidualization may be used to describe any change due to progesterone, including the eosinophilic proliferation around arterioles after ovulation.

8. **(C)** Adenomyosis is a condition in which endometrial glands and stroma are found within the myometrium on histologic examination. These structures must be one or more low-power microscopic fields below the surface. It is not malignant. Endometrial glands do not undergo metaplasia to muscle, nor does muscle undergo metaplasia to glands. Endometriosis is the term that refers to ectopic endometrium in any location outside the uterus. Adenomyosis used to be referred to as endometriosis interna.

9. **(D)** Leiomyomas are common benign neoplasms of uterine smooth muscle. They are usually discrete, very firm, smooth masses that

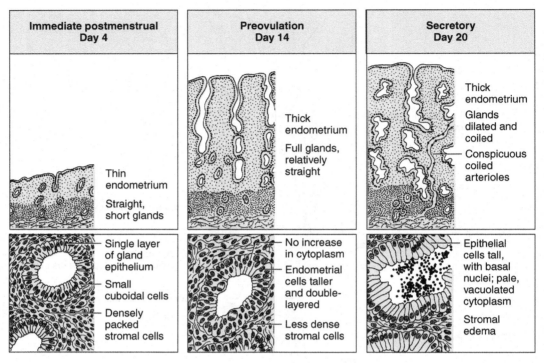

Figure 2–2.

are tan in color. They are found most commonly attached to the uterus, though they can occur at other sites. They are also called fibroids, fibromyoma, myomas, and other colloquial terms. They are not premalignant and are rarely tender or inflamed. Most patients who have them are asymptomatic.

10. **(B)** Endometrial hyperplasia is a condition with increased numbers of endometrial glands and a decrease (but not an absence) in the amount of intervening stroma. The cells lining the glands also build up and overlap (see Figure 2–3). Hyperplasia with atypical cells is often a precursor to endometrial carcinoma. Distractor C is a description of decidualization. Distractor D describes secretory endometrium and E is a description of an endometrial polyp.

11. **(D)** Each portion of the female genital tract has a characteristic epithelial lining. The fallopian tube is lined by ciliated columnar epithelium. Many of the tubal cells appear ciliated, while others are secretory or absorptive. The cilia and mucus facilitate egg transport. The secretory cells provide additional nutrients to the blasto-

cyst as it works its way to the endometrial cavity. However, this columnar epithelial also increases the easy of either Chlamydia or GC being able to establish an infectious process.

12. **(D)** Ova were thought to arise from this lining. Though they do not, the older terminology persists. The medulla is the central core of the ovary and is continuous with the hilum, where blood vessels and lymphatics gain entrance. The

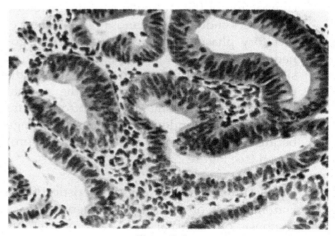

Figure 2–3.

cortex is the outer layer, containing primary oocytes and stroma. The ovary is covered by a thin "germinal" epithelium, which is not derived from germ cells but from the peritoneum. Understanding this anomalous terminology is important when using embryology to classify ovarian tumors.

13. **(A)** The oocyte is surrounded by the zona pellucida, the granulosa, and the theca. During each menstrual cycle, the follicles selected for ovulation grow until an egg is ovulated by erupting through the surface of the ovary surrounded by some of the follicle cells. If the early eggs are not surrounded by follicular cells to form primordial follicles, they resorb.

14. **(C)** A woman is born with all of the gametes she will have for her lifetime. Of the many follicles present at birth, only about 400 to 600 ever mature and extrude an ovum. Many become atretic and disappear without developing, and others that start to develop become atretic. Only a small proportion will ovulate, form a corpus luteum, and produce progesterone.

15. **(B)** The outer cell layer surrounding the follicle (outside the granulosa) is called the theca. Cells closest to the granulosa are called theca interna. All these cells develop and convert their cytoplasm to become efficient producers of both estrogen and progesterone. Cholesterol is stored within them, imparting a yellow color. The whole structure is known as the corpus luteum. High levels of human chorionic gonadotropin (HCG) as seen in multiple pregnancies or hydatidiform moles can stimulate abnormal luteinization and the production of many luteinized cysts (theca lutein cysts). These cysts can make the ovaries very large.

16. **(E)** In serous cystadenocarcinoma, more than three cell layers of stratification exist in the epithelial cell lining. The individual cells are atypical, and there is invasion of the ovarian stroma and/or protrusion from the capsule (excrescences). A borderline malignant tumor has three or fewer cells in the lining of the cyst and no evidence of invasion. It is the thickness of the lining, invasion, and atypia that makes the di-

agnosis of ovarian carcinoma. The calcifications are called psammoma bodies and are suggestive but not diagnostic of an ovarian malignancy (see Figure 2–4).

17. **(C)** Immature teratomas are malignant, containing embryonic-like tissues. Mature teratomas may contain all three germ lines but they may or may not be malignant. Mature teratomas can be malignant, usually because they have malignant elements of mature skin (squamous epithelium) and neural ectoderm. The neural tissue is most useful in grading the virulence of the tumor (those with large areas of neuroblast are most virulent).

18. **(E)** The fascia of the superficial chest muscles becomes condensed into bands called Cooper's ligaments. These bands run from the base of the breast to the skin to provide support for the breast. Distortion of these bands by a tumor may cause dimpling of the skin overlying the breast. Such dimpling is considered a sign of malignancy.

19. **(A)** After menopause, the breast undergoes involution. There is a decrease in the acinar and ductal elements and generalized atrophy. Parenchymal elements decrease and are replaced by fat, making the breast appear less dense on mammography.

20. **(A)** The pathologic types of breast cancer are identified by their histologic appearance. About 75% of breast cancers will arise from ductal epithelium. No other cell type in the breast accounts for more than 10% of pathologic types. The histologic subtype has less bearing on prognosis than stage of the cancer at treatment, which is the most important prognostic factor for survival.

21. **(B)** The biopsy showing atypical hyperplasia indicates a risk greater than the general population for developing breast cancer, but it is not a malignancy. It indicates a need for close surveillance, as approximately 8% of these women will develop breast cancer within 15 years. If other risk factors were present, such as two or more first-degree relatives with breast cancer or a

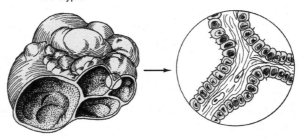

Benign serous cystadenoma
• Single layer of epithelial cells
• No atypia

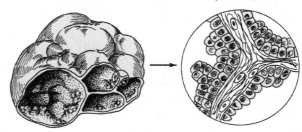

Serous tumor of low malignant potential
• Mild atypia
• Stratification of cells less than three layers deep

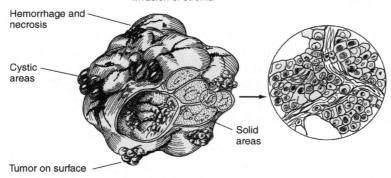

Malignant serous cystadenocarcinoma
• Stratified epithelium with marked cytologic atypia
• Invasion of stroma

Hemorrhage and necrosis

Cystic areas

Solid areas

Tumor on surface

**Figure 2–4.**

previous carcinoma in the other breast, other plans or treatment modalities might be considered, but usually not on the basis of this biopsy result alone.

22. **(C)** Fibrocystic breast changes are common in women 30 to 50 years old and are often asymptomatic. When symptomatic, they often present as a painful mass that changes with menses. The histology may be imprecise, and these changes may represent a normal process in the breast. It is thought not to be a risk factor for most women (Figure 2–5).

23. **(E)** By definition, fibrous tissue and glands should be a fibroadenoma. It is most common in women younger than 35 years. It is generally asymptomatic and presents as a 1- to 5-cm mass. Local excision may or may not be necessary, depending on patient reliability. Cystosarcoma phyllodes is a type of fibroadenoma with a cellular stroma. It can grow quickly and may recur and act like a malignancy unless completely excised. Macromastia is simply large breasts. This may or may not be a problem for the patient. Mastitis is an infection of the breast almost always secondary to breast-feeding.

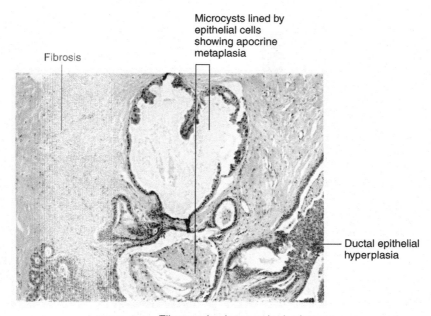

Fibrosis

Microcysts lined by
epithelial cells
showing apocrine
metaplasia

Ductal epithelial
hyperplasia

**Figure 2–5.** Fibrocystic changes in the breast.
(Reproduced with permission from Chandrasoma P, Taylor CR. *Concise Pathology*, 3rd ed. New York: McGraw-Hill, 1999.)

Fat necrosis is usually secondary to injury and may or may not produce a mass. It does not need treatment if the condition can be accurately identified.

24. **(B)** One of the distinctions between complete mole and normal placenta is the lack of blood vessels in the moles. In most cases, complete moles are 46,XX with euploidy and are therefore sex-chromatin positive. One-half of normal placentas are sex-chromatin positive. Microscopically, moles have edematous villi (hydropic degeneration) and both moles and placentas have proliferating syncytiocytotrophoblast, although random mix of cyto- and syncytiotrophoblast is more common in moles. However, some placentas, especially of hydropic fetuses, can show this also. Cellular atypia is common in both normal and molar placentas.

25. **(D)** Grossly, a condyloma is a raised white lesion of the vulva with an irregular appearance. Histologic section shows a papilliform shape to the epithelium. The section is acanthotic, with increased keratin and parakeratosis. The surface is irregular and spiked in appearance. This is a classic description of a wart.

26. **(A)** Molluscum contagiosum lesions appear as waxy, raised, dome-shaped papules with an umbilicated center. Microscopically, there are eosinophilic inclusions contained in a central cistern of a raised lesion.

27. **(C)** Lichen sclerosis is a chronic lesion that is common on the vulva. It is often pruritic and has a smooth and atrophic appearance. The epidermis is usually thin and may have a significant keratin layer. Pathologic characteristics are a lack of rete pegs and a pink hyaline appearance with lack of cellularity in the dermis.

28. **(B)** Vulvar intraepithelial neoplasia can involve a small fraction or the entire thickness of the epithelium. It may appear as a discrete or diffuse lesion. It can be unifocal or multifocal. It may be white, red, brown, or black. Histologic sections will show a lack of normal differentiation of cells. Large basal cells are not confined to the basal-most layers but extend well up into the epithelium. Cellular density and mitotic activity are increased. Some of the mitoses may be abnormal. Multinucleation and nuclear hyperchromasia are common features.

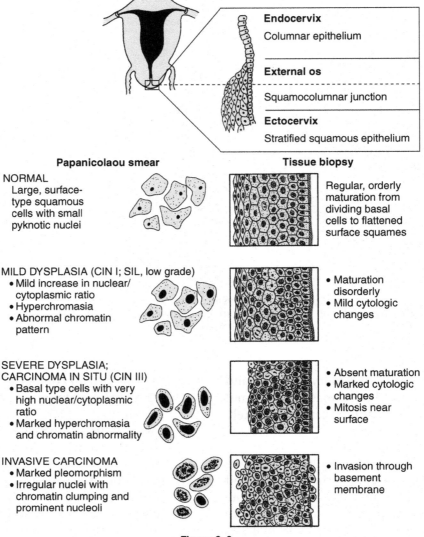

**Figure 2–6.**

**29. (B)** Dysplastic cells make up CIN. They have large, irregular nuclei and abnormal mitoses. They are also likely to be aneuploid. Gross clinical examination, however, will not reveal this.

**30. (A)** Squamous metaplasia is commonly found in cervical epithelium. It is a physiologic process by which squamous epithelium replaces columnar epithelium. Squamous metaplasia is found within the transformation zone of the uterine cervix (see Figure 2–6).

**31. (B)** CIN is graded as I, II, or III. It refers to dysplastic cells with a defect in their nuclear/cytoplasmic ratio and chromatin abnormalities of the nucleus. These abnormally maturing cells may progress from CIN I to CIN II to CIN III as they encompass greater amounts of the epithelial thickness. CIN does not include specimens with any evidence of invasion below the basement membrane. Such invasion denotes cancer, not a precursor (see Figure 2–6).

---

# CHAPTER 3

# **Embryology**

## Questions

**DIRECTIONS (Questions 1 through 22): For each of the multiple choice questions in this section, select the lettered answer that is the one best response in each case.**

1. You are counseling a couple about infertility. In your discussion about conception, tubal disease, and implantation, you explain to them that implantation in the uterus occurs at which stage of development?

   (A) eight-cell embryo
   (B) zygote
   (C) morula formation
   (D) blastocyst
   (E) embryonic disk

**Questions 2 and 3 apply to the following patient:**

A 25-year-old G2 P1 had a previous child with ambiguous external genitalia including hypertrophied clitoris and labial fusion. She and her partner are carriers of 21-alpha hydroxylase deficiency.

2. In this pregnancy you counsel her that her fetus has what chance of recurrence?

   (A) 50% chance of recurrence
   (B) 25% chance of recurrence
   (C) <5% chance of recurrence
   (D) 100% chance of recurrence
   (E) Impossible to predict recurrence because of incomplete penetrance

3. She would like to prevent a recurrence. You offer her maternal dexamethasone in order to do which of the following?

   (A) calm her anxiety
   (B) suppress fetal adrenal glad
   (C) block fetal genital steroid receptors
   (D) provide negative feedback to the maternal pituitary
   (E) block transplacental passage of maternal androgens

4. In counseling a woman about an alcohol binge she had at 6 weeks after her last menstrual period you explain that, with the exception of the brain, organogenesis is completed within how many weeks after her last period?

   (A) 4 weeks after ovulation
   (B) 10 weeks after ovulation
   (C) 18 weeks after ovulation
   (D) 26 weeks after ovulation
   (E) 38 weeks after ovulation

5. A couple of Southeast Asian ancestry are both thalassemia carriers. In counseling them you explain that the main form of hemoglobin in the normal fetus is which of the following?

   (A) Gower 1
   (B) hemoglobin A (HbA)
   (C) Gower 2
   (D) hemoglobin F (HbF)
   (E) Bart's hemoglobin

**6.** A woman has had a previous child with renal agenesis. She is a middle school biology teacher and wants to understand more about development of the kidneys. Which of the following best describes the function of pronephros?

  (A) They begin the developmental sequence that forms the permanent excretory ducts and kidneys.
  (B) They are the primitive kidney and ureter that will mature into the adult urinary tract.
  (C) They develop as the primitive kidney and migrate caudally and laterally to form the mesonephros.
  (D) They will serve as the fetal kidney until 16 weeks and the development of the metanephros.
  (E) They form the primitive kidney and primitive upper genital ducts.

**7.** An amniocentesis results show a fetus with 45XO. In counseling the parents, how would you explain that the genetic sex is determined?

  (A) at ovulation
  (B) at conception
  (C) by the presence or absence of testosterone
  (D) in the absence of Müllerian-inhibiting factor
  (E) psychosocially after birth

**8.** A women is worried because she has been taking "body-building steroids" through week 10 of her pregnancy. One of the steroids has a strong proportion of androgens. You explain that androgens can cause which of the following?

  (A) paramesonephros to differentiate into the proximal urinary duct system
  (B) Wolffian ducts to develop
  (C) Müllerian ducts to regress
  (D) the primitive vaginal tube to regress
  (E) the gonadal ridge to differentiate into a testis

**9.** Germ cells arise in which of the following?

  (A) germinal epithelium of the gonad
  (B) endoderm of the primitive gut

  (C) Müllerian duct
  (D) mesonephros
  (E) ovarian cortex

**10.** You are counseling a 32-year-old nulligravida with breast cancer about preserving fertility. You explain that the maximal number of oogonia is found at what age?

  (A) 1 month's gestational age
  (B) 5 month's gestational age
  (C) birth
  (D) puberty
  (E) 21 years of age

**11.** The paramesonephric ducts will form which of the following?

  (A) the prostatic utricle
  (B) seminal vesicles
  (C) oviducts, uterus, and upper vagina
  (D) upper vagina only
  (E) the ureters

**12.** Vaginal epithelium and the fibromuscular wall of the vagina originate from which of the following, respectively?

  (A) mesonephric duct and endoderm of the urogenital sinus
  (B) mesonephric duct and the uterovaginal primordium
  (C) endoderm of the urogenital sinus and the mesonephric duct
  (D) endoderm of the urogenital sinus and the uterovaginal primordium
  (E) endoderm of the urogenital sinus and the paramesonephric ducts

**13.** The urogenital sinus is derived from which of the following?

  (A) invagination of the genital ridges
  (B) proliferation of the hindgut
  (C) partitioning of the endodermal cloaca
  (D) a track developing in the genital mesoderm
  (E) hyperplasia of the metanephros

**Questions 14 and 15 apply to the following scenario:**

In counseling a mother with congenital adrenal hyperplasia, you explain in utero masculinization of female fetuses.

14. The labia majora are homologous to which male body part?

 (A) penis
 (B) testicle
 (C) foreskin
 (D) scrotum
 (E) gubernaculum testes

15. The female clitoris is homologous to which of the following male body parts?

 (A) scrotum
 (B) frenulum
 (C) prostate
 (D) foreskin
 (E) penis

16. The absence of the vagina is common in which of the following?

 (A) congenital adrenal hyperplasia in a female infant
 (B) Turner's syndrome
 (C) association with an absent or rudimentary uterus
 (D) medication-induced fetal masculinization of a female infant
 (E) gonadal dysgenesis

17. Which of the following is the result of lack of fusion of the Müllerian duct system?

 (A) uterine didelphys
 (B) transverse vaginal septum
 (C) unilateral renal agenesis
 (D) imperforate hymen
 (E) ovarian remnant syndrome

18. During early embryonic development the germ cells must migrate. If germ cells fail to enter the developing genital ridge, which of the following is most likely to occur?

 (A) ovarian teratomas
 (B) ectopic pregnancy
 (C) ovarian choriocarcinoma
 (D) gonadal agenesis
 (E) testicular feminization

19. You are giving a lecture to a college physiology class. They are fascinated with the genetics and development of hermaphrodites. You explain that true hermaphrodites have which of the following?

 (A) ovaries and testicular remnants
 (B) the absence of any Müllerian tissue due to Müllerian-inhibiting factor (MIF)
 (C) 46,XY karyotype
 (D) ambiguous genitalia
 (E) external genitalia that are responsive to both adrenal and testicular androgens

20. In the examination of the newborn infant with ambiguous genitalia, which of the following is true?

 (A) gonads that are palpable in the lower inguinal canal are always testes
 (B) the presence of descended gonads rules out high testosterone virilization in an otherwise normal female infant
 (C) pelvic ultrasound is usually not helpful as a method of assessing a newborn with ambiguous genitalia
 (D) the presence of a normal uterus rules out the possibility of dysgenetic testes
 (E) if the urethra is superior to the phallus, the infant is a male

**21.** On ultrasound, a large isolated cyst is seen in the fetal pelvis. At birth a cloaca is seen in a female fetus. You explain to the parents that urorectal septum did not form thus resulting in which of the following?

(A) The single-chambered cloaca did not divide into the urogenital sinus and anorectal canal.

(B) The junction of the cloacal membrane and urorectal septum become the labia.

(C) The cloacal membrane differentiated into the urogenital membrane and the anal membrane.

(D) The urogenital sinus did not form the vagina and the lower bladder wall to the ureterovesical junction.

(E) The urorectal septum did not form a rectum and lower third of the sigmoid colon.

**22.** Of the following anomalies, which is (are) most likely to proceed to a term pregnancy?

(A) uterus didelphys

(B) bicornuate uterus with a rudimentary horn

(C) unicornuate uterus

(D) longitudinal vaginal septum

(E) Gartner's duct cysts

**DIRECTIONS (Questions 23 through 30): The following groups of questions are preceded by a list of lettered options. For each question, select the one lettered option that is most closely associated with it. Each lettered option may be used once, multiple times, or not at all.**

**Questions 23 through 27**

(A) morula

(B) blastocele

(C) trophoblast

(D) embryo

(E) zygote

(F) primitive streak

(G) blastocyst

(H) chorionic plate

(I) fetus

(J) gamete

**23.** The name applied to the 16-cell mass that precedes the blastocyst

**24.** A fertilized ovum

**25.** The name applied to the cells capable of invading endometrium

**26.** The name applied to the products of conception from the third to the eighth week after ovulation

**27.** The name applied to the cell or cells capable of uniting to reproduce

**Questions 28 through 30 apply to the following patient:**

A 16-year-old girl presents with primary amenorrhea. She has normal breast development, pubic hair, and axillary hair. Match the diagnosis with the physiologic explanation.

(A) anomalous partitioning of the vagina

(B) secondary to incomplete or partial canalization of the vaginal plate

(C) anomaly of caudal fusion

(D) Müllerian duct aplasia

(E) in utero exposure to androgenic hormones

(F) anomalous development of the pronephros at 8–10 weeks after ovulation

(G) maternal viral infection during the first trimester

**28.** Transverse vaginal septum

**29.** Absent vagina

**30.** Imperforate hymen

# Answers and Explanations

1. **(D)** It is important to recognize that implantation occurs 6 to 7 days after ovulation and that the embryo is actively growing during this time. Progestin-only contraceptives and the so-called "morning-after pill" may prevent the implantation of a growing blastocyst by their effect on the endometrium during the days between fertilization and implantation. Zygote is a term for the single fertilized cell with two pronuclei present. An embryo divides to become eight cells during its transportation through the fallopian tube.

2. **(B)** Congenital adrenal hyperplasia-21 alpha hydroxylase deficiency is an autosomal recessive condition. Thus each parent has a 1:2 chance of passing it on. Each child has a 25% (1:4) chance of having the disease.

3. **(B)** Dexamethasone, given to the mother, crosses the placenta and suppresses ACTH secreting cells in the fetal pituitary. This inhibits fetal adrenal androgen secretion and prevents masculinization. The drug does not block fetal genital receptors. The purpose is not related to maternal androgens or maternal pituitary since these are not causative of the syndrome. Once the sex of the fetus is known and if the fetus is male, the androgen treatment can be stopped.

4. **(B)** Fifty-six days' gestational age or 10 weeks after the last menstrual period is generally accepted as ending the embryonic period. Prior to this time teratogens can cause severe defects, with partial to complete absence of organ structures, depending upon the stage of development when the teratogen was present. Beyond this time period, fetal effects of teratogens are significantly less.

5. **(E)** All these types differ in the globin moiety and can be differentiated by electrophoresis. Fetal hemoglobin (HbF) has more oxygen-binding capacity than adult hemoglobin (HbA). Gower 1 and Gower 2 are embryonic hemoglobins and the most primitive of human hemoglobins. They are less efficient oxygen carriers than HbF.

6. **(A)** The pronephros and the mesonephros are two primitive urinary systems that precede the development of the metanephros which will develop into the mature urinary system. The mesonephric ducts grow caudally, and by week 5 of development they open into the lateral wall of the cloaca. The pronephros degenerate by the end of the fourth week (2 weeks embryologic age) but do initiate the events that will lead to the formation of the adult kidney and collecting ducts.

7. **(B)** Genetic sex is determined at fertilization by the complement of sex chromosomes in the fertilizing sperm. If the sperm bears an X, a female is conceived. If it bears a Y, a male is conceived. The other options pertain to genital or phenotypical gender that may be different from genetic sex due to influence of the presence or absence of critical hormones.

8. **(E)** Stimulation by testosterone causes the male mesonephric ducts (Wolffian ducts) to differentiate. Anti-Müllerian factor (MIF) produced by the testes causes the Müllerian (paramesonephric) ducts to regress. Absence of

these hormones causes the Müllerian ducts to persist and develop independently of the presence of estrogen. Genital sex is therefore determined by the presence or absence of functional androgen and MIF.

9.  **(B)** Primordial germ cells are visible early in the fourth week among the endodermal cells of the wall of the yolk sac near the origin of the allantois. Migration of primordial germ cells (which will become ova) to the gonadal ridge occurs early in embryonic life (5–6 weeks). Germ cells migrate from the primitive yolk sac to the gonadal ridge by an unknown mechanism.

10. **(B)** An oogonium becomes an oocyte when it enters the first stage of meiosis. This occurs prior to birth. After birth there is a slow decrease in the number of oocytes. By menopause none can be found. By 5 months' gestation there is a maximum number of oocytes, of about 4 to 7 million! At birth, the number of oocytes has decreased to 1 or 2 million. There continues to be attrition of oocytes during childhood so that by the onset of puberty fewer than 500,000 oocytes remain.

11. **(C)** The genital ducts (mesonephric or Wolffian and paramesonephric or Müllerian) are present in both sexes. The mesonephric ducts will become the male ducts and seminal vesicles. The female paramesonephros will form the oviducts, uterus, and upper two-thirds of the vagina. The lining of these ducts becomes the epithelial lining of the adult structures. Muscle and connective tissue originate from the adjoining mesenchyme. The prostatic utricle and the appendix testis in the male may indeed be remnants of paramesonephric duct but are not really formed by the ducts (see Figure 3–1).

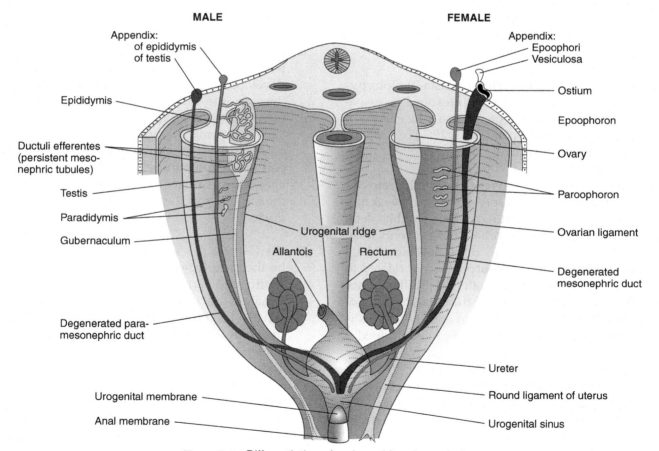

**Figure 3–1.** Differentiation of male and female genitalia.
(Reproduced, with permission, from DeCherney AH, Nathan L. *Current Obstetric and Gynecologic Diagnosis and Treatment*, 9th ed. New York: McGraw-Hill, 2003.)

12. **(D)** The vaginal epithelium is derived from the endoderm of the urogenital sinus while the fibromuscular wall of the vagina develops from the uterovaginal primordium. In the female, parts of the mesonephric duct persist as the duct of Gartner in the broad ligament along the lateral wall of the uterus. Occasionally, women may develop Gartner's duct cysts in the lateral vaginal walls. The paramesonephric duct develops into the uterus, fallopian tubes, broad ligament structures, and occasionally hydatid cysts of Morgagni.

13. **(C)** The urogenital sinus is derived from partitioning of the endodermal-derived embryonic cloaca. It is the precursor to the urinary bladder and the genitalia in each sex. The cloaca is a pouch on the caudal end of the hindgut that was formed by folding of the caudal region of the embryonic disk.

14. **(D)** In infants with ambiguous external genitalia, confusion may arise as to whether this rugated structure is a scrotal sac or a fused labia. The most common cause of ambiguous genitalia in the newborn is congenital adrenal hyperplasia (see Figure 3–2).

15. **(E)** The clitoris is a small, erectile body that responds to androgen stimulation with increased growth. Increasing clitoral size is one sign of virilism. Virilization can be caused by internal

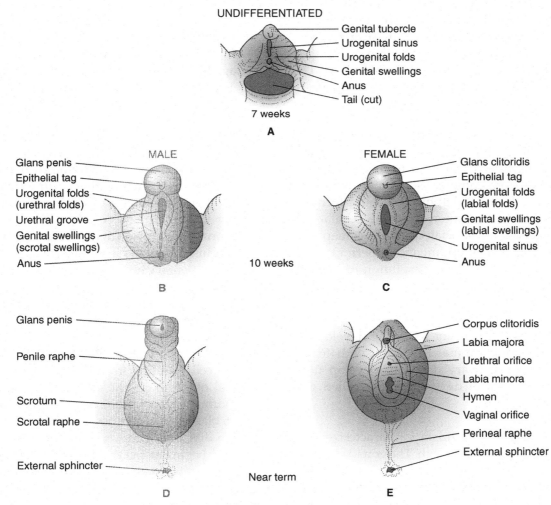

**Figure 3–2.** Differentiation of the external genitalia.
(Reproduced, with permission, from DeCherney AH, Nathan L. *Current Obstetric and Gynecologic Diagnosis and Treatment*, 9th ed. New York: McGraw-Hill, 2003.)

(adrenal or ovarian) androgens or by androgenic substances such as some progestins that are ingested by the mother.

16. **(C)** The frequency of vaginal agenesis is about 0.025%. It is due to failure of the uterovaginal primordium to contact the urogenital sinus. The uterus is usually absent. Ovarian agenesis is rarely associated with vaginal agenesis. When the vagina is absent, the greater vestibular glands are still present in most cases. In Müllerian aplasia, most of the vagina and uterus are absent. It is thought that 80% to 90% of individuals without a vagina have Müllerian aplasia rather than atresia. One embryologic defect is apt to be associated with others. You should also look for abnormalities of the urinary tract. In the absence of Müllerian Inhibitory Factor from testes, the fetus will develop a uterus and vagina as a default program. In Turner's syndrome (XO), which is a form of gonadal dysgenesis, the uterus and vagina are present. Also in a genetically XY fetus with gonadal dysgenesis a female phenotype will be formed.

17. **(A)** The fusion of the Wolffian duct system gives rise to the uterus, cervix, and upper vagina. Incomplete fusion may lead to several uterine anomalies from complete separation with two cervices—uterine didelphys to a mild form of incomplete fusion—uterine septae. Unilateral renal agenesis is associated with metanephros failure. Transverse septum and imperforate hymens are due to lack of dissolution of the cell cord of the fused Mullerian ducts and the urogenital sinus.

18. **(D)** If germ cells do not reach the developing ovary, gonadoblastomas may form with 46,XY karyotype. The ovary does not develop normally. This lack of development is called gonadal dysgenesis.

19. **(D)** True hermaphroditism is characterized by ambiguous genitalia at birth. The gonads may be any combination of ovary, testis, or ovotestis. Interestingly, a testis or ovotestis is usually located on the right side. Müllerian structures are usually present on the side ipsilateral to an ovary or ovotestis. Most true hermaphrodites are 46,XX with no identifiable Y chromosome but rather small portions of the Y chromosome incorporated into their genome.

20. **(B)** The physical examination of the newborn with ambiguous genitalia may reveal gonads that are palpable in the scrotum or lower inguinal canal. These gonads may be testes or ovotestes. High circulating androgens in the female fetus are not sufficient to cause descent of normal ovaries and therefore descended gonads cannot be ovaries. Pelvic ultrasound is frequently useful in identifying Müllerian structures while the presence of a normal uterus rules out the possibility of normal testicular tissue.

21. **(A)** Only the distal one-third of the vagina is formed from the urogenital sinus. The proximal vagina is formed by fusion of the Müllerian ducts. This explains why, in cases of Müllerian agenesis, patients have a rudimentary vagina. The bladder and rectum are formed from endodermal tissue not the urogenital sinus.

22. **(E)** Abnormalities of fusion of the paramesonephric ducts often cause pregnancy wastage. The various types of uterine duplication and vaginal malformation that occur with improper fusion include uterus didelphys, which is a double uterus with a double vagina, bicornuate uterus with a fusion defect isolated to the uterine fundus but not vagina, unicornuate uterus with a rudimentary horn, and a longitudinal septum where a caudal fusion problem exists but uterine fusion is adequate. Gartner's duct cysts do not affect pregnancy in general.

23–27. **(23-A, 24-E, 25-C, 26-D, 27-J)** The zygote is the cell resulting from the union of the sperm and ovum (egg), the gametes, or the fertilized ovum. Blastocele is the name applied to the 12 to 16 blastomeres composing the ball of cells from the division of the zygote. The embryonic period begins at the third week of development. During this time, most of the major structures are formed, and the greatest risk from teratogens exists. The fetal period begins in the ninth developmental week and extends to birth. The ninth week to birth is more remarkable for rapid growth than for major developmental change. This is a period of growth and maturation of the existing structures. Trophoblastic invasion is the process by which the embryo implants into the uterine lining at the blastocyst stage. The blastocele is the fluid-filled cavity that forms immediately prior to blastocyst formation.

**28–30.   (28-B, 29-D, 30-B)** A transverse vaginal septum and an imperforate hymen imply that canalization of the vaginal plate at its junction with the sinusal (Müllerian) tubercle did not proceed completely. A longitudinal septum implies that the caudal fusion of the Müllerian ducts did not result in complete canalization of the uterovaginal primordium. When the vagina is absent, in most cases it will be due to aplasia of the Müllerian ducts. When the urogenital sinus persists, it causes any number of anomalies, most representing either no opening for the anus or an aberrant opening.

# CHAPTER 4

# Genetics and Teratology

## Questions

**(Questions 1 through 25):** For each of the multiple choice questions in this section, select the lettered answer that is the one *best* response in each case.

**Questions 1 through 4 apply to the following patient:**

You are counseling a 16-year-old G1P0 girl and her 16-year-old boyfriend. Two weeks ago they received a quad screen result with a 1:50 risk for Down syndrome. She has noninformative family history and medical history.

1. You begin counseling by explaining that the number of chromosomes in a fetus is how many?
   - (A) 23
   - (B) 46
   - (C) 48
   - (D) 47 for a female fetus
   - (E) 21 for Down syndrome

2. You counsel that the quad screen does which of the following?
   - (A) measures chemicals from the baby's blood
   - (B) looks at the four aspects of Down syndrome
   - (C) is less predictive than ultrasound screens
   - (D) predicts with 85–90% certainty whether the baby has Down syndrome
   - (E) has different levels of sensitivity depending on the mother's age

3. You perform an ultrasound that places the fetus currently at 15½ weeks' gestation. You should counsel which of the following?
   - (A) The quad screen was drawn too early.
   - (B) The small fetus makes it more likely the baby has a chromosome problem.
   - (C) In light of an abnormal ultrasound and a worrisome quad screen she should have an amniocentesis.
   - (D) It would be safe to wait until 22 weeks for her amniocentesis.
   - (E) She should consider termination as an option considering significant intrauterine growth restriction (IUGR) and the worrisome quad screen.

4. If she decides she would like amniocentesis, you counsel her the complications would include which of the following?
   - (A) 1–250 risk of fetal injury
   - (B) 1–250 risk of miscarriage
   - (C) 1:500 to 1:1000 risk of miscarriage
   - (D) 1–250 risk of bleeding and abruption
   - (E) 1–100 risk of growth lay with 1–250 risk of ruptured membranes

**Questions 5 through 7 apply to the following patient:**

A 25-year-old G1P0, 20 weeks' gestation has a family history of classic hemophilia. Her uncle on her mother's side and her brother are affected. A perinatal ultrasound notes a male fetus.

5. What is the chance that her son (in utero) will inherit hemophilia?

    (A) 25%
    (B) 50%
    (C) 33%
    (D) 100%
    (E) Impossible to say

6. If her son does have the disease, he would be classified as which of the following?

    (A) codominant
    (B) heterozygous
    (C) hemizygous
    (D) homozygous
    (E) intermediate

7. In counseling this patient, she asks why her uncle died when he was 4 and her brother, now 17, has had little problem with the disease. You explain that the different expression of the gene relates is a result of which of the following?

    (A) percentage of individuals who have a gene in which there is an effect
    (B) percentage of individuals in a population who have a gene
    (C) phenotypic variation among the individuals who have a gene
    (D) change in the form of a gene with chromosomal aging
    (E) shape and number of chromosomes

8. A female who possesses an X-linked trait may do so because either she inherited a recessive gene from both her mother and her father or which of the following?

    (A) She inherited a recessive gene from one of her parents and may express the recessive characteristic as a function of the Lyon hypothesis.
    (B) She has undergone spontaneous mutation from an environmental source.
    (C) She is really a testicular feminization patient.
    (D) She lacks the genetic expressor gene for dominance.
    (E) She has a translocated Y determinant on one of her autosomes.

9. You are seeing a patient who has been exposed to a medication. You look it up in the register of pregnancy medications. It is listed as category C. The patient asks you what this means. Which of the following is your best response?

    (A) The drug has been evaluated in well-controlled human studies and no fetal risk has been shown.
    (B) Animal studies have not shown any fetal risk, or suggested some risk not confirmed in humans, or there are not adequate studies in women.
    (C) Animal studies have shown adverse effects, but there are no adequately controlled studies in humans.
    (D) There are some fetal risks, but benefits may outweigh risks under certain circumstances; thus, patients should be warned.
    (E) Fetal abnormalities have occurred in animal and human studies, the risk is greater than the benefit, and the drug is contraindicated in pregnancy.

10. Approximately what percentage of spontaneous first-trimester abortions shows chromosomal abnormalities?

    (A) 1
    (B) 10
    (C) 25
    (D) 50
    (E) 75

11. Live births of infants would demonstrate approximately what percentage of chromosomal abnormalities?

(A) less than 1
(B) 1–5
(C) approximately 10
(D) 15–20
(E) 40–50

12. A 22-year-old woman and her husband are being counseled after a first-trimester miscarriage. She has no significant medical problems. Her physical examination is unremarkable and in counseling her you explain in lay terms that the most likely cause of her miscarriage is aneuploidy. Which of the following is the most common aneuploidy causing miscarriage?

(A) trisomy 18
(B) 45,XO
(C) triploidy
(D) unbalanced translocation
(E) tetraploidy

**Questions 13 and 14 apply to the following patient:**

A 19-year-old woman with a complaint of never having had menses comes to your office. Physical examination shows that she is 1.37 m tall and weighs 94 lb. She lacks breast and pubic hair development. There is webbing of her neck and cubitus valgus.

13. Which of the following would be the simplest, yet most useful, initial test to begin her evaluation?

(A) serum estrogen level
(B) prolactin
(C) thyroid index
(D) serum follicle-stimulating hormone (FSH) and luteinizing hormone (LH)
(E) a cardiogram

14. Given the description of this patient, which of the following is her most likely diagnosis?

(A) testicular feminization
(B) Klinefelter's syndrome

(C) Turner's syndrome
(D) congenital adrenal hyperplasia (CAH)
(E) normal but delayed development

15. Patients with a 45,XO karyotype are invariably of short stature because the locus responsible for short stature is located where?

(A) long arm of X
(B) short arm of X
(C) centromere of the O chromosome
(D) long arm of chromosome 45
(E) short arm of chromosome 45

16. Your patient's previous child died at 8 weeks of age. Her family called it crib death, but the autopsy suggested a metabolic disease. Which of the following most commonly describes inborn errors of metabolism that are diagnosable in utero?

(A) not genetic diseases
(B) autosomal dominants
(C) autosomal recessives
(D) sex linked
(E) polygenic in origin

17. A couple is concerned about the safety of antenatal ultrasound. What should you counsel them regarding the procedure?

(A) Ultrasound has been in use for almost 40 years with no noted side effects.
(B) The reason it is called ultrasound is that it is safe, as verified by the Food and Drug Administration (FDA).
(C) Ultrasound is done only by trained sonographers to ensure safe practice.
(D) Ultrasound may be associated with cataracts and hearing loss in animals, if used continually, and thus it is used only when indicated.
(E) Antenatal ultrasound may be associated with heating in tissue and thus is used only when indicated.

18. A woman with blood type O gave birth to an AB infant. She and her partner are quite concerned that there may be a mix-up in the nursery. What is the most likely diagnosis?

(A) Lyon hypothesis
(B) chimerism
(C) Bombay phenotype
(D) laboratory error
(E) a maternal blocking antibody

19. A baby presents with ambiguous genitalia. A full chromosome count is sent and will return in 72 hours. Your laboratory can perform a test for Barr body so you can provide a preliminary answer sooner. What is the Barr body?

(A) the condensed, nonfunctioning X chromosome
(B) the darkest, widest band found on chromosomes
(C) an extra lobe on the female polymorphonuclear leukocytes
(D) found only in the female
(E) the largest chromosome in the female genotype

**Questions 20 and 21 apply to the following patient:**

A couple presents to your office during the ninth week of pregnancy. Their previous child was diagnosed with trisomy 18, so they are extremely anxious and would like prenatal diagnosis as early as possible. They have many questions about chorionic villus sampling (CVS).

20. Which of the following would be the best response to their questions about CVS? Which is the best answer?

(A) CVS may be performed anytime in pregnancy after 9 weeks.
(B) CVS done in the 9- to 10-week range has a very small association (less than 1:1000) with limb malformations.
(C) CVS provides a preliminary answer within 48 hours; a definitive answer needs the 16-week amniocentesis.
(D) CVS cannot be performed in multiple gestations.

(E) CVS may be used to detect open neural tube defects after 12 weeks' gestation.

21. You explain to the couple that complications of CVS include which of the following?

(A) amniotic band syndrome
(B) IUGR
(C) rupture of the umbilical cord
(D) vaginal bleeding
(E) VATER syndrome

22. A mother with blood group AB has an AB child. She would like to establish paternity through blood typing. Which blood type excludes a male from being the potential biologic father?

(A) AA
(B) BB
(C) BO
(D) AO
(E) OO

23. A woman presents from prenatal diagnosis requesting amniocentesis. Of the following issues in a patient history, which would be better diagnosed with ultrasound over amniocentesis?

(A) maternal age over 41 years
(B) previous chromosomally abnormal child
(C) family history of open neural tube defect
(D) abnormal serum marker for trisomy 18
(E) possible female carrier of 21 hydroxylase deficiency

24. A pregnant woman presents to your clinic with a history of a previous child who was diagnosed with phenylketonuria (PKU) as a neonate. Her partner is not the father of the first child. The mother remembers that she had to have a special diet when she was a child. In counseling her, you should explain which of the following?

(A) PKU is an autosomal dominant disease, thus this child has a 50% chance of being affected.
(B) Because this is a new father, the pregnancy cannot result in an affected child although the child may be a carrier.

(C) If the father's phenotype is normal, the fetus cannot have the disease.

(D) The fetus may be affected in utero if the mother has PKU.

(E) Unless the first baby's father can be tested, we cannot test the neonate.

25. A couple presents wanting to know the likelihood of recurrence of certain inherited traits. Which of the following is an autosomal dominant inheritance that gives the couple a 50/50 chance of recurrence with their next pregnancy?

(A) cleft lip
(B) tetralogy of Fallot
(C) pyloric stenosis
(D) achondroplasia
(E) clubfoot (talipes equinovarus)

**DIRECTIONS (Questions 26 through 47): The following groups of questions are preceded by a list of lettered options. For each question, select the one lettered option that is most closely associated with it. Each lettered option may be used once, multiple times, or not at all.**

**Questions 26 through 33**

(A) mosaicism
(B) polyploidy
(C) aneuploidy
(D) deletion
(E) translocation
(F) isochromosome
(G) inversion
(H) insertion
(I) nondisjunction
(J) linkage
(K) codominance
(L) translational errors

26. Amniocentesis with an ambiguous result showing more than one cell line present

27. $2n + 1$ or $2n - 1$

28. Anomalous fetus with FISH results of three signals for chromosome 13, 18, and 21, and signals for X

29. May be either reciprocal or Robertsonian

30. Results when a chromosome divides by horizontal rather than longitudinal split at the centromere

31. May be either paracentric or pericentric

32. May result in a ring chromosome

33. The most common cause of chromosomal abnormalities

**Questions 34 through 39**

Match the chromosomal complement with the phenotype.

(A) 45,XO
(B) 46,XY
(C) 47,XXY
(D) 46,XX t(14q21q)
(E) 46,XX, 5p–
(F) 46,XX/XY

34. A male that appears with tall stature, eunuchoidism, sometimes gynecomastia

35. A newborn female with edema of the hands and feet

36. Epicanthic folds, hypertelorism, mental deficiency, single palmar crease

37. Large breasts, scanty axillary hair, absent uterus

38. Microcephaly, severe mental retardation

39. True hermaphrodite

**Questions 40 through 47**

(A)  autosomal dominant

(B)  autosomal recessive

(C)  X-linked

(D)  polygenic or multifactorial

(E)  not a genetic disease

40.  Diabetes mellitus

41.  Sickle cell anemia

42.  Hemophilia

43.  Fragile X syndrome

44.  Transmitted through the daughter to half of the grandsons

45.  Most such diseases have a carrier rate in the general population of less than 1%

46.  CAH

47.  Neurofibromatosis

**DIRECTIONS (Questions 48 through 55): For each of the multiple choice questions in this section, select the lettered answer that is the one *best* response in each case.**

48.  A 24-year-old G2P0 comes to you at 17 weeks' gestation. She has epilepsy with grand mal seizures that developed after motor vehicle trauma. She is currently on valproic acid, which puts her fetus at risk for which of the following?

(A)  aplasia actuis

(B)  neural tube defect

(C)  diaphragmatic hernia

(D)  club feet

(E)  hypospadias

49.  A 28-year-old G6P1 A4 comes to you for consultation at 14 weeks. She is being treated for a diagnosis of bipolar disease. She was on paroxetine (Paxil); however, her primary care provider had taken her off at 8 weeks. She is extremely anxious, her family tells you she is not sleeping well and is "doing poorly head wise." What is your most appropriate course of action?

(A)  start her on a tricyclic antidepressant

(B)  start a more long-acting antidepressant, such as fluoxetine (Prozac)

(C)  use a benzodiazepine to decrease anxiety

(D)  restart Paxil

(E)  try a 4-week course of Depakote (valproic acid)

50.  A 29-year-old G5P0 SAB4 woman is taking Coumadin for a DVT she suffered 3 months ago. She is now 8 weeks' pregnant. What is the most appropriate course of action?

(A)  stop Coumadin until after pregnancy

(B)  stay on Coumadin until 12 weeks and then switch to heparin

(C)  switch to heparin at this time

(D)  recommend termination of the pregnancy

(E)  stop Coumadin now and treat with heparin for the last trimester and 6 weeks postpartum

51.  Which of the following is the most common complication of full anticoagulation with low-molecular-weight heparin?

(A)  osteoporosis

(B)  ulcers

(C)  renal stones (nephrolithiasis)

(D)  bleeding

(E)  thromboembolism

52.  In giving a lecture to a pregnancy class about medications during pregnancy and lactation, which of the following accurately describes drug interaction?

(A)  Antidepressants do not cross into the breast milk.

(B)  Oral diabetic agents and insulin (sulfonylureas) do not cross into breast milk.

(C)  The only major antibiotics contraindicated with lactation include erythromycin and tetracycline.

(D) Selective serotonin reuptake inhibitor (SSRI) is contraindicated during breastfeeding.

(E) Women may use anti-herpes medicine such as Valtrex or acyclovir during pregnancy.

53. A 37-year-old G1P0 at 11 weeks' gestation has a fetus with a nuchal thickness of 2.9 mm. How should you counsel your patient at this time?

(A) consider termination if morally acceptable

(B) recheck in 2 weeks, since she is only 11 weeks' pregnant

(C) consider CVS

(D) consider amniocentesis

(E) wait until 15 weeks and draw a quad screen

54. A 21-year-old G2P1 comes to see you at 5 weeks' gestation. She has returned from spring break 3 weeks ago at which time she spent several nights partying and she states she may have gotten drunk once or twice. She has not gotten drunk since then. What should you counsel your patient?

(A) She most likely does not have to worry.

(B) She should have a targeted ultrasound at 16 weeks and quad screen.

(C) She should consider a CVS or amniocentesis to rule out fetal alcohol syndrome.

(D) She should consider termination if it is morally acceptable.

(E) You should draw serial HCG levels to check their rise.

55. A 33-year-old G3P0A2 had a quad screen drawn with an alpha-fetoprotein (AFP) level that was 3.4 multiple of the median (MOM) at 15 weeks. The rest of the values were unremarkable. What is the most appropriate next step?

(A) redraw the AFP only

(B) redraw the quad screen

(C) perform a fasting blood draw of AFP

(D) perform an ultrasound at this time

(E) schedule a level 2 ultrasound at 19–20 weeks' gestation

**DIRECTIONS (Questions 56 and 57):** The following group of questions is preceded by a list of lettered options. For each question, select the one lettered option that is most closely associated with it. Each lettered option may be used once, multiple times, or not at all.

Of the following medications, pick the medication with the best safety profile for the fetus.

(A) hydantoin (Dilantin)

(B) carbamazepine (Tegretol)

(C) valproic acid (Depakote)

(D) lamictogene (Lamictal)

(E) phenobarbital

(F) paroxetine (Paxil)

(G) citalopram (Celexa)

(H) sertraline (Zoloft)

(I) valproic acid (Depakote)

(J) fluoxetine (Prozac)

56. A mother with grand mal seizures

57. A mother with bipolar depression

**DIRECTIONS (Questions 58 through 65):** For each of the multiple choice questions in this section, select the lettered answer that is the one *best* response in each case.

58. A woman with a severe ankle sprain was prescribed ibuprofen for 72 hours. At what gestational age should she avoid this medication?

(A) any gestational age

(B) before 12 weeks and after 26 weeks

(C) after 36 weeks

(D) after 32 weeks

(E) during lactation

59. A woman was being treated for polycystic ovary disease with metformin (Glucophage). During her first visit at 10 weeks' gestation, you should do which of the following?

    (A) stop immediately and order a nuclear thickness measurement and ultrascreen
    (B) stop immediately and place her on insulin
    (C) recommend amniocentesis targeted ultrasound at 16 weeks
    (D) stop the medication at 20 weeks' gestation
    (E) allow her to continue until delivery

60. During pregnancy, what is the safest analgesic with the least fetal affect?

    (A) aspirin
    (B) acetaminophen
    (C) ibuprofen
    (D) gabapentin
    (E) oxycodone

61. A 35-year-old woman at 18 weeks' gestation is found to have choroid plexus cysts, and a fetus 9 days' size less than dates. You should do which of the following?

    (A) consider termination if it is morally acceptable
    (B) consider CVS
    (C) consider amniocentesis
    (D) repeat the ultrasound in 4 weeks
    (E) counsel that isolated choroid plexus cysts are not of concern

62. A 35-year-old G4P3 at 18 weeks with an unremarkable family history has a risk after sequential screening of 1:170 for Down syndrome. You should do which of the following?

    (A) offer CVS
    (B) offer amniocentesis
    (C) perform a targeted ultrasound
    (D) offer genetic counseling
    (E) advise her the risk is quite small for aneuploidy

63. A 24-year-old Jewish woman presents for prenatal diagnosis, at 16 weeks' gestation. Her family history is unknown since she is adopted. The father of the baby is half Jewish. What should you counsel your patient?

    (A) amniocentesis
    (B) maternal screening for Tay-Sachs disease
    (C) CVS
    (D) targeted ultrasound and quad screen instead of screening for Tay-Sachs disease
    (E) not to worry since she is adopted and her husband is only half Jewish

64. A 26-year-old woman is trying to quit smoking. She was using the nicotine patch (28 mg/d) with nicotine gum for breakthrough when she found out she was pregnant. She immediately stopped the patch and is back to smoking 1 to 1.5 packs a day. She is 11 weeks' pregnant. What should you advise your patient?

    (A) she should consider termination if morally acceptable
    (B) consider CVS
    (C) consider first-trimester screening and targeted ultrasound
    (D) consider amniocentesis at 16 weeks
    (E) the patch and gum are of very low concern for birth defects

65. A 24-year-old G2P1, living children 0, came to see you at 12 weeks' gestation. Her previous child died at 1 day of age with hypoplastic left heart. In this pregnancy you should advise which of the following?

    (A) CVS at this time
    (B) amniocentesis at 16 weeks' gestation
    (C) sequential screening now and at 15 weeks
    (D) fetal cardiac echo in the mid-second trimester
    (E) regular pregnancy care since the risk of recurrence is quite small

# Answers and Explanations

1. **(B)** There are 23 pairs of chromosomes in the normal human cell. Twenty-two are alike in males and females and are called autosomes. The remaining pair are sex chromosomes, the X and the Y, and determine genetic sex. In Figure 4–1, a 47,XX + 21 chromosome complement is illustrated.

2. **(E)** The quad screen, drawn from maternal blood at 15 to 21 weeks, combined with the mother's age will give a risk ratio for the likelihood of Down syndrome. The four blood chemicals come from the placenta and fetus that diffuse into the maternal circulation. The sensitivity is increased as the incidence increases, thus it is affected by the mother's age.

3. **(A)** A QUAD screen drawn at 13½ weeks would not be valid. She is currently at 15½ weeks' gestation and the test was drawn 2 weeks ago. It would be extremely unlikely to have that significant of an IUGR infant to be 2+ weeks difference without other marked anomalies on ultrasound. The most common cause is misdating.

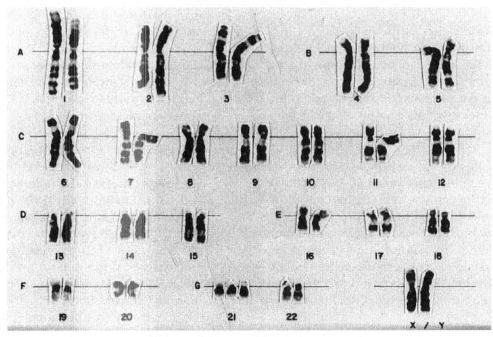

**Figure 4–1.** Abnormal female karyotype.
(Reproduced, with permission, from Cunningham FG, Gant NF, Leveno KJ, Gilstrap LC, Hauth JC, Wenstrom KD. *Williams Obstetrics*, 21st ed. New York: McGraw-Hill, 2001.)

4. **(C)** The risk of miscarriage is 1:500 to 1:1000. This risk was previously quoted at 1:250, but in the hands of an experienced individual, and with the use of ultrasound, it has been decreased by two- to fourfold.

5. **(A)** Classic hemophilia is X-linked. The mother has a 50% chance of being a carrier. Since her brother has the disease, we know the patient has the potential of being positive. Since the fetus is a male, it has a 50% chance of getting the affected X chromosome. Thus 50% chance of 50% is 25%.

6. **(C)** The female, having two X chromosomes, can be either heterozygous or homozygous for an X-linked gene. The male with only one X will express all the characteristics of the lone X, hence the term hemizygous, rather than heterozygous. In this form of inheritance (X-linked or sex-linked), the condition occurs more commonly in males. If both parents do not possess the trait and an affected male is born, the mother is a carrier. If the father is affected and an affected male is born, the mother is a heterozygote. While a characteristic linked to a Y chromosome is possible, there seems to be none of real clinical significance.

7. **(C)** Expressivity means the gene has a different effect or appearance in different kindreds. Sometimes the gene may be expressed in mild, moderate, or severe forms. It is an example of how the entire genome must be taken into account when considering the effect of some genes.

8. **(A)** All females are mosaics (have more than one cell line) for the X chromosome. It is believed that this occurs because as an embryo, every female cell selects one X to be expressed and the other to become inactive. The selection is more or less random. By chance, a genotypical heterozygote could express a recessive trait phenotypically. The inactive material of each X appears in the cell as a clump of chromatin called the Barr body.

9. **(C)** Teratogenicity drug labeling is required by the FDA. The FDA has established five categories of drugs based on their potential for causing birth defects. The categories are A through D, which correspond directly to distractors A through D in this question. The fifth category is X and corresponds to distractor E. The FDA is working to change this system to one that provides more data. In the current system there is little clinical difference between category B and C drugs in actual risk. There is a difference in amount of information available.

10. **(D)** The 50% number represents testable products of conception in the first trimester. Second-trimester losses are to a much lower degree by chromosomal anomalies caused.

11. **(A)** Elective abortions and term births have approximately the same incidence of chromosomal abnormalities: 1 per 200 (less than 1%). Spontaneous abortions may have 50 to 75 times the incidence, according to some studies.

12. **(A)** Of abortuses that are abnormal, more than one-half are trisomic. One-third of the trisomies are trisomy 16, which does not occur in the liveborn since all such fetuses die. Then trisomy 18 or 21. Next is 45,XO, which occurs in about roughly 20% of chromosomally abnormal abortuses. Triploidy (69 chromosomes) or tetraploidy are less than 5% of cases.

13. **(D)** An evaluation of serum gonadotropins would demonstrate ovarian failure, one of the hallmarks of this syndrome. Karyotyping is not always necessary.

14. **(C)** The initial three anomalies described by Turner's were short stature, cubitus valgus, and webbing of the neck. Lymphedema of the hands and feet is a sign often present at the birth of these infants and may be the first diagnostic sign. Clogging of lymphatics causes webbing of the fetal neck with the resultant skin bridges and edema of the extremities. Coarctation of the aorta and absence of a kidney may also be present. Normal fertility is not possible since the gonads are dysfunctional (gonadal dysgenesis). Only two-thirds of the patients, however, have the classic 45,XO chromosomal complement. The syndrome is synonymous with the term of gonadal dysgenesis. Patients with pure

gonadal dysgenesis lack the associated physical findings of Turner's syndrome.

In Klinefelter syndrome (47,XXY), boys are typically tall but do not virilize in puberty and thus require testosterone replacement. They have small testes, are infertile as a result of gonadal dysgenesis, and may have gynecomastia. CAH would cause female virilization and ambiguous genitalia at delivery. Testicular feminization would give an individual with a very normal female phenotype except with puberty when they will get breast development and increased growth but no pubic hair or menses.

15. **(B)** Patients who lack an X (such as XO) or have Xp (short arm of X) missing will be short. X inactivation (Lyons) appears to be incomplete. More specifically, those missing the distal-most portion of the short arm of X are of short stature.

16. **(C)** Many of these enzyme defects lend themselves to biochemical determinations, either on the amniotic fluid itself or on cells cultured from it. Unfortunately, in most instances you must know prospectively which defect to screen. Many metabolic diseases are screened for at birth.

17. **(A)** Ultrasound has been available for more than 40 years and no ill effects are noted, because the frequency and importantly the power are not in a harmful range. Thus heating (as for physical therapy use) or cavitation (as for kidney stones) is not an issue.

18. **(C)** The Bombay phenotype is very rare and has inactive alleles for H antigen. If no H is formed, neither A nor B antigen can be formed, and the patient's blood will be type O even if the A or B gene is present. Laboratory error is always possible, but given the caution with which blood typing is done, it is unlikely. Blocking antibodies will not disguise a blood type.

19. **(A)** The Barr body is the inactivated X chromosome and is also known as the sex chromatin. The number of Barr bodies is generally one less than the number of X chromosomes. It tells nothing about the number of Y chromosomes. It

equals the total number of X chromosomes minus one.

20. **(B)** CVS, also known as chorionic villus biopsy, has been performed in the United States for the past 25 years. It is associated with a 1 per 500 pregnancy loss rate. One complication is the very small risk of less than 1 per 1000 limb malformations when CVS is performed at 9 to 10 weeks. Thus, many centers will perform CVS only around $10\frac{1}{2}$ to $12\frac{1}{2}$ weeks. CVS is performed by placing a small catheter or needle into the placenta (not into the chorionic membranes or into the amniotic fluid) and removing a small bit of villus through suction aspiration. The chorionic villus is then dissected, and cells are harvested for chromosomal analysis. The analysis made from CVS can essentially give the same information as the chromosomal analysis from amniocentesis CVS cannot be used to evaluate structural lesions that is best done with ultrasound. CVS may be used in most circumstances with multiple gestations.

21. **(D)** Complications, besides the small risk of limb defects, include bleeding and miscarriage. Bleeding occurs in up to $\frac{1}{3}$ of women. VATER syndrome is an association of vertebral defects, anal atresia, tracheoesophageal fistula with esophageal atresia, and radial dysplasia. This is a group of anomalies that occur together frequently but do not seem to be linked etiologically. It is not associated with CVS.

22. **(E)** The father could not be type O, unless of the very rare Bombay phenotype, since the child would have been AO or BO and could not be AB.

23. **(C)** Since developed by Liley in 1962, amniocentesis and CVS for prenatal diagnosis and therapy have become very common. There are now several hundred diagnosable diseases. Structural lesions are usually best diagnosed by ultrasound.

24. **(D)** PKU is an autosomal recessive disease in which an affected individual lacks the enzyme phenylalanine hydroxylase. When excessive amounts of phenylalanine accumulate, mental retardation usually occurs. The disease

may be treated with a low phenylalanine diet in childhood. If a woman with PKU becomes pregnant and is not on a special diet, the maternal phenylalanine levels may cause fetal abnormalities, growth retardation, and microcephaly. Thus, her fetus may be affected even though the fetus does not have the disease. Because individuals who carry one gene are asymptomatic, the father of this pregnancy may be a carrier and still have an affected infant. In addition, testing the previous child's father has no bearing on this pregnancy.

25. **(D)** Polygenic/multifactorial inheritance is involved in many abnormalities. These inheritance patterns present with a greater than expected recurrence rate than that seen at random, usually 2% to 5%. Many structural abnormalities, including cleft lip and palate, tetralogy of Fallot, pyloric stenosis, and clubfoot, are examples of such inheritance. Achondroplasia is an autosomal dominant inheritance.

26. **(A)** Chromosomal abnormalities may be numerical or structural and may involve autosomes, sex chromosomes, or both simultaneously. The abnormality may be present in all body cells or only in some of the cells, producing what is called mosaicism (or more than one cell line).

27. **(C)** Each species has a characteristic number of chromosomes (ploidy). In humans, this $2n$ number is 46. Any multiple of the haploid number ($1n$) is called euploid. Polyploid means any exact multiple greater than $2n$ ($3n$, $4n$, and so forth). Aneuploid means any number of chromosomes that is not an exact multiple of $1n$.

28. **(B)** The FISH signal, fluorescent in situ hybridization, in the fetus shows signals for three separate chromosomes and three sets for XX (six total). The preliminary diagnosis would be 69XX or polyploidy.

29. **(E)** Translocations consist of two chromosomes breaking and exchanging material between them. They may be of two types, either reciprocal (the exchange of chromatin between two nonhomologous chromosomes) or Robertsonian (fusion of two chromosomes at the cen-

tromere with loss of their heterochromatic short arms).

30. **(F)** A chromosome divides such that the two arms separate, rather than the two chromatids. This is an isochromosome. The most common isochromosome involves the long arm of the X, i(Xq). Fifteen to twenty percent of Turner's syndrome patients have this karyotype.

31. **(G)** Breakage and rearrangement of a chromosome such that a fragment ends up rotated 180 degrees. If the rearrangement takes place in a single arm, the inversion is called paracentric. If it involves the region of the centromere, it is called pericentric.

32. **(D)** A ring chromosome is a type of deletion chromosome in which two broken ends are reunited to form a ring-shaped chromosome. As long as the ring chromosome retains a centromere, it is capable of division.

33. **(I)** Nondisjunction is the failure of paired chromosomes to separate in anaphase. It is the most common cause of an error in chromosome number.

34. **(C)** Klinefelter's syndrome can also be found with 48,XXXY. This patient would have two Barr bodies per cell, yet still be male.

35. **(A)** 45,XO is the karyotype for Turner's syndrome. Early diagnosis is important, as other developmental defects such as coarctation of the aorta and renal abnormalities are also associated. Any child born with lymphedema of the extremities should be thoroughly investigated for possible Turner's syndrome.

36. **(D)** Translocation can cause Down syndrome with 46 chromosomes present. The occurrence of this entity does not increase with age and is rarely transmitted by the male. The current terminology for this condition would be t(14q 21q)–.

37. **(B)** Testicular feminization patients have a normal male chromosome pattern and target organs that are insensitive to testosterone. They are

generally of a normal female phenotype but with the potential for gonadal malignancy.

38. **(E)** Cry of the cat, or cri du chat, syndrome is due to deletion of the short arm of chromosome 5. It can also occur because of a parental translocation. It, however, is the most common human chromosomal syndrome caused by deletion.

39. **(F)** In the true hermaphrodite, both testicular and ovarian tissues (ovotestes) must be present. The external genitalia may resemble either a male or a female, depending on the ratio of estrogens and androgens present. Some are XX, some XY, while others are chimeras (XX/XY).

40. **(D)** Diabetes mellitus is another entity that has no single known genetic defect and no definite age of onset. It does exhibit characteristics indicating multifactorial genetic inheritance with associated human lymphocyte antigen types.

41. **(B)** Sickle cell anemia is caused by an abnormal hemoglobin resulting from a change in the amino acid sequence of the globin chain. The abnormality is the result of a single amino acid in the sixth position on the 146 amino acid chain being substituted.

42. **(C)** Hemophilia is due to a defect in the production of antihemophilic globulin. Fortunately, it is rare, occurring in about 1 in 10,000 male births. One-third of all cases arise from new mutations in lethal X-linked diseases but are much less common in nonlethal diseases such as hemophilia.

43. **(C)** Fragile X is the most common cause of mental retardation in males. It is caused by (repetitive sequences) of the genome; usually these missense sequences increase in size and thus become worse in subsequent generations.

44. **(C)** This sequence is characteristic of X-linked recessive inheritance. In X-linked dominant inheritance, an affected male transmits the disease to all of his daughters and none of his sons. This is a rare situation.

45. **(B)** Dominant inheritance diseases do not have a carrier state, and sex-linked recessives occur only in males. The incidence may be as low as one in a thousand.

46. **(B)** This disease is usually discussed under the heading of intersex or ambiguous genitalia. Its genetic etiology may be overlooked. It can be lethal within the first few days of life or produce adrenal insufficiency and short stature in other cases. It is the most common cause of female pseudohermaphroditism, causing virilization of female infants. It is the most common cause of ambiguous genitalia in the newborn. These patients have normal XX chromosomes but lack an enzyme needed for normal steroid metabolism. They are deficient in 21, 17, or 11 hydroxylase enzymes. The site of the block determines the manifestations of the disease.

47. **(A)** The defect resulting in neurofibromatosis (von Recklinghausen disease) is autosomal dominant. It is one of the genetic diseases that increase (shows evidence of greater mutation) with increasing paternal age. It shows a very high mutation rate in man and also shows extremely variable patterns of inheritance. Duchenne's muscular dystrophy has similar patterns of transmission.

48. **(B)** Valproic acid (Depakote) is associated with many anomalies. Neural tube defects are among the most severe.

49. **(D)** The use of antidepressant is based on an assessment of risk/benefit ratio. In this woman's case she is beyond the first trimester and at risk of fetal anomalies. She is having significant problems. The lowest effective dose should be used. The drug that worked before should be used as well.

50. **(C)** As soon as pregnancy is verified, a patient should be changed to heparin. Heparin either unfractionated or low-molecular-weight does not cross the placenta. Coumadin may be restarted after delivery. It does not cross in breast milk. Coumadin during pregnancy not only causes birth defects in the first trimester but it may also cause fetal death in the second and third trimesters as well.

51. **(D)** Bleeding is the worst common complication. Heparin will cause calcium loss from bones, and most authorities recommend calcium and vitamin D supplementation.

52. **(E)** Most medicines cross to some extent including oral diabetic agents and antidepressants. For the later they are still safe to use during lactation. Anti-herpetic agents are safe in pregnancy and lactation.

53. **(C)** CVS is a consideration at 11 weeks for any nuchal thickness more than 2.5 mm. There is no reason to terminate at this point or wait for later screening. Amniocentesis is contraindicated at 11 weeks. Lastly, 11 weeks is a correct time to assess nuchal thickness.

54. **(A)** Her alcohol exposure was prior to conception and thus it should not have affected the pregnancy. However, since the history may have been influenced by guilt, it would be valuable to follow her closely, even ordering a follow-up ultrasound in 3 to 4 weeks.

55. **(D)** Elevated AFP is associated with fetal malformations, twins, and fetal distress. At 3 to 4 times normal (3.4 MOM) an ultrasound should be performed now. AFP elevations of 2 to 2.5 MOM may be repeated.

56. **(D)** Most of all anti-seizure medications are problematic. Also having grand mal seizures is problematic. Lamictal appears to be the safest of those listed. Multiple medications are associated with the most problems and fetal abnormalities.

57. **(H)** Sertraline has the best safety record in pregnancy and lactation of the medications listed. All of the serotonin reuptake inhibitors (SRIs) may be associated with a very low incidence of neonatal irritability and poor transition. Of those listed, paroxetine (Paxil) is the most troublesome.

58. **(D)** Nonsteroidal anti-inflammatory agents may be used for short courses prior to 32 weeks' gestation. If they are used for longer times, they may lead to oligohydramnios, and premature closure of the ductus.

59. **(D)** Current studies have shown that women using metformin do better if they stay on the medication through 20 weeks. It is not associated with specific fetal anomalies.

60. **(B)** Acetaminophen is the analgesic of choice. Short courses of nonsteroidal anti-inflammatory drugs (NSAIDs) are safe prior to 32 weeks. However, the pregnancy should be monitored. Gabapentin is probably safe, but we have little information.

61. **(C)** Choroid plexus cysts are associated (weakly) with trisomy 18. Her age, 35, and the small fetal size are also warning signs. It is too late for CVS, and since most likely the fetus is normal, termination is not indicated at this time. If the chromosomes are normal then the choroid plexus cysts are of no concern.

62. **(D)** This patient at age 35 should be offered genetic counseling. She and her partner must assess the risk they feel comfortable with. Amniocentesis, prior to counseling, is not as helpful. CVS is not appropriate at 18 weeks' gestation.

63. **(B)** Best option is Tay-Sachs carrier status screening in maternal blood. If she is not a carrier then the matter is moot. Many adopted children are of the same religion as the parents who adopt them, particularly when they are of similar race. Thus, it is common for Jewish parents to adopt a Jewish child. Thus, we cannot assume anything about her Tay-Sachs status. CVS and amniocentesis are not appropriate until we know her status.

64. **(E)** In this patient's case we should work with her to quit smoking. However, she is not at increased risk for fetal birth defects. However, if she continues to smoke she is at increased risk of pregnancy complications.

65. **(D)** The risk of recurrence is approximately 6% to 10% if there is a previous child or first-degree relative with left-sided disease. The recurrence though falls into a spectrum from hypoplastic left heart to bicuspid aortic valve. Structural evaluation with ultrasound, and in particular fetal cardiac echo, is the modality of choice for screening.

# CHAPTER 5

# Physiology of Reproduction

## Questions

**(Questions 1 through 34): For each of the multiple choice questions in this section, select the lettered answer that is the one *best* response in each case.**

**Questions 1 and 2 apply to the following topic:**

In the female endocrine system, gonadotropin-releasing hormone (GnRH) is able to modulate two hormones to result in the release of a single ovum. This complex system is vulnerable to disruption with resulting abnormal uterine bleeding and infertility.

1. Gonadotropin-releasing hormone (GnRH) stimulates the release of follicle-stimulating hormone in addition to which of the following?

   (A) adrenocorticotropic hormone (ACTH)
   (B) growth hormone (GH)
   (C) luteinizing hormone (LH)
   (D) opiate peptide
   (E) thyroid-stimulating hormone (TSH)

2. The GnRH secretion can be disrupted by a number of neuropsychiatric medications because which of the following substances stimulates GnRH secretion?

   (A) beta-endorphin
   (B) dopamine
   (C) dynorphin
   (D) norepinephrine
   (E) serotonin

3. X-rays on a 35-year-old man after a motor vehicle accident reveal a basilar skull fracture and raise a concern about an interruption of the hypophyseal portal circulation. This would cause a decline in circulating which of the following?

   (A) arginine vasopressin (AVP)
   (B) dopamine
   (C) gonadotropins
   (D) oxytocin
   (E) prolactin (PRL)

4. A patient presents with amenorrhea and galactorrhea. Her PRL levels are elevated. She is not and has never been pregnant. In addition to evaluating her for a prolactinoma, one also needs to evaluate for other causes that would increase PRL such as elevated level of which of the following?

   (A) corticotropin-releasing hormone (CRH)
   (B) dopamine
   (C) gamma-aminobutyric acid (GABA)
   (D) histamine type II receptor activation
   (E) thyrotropin-releasing hormone (TRH)

5. Since the workup of an elevated PRL level can be expensive, it is recommended that PRL levels are drawn when the lowest values are to be expected. Which of the following is true about PRL levels?

   (A) decrease after exercise
   (B) decrease during surgery
   (C) decrease shortly after sleep
   (D) decrease after a breast examination
   (E) increase during stress

6. It is now possible to administer GnRH in either a brief pulse or continuously. This allows diagnostic and therapeutic interventions in the hypothalamic–pituitary axis. To anticipate a normal response to GnRH stimulus one must understand how GnRH controls LH and FSH release. Which of the following is true concerning GnRH-stimulated LH secretion?

   (A) associated with steady LH release
   (B) enhanced by gonadotrope exposure to continuous GnRH
   (C) enhanced by gonadotrope exposure to estrogen
   (D) enhanced by gonadotrope exposure to progesterone
   (E) increased by gonadotrope exposure to testosterone

7. In the 1950s to 1960s physicians commonly used various compounds in an attempt to hormonally support a pregnancy and avoid a miscarriage. A popular preparation was found to cause vaginal adenosis in female offspring often 20 to 30 years later. Which of the following compounds that were used to prevent miscarriages had this unfortunate complication?

   (A) dehydroepiandrosterone
   (B) diethylstilbestrol (DES)
   (C) estradiol
   (D) estrone
   (E) testosterone

8. The development of the oral contraceptive pill was a milestone for reproductive gynecology. Addition of an ethinyl group at the 17C position of estradiol was critical in the development of the oral contraceptive pill because it does which of the following?

   (A) decreases biological activity
   (B) increases androgenic activity
   (C) increases hepatic degradation
   (D) increases sex hormone-binding globulin (SHBG) affinity
   (E) maintains biological activity after oral absorption

9. A 50-year-old menopausal patient wishes to stay on her oral contraceptive pill (ON 1+35). Her health care provider tries to explain that this provides more estrogen than she needs postmenopausally and in turn increases her risks of side effects and complications. What dose of ethinyl estradiol is roughly biologically equivalent to the typical postmenopausal dose of 0.625 mg of conjugated estrogens?

   (A) 0.005–0.010 mg
   (B) 0.05–10.0 mg
   (C) 0.50–1.0 mg
   (D) 5.0–10.0 mg
   (E) 50.0–100.0 mg

10. A patient with polycystic ovarian syndrome will often have an increase in insulin resistance (commonly known as metabolic X syndrome). The subsequent menstrual irregularities are a result of an increase in which of the following?

    (A) free estradiol level
    (B) follicle-stimulating hormone (FSH)
    (C) free testosterone level
    (D) hepatic production of SHBG
    (E) suppression of the action of LH on theca cells

11. Given that prostaglandins (PGs) appear to be involved in preterm labor, which of the following medications might provide some help through interference with PG synthesis or release in stopping preterm labor?

    (A) ACTH
    (B) indomethacin
    (C) progesterone
    (D) dopamine agonist
    (E) thyroid hormone

12. The change necessary to develop a phenotypic male fetus is an active process that involves the presence of key hormonal triggers. The development of a phenotypic female fetus is a more passive event due to the lack of these hormonal triggers. A patient presents at approximately 12 weeks' estimated gestational age. She is concerned that she had been exposed to testosterone prior to realizing she was pregnant. If she has a genetically female fetus, which of the following statements best describes the impact of testosterone given its role in developing a phenotypic male fetus?

    (A) causes elongation of the genital tubercle into the phallus

    (B) is mainly responsible for corpus spongiosum development

    (C) is mainly responsible for paramesonephric duct development

    (D) secretion is stimulated by maternal circulating gonadotropins

    (E) secretion is stimulated by human chorionic gonadotropin (hCG)

13. A mother brings her 2-month-old daughter to the pediatrician because she feels a lump in her abdomen. On pelvic ultrasound the infant has an ovarian mass. When counseling the mother, you inform her that the most common ovarian lesion associated with the transient elevated gonadotropins in a female newborn during the first 6 to 12 months of life is which of the following?

    (A) granulosa cell tumor

    (B) leiomyoma

    (C) serous cystadenoma

    (D) single large follicular cyst

    (E) theca cell tumor

**Questions 14 through 16 apply to the following patient:**

A mother and her 16-year-old daughter present to your office because the daughter has not yet menstruated. They are very concerned that something is wrong. By applying principles of puberty to this patient, it is possible to determine if the teen is simply undergoing a slightly delayed puberty versus potentially manifesting a significant endocrine or anatomical problem.

14. Which of the following best describes the normal sequence of pubertal changes in the female?

    (A) maximal growth velocity, menarche, thelarche

    (B) maximal growth velocity, thelarche, menarche

    (C) menarche, maximal growth velocity, thelarche

    (D) thelarche, maximal growth velocity, menarche

    (E) thelarche, menarche, maximal growth velocity

15. Menarche usually occurs between which years of age?

    (A) 8 and 10 years

    (B) 11 and 13 years

    (C) 14 and 16 years

    (D) 17 and 18 years

16. Which of the following pubertal events is not mediated by gonadal estrogen production and therefore would occur even in the absence of estrogen production?

    (A) breast development

    (B) menstruation

    (C) pubic hair growth

    (D) accelerated skeletal growth

    (E) vaginal cornification

17. A 16-year-old girl is brought to clinic by her mother with concerns regarding the lack of any signs of puberty. The appearance of external genitalia is of a normal prepubertal female. Laboratory studies show markedly elevated FSH and LH levels. Which of the following causes of delayed puberty accompanies elevated circulating gonadotropin levels?

    (A) chronic illness

    (B) gonadal dysgenesis

    (C) hypothalamic tumors

    (D) Kallmann syndrome

    (E) malnutrition

**18.** A 7-year-old girl is brought in for evaluation. On examination, she has well-developed pubic hair and breasts and she is 99% of height for her age. Her mother recently noted some bloodstains on her underwear. Which of the following conditions is most likely the cause of these findings?

(A) estrogen-producing ovarian cyst

(B) hepatoma

(C) hypothalamic tumor

(D) sex steroid-containing medication

(E) thecal/Leydig cell tumor

**19.** A 24-year-old patient presents with amenorrhea for more than 6 months. Prior to the amenorrhea she had had oligomenorrhea for a number of months. She is not pregnant, her weight has been stable with body mass index (BMI) of 23, and there is no evidence of hirsutism or galactorrhea. On the basis of clinical evaluation, it appears that she has GnRH suppression. A detailed history needs to be considered regarding medication use since the inhibitory action of sex steroids on GnRH secretion is primarily mediated by which of the following?

(A) dopamine

(B) melatonin

(C) norepinephrine

(D) opioid peptides

(E) serotonin

**Questions 20 through 23 apply to the following topic:**

Unlike male gonadotropins, female gonadotropins are able to promote the development of a single optimal dominant follicle during most cycles with the release of a single gamete from an LH surge and then optimization of the uterine environment for implantation. To understand pathologies in this complex system, one must understand the ideal steps within the normal menstrual cycle.

**20.** Which of the following statements best describes the role of FSH in menstruation?

(A) FSH increases its own receptor numbers on theca cells.

(B) FSH induces granulosa cell LH receptors within the dominant follicle.

(C) FSH induces theca cell aromatase.

(D) FSH stimulates follicular growth only in the early preantral stage.

(E) FSH stimulates granulosa cell androgen production.

**21.** Which statement best describes estrogen-positive feedback on LH release?

(A) It is affected by the level of circulating estrogen.

(B) It is enhanced by testosterone.

(C) It is increased by opioid peptides.

(D) It is unaffected by progesterone.

(E) It is unaffected by the duration of estrogen stimulation.

**22.** Which of the following gametes is released from the Graafian follicle during ovulation?

(A) primary oocyte

(B) primary oocyte and first polar body

(C) secondary oocyte

(D) secondary oocyte and first polar body

(E) secondary oocyte and second polar body

**23.** Which of the following hormone(s) is/are produced by the corpus luteum?

(A) progesterone only

(B) progesterone and estrogen only

(C) progesterone, estrogen, and inhibin only

(D) progesterone, estrogen, inhibin, and relaxin only

(E) progesterone, estrogen, inhibin, relaxin, and contractin

**24.** During an evaluation for infertility, a woman may have an endometrial biopsy to evaluate the quality of her ovulation, since the optimal development of the corpus luteum is most closely associated with which of the following?

(A) fertilization of an ovum

(B) follicular phase of the endometrium

(C) proliferative phase of the endometrium

(D) secretory phase of the endometrium

(E) shedding phase of the endometrium (menstruation)

**Questions 25 through 27 apply to the following topic:**

Fertility awareness method of contraception emphasizes the monitoring of normal physiologic changes due to hormonal changes throughout the cycle. The patient must be able to predict when she is likely to ovulate and when she has completed ovulation.

25. The consistency of the cervical mucous is an indicator of phase of the menstrual cycle and hence fertility. The presence of ferning depends on which of the following hormones?

(A) estrogen

(B) estrogen and progesterone

(C) hCG

(D) LH

(E) progesterone

26. Spinnbarkeit describes which of the following?

(A) amount of cervical mucus

(B) clarity of cervical mucus

(C) elasticity of cervical mucus

(D) ferning of cervical mucus

(E) viscosity of cervical mucus

27. Which of the following is mediated by progesterone thus implying successful ovulation?

(A) mammary ductal development

(B) proliferative endometrium

(C) shortened GnRH pulse interval

(D) thermogenic effect

(E) thin, stretchy cervical mucus

28. A patient with an infected incomplete abortion presents to the emergency department. During the dilatation and curettage (D&C) excessive bleeding develops that requires vigorous curetting to control. She returns to her physician 6 months later complaining that she has not had a menstrual cycle since. She has all the symptoms

of getting ready to start a period but never sees any bleeding. This history implies what layer of endometrium is damaged?

(A) arteriole zone

(B) basalis zone

(C) compact zone

(D) functional zone

(E) spongy zone

29. Women perceive the menstrual flow as an indication that the reproductive system is functioning well. In fact the actual menstrual flow is associated with which of the following?

(A) prolonged maintenance of estrogen

(B) prolonged maintenance of progesterone

(C) withdrawal of FSH

(D) withdrawal of LH

(E) withdrawal of progesterone

30. A 43-year-old patient presents with complaints of two menstrual cycles with heavy vaginal bleeding that included 2- to 3-cm clots associated with severe cramping which is unusual for her. The presence of the clots supports her report that the amount of blood loss is greater than usual. Menstrual blood is usually nonclotting because of which of the following?

(A) heparin

(B) organ hemophilia

(C) prior clotting and liquefaction

(D) toxins that inhibit clotting

(E) von Willebrand variant

31. Even after menopause, most women have circulating estrogen. In high enough levels, this can promote the development of endometrial cancer. It mainly originates from the aromatization of which of the following?

    (A) androstenedione to estradiol by ovarian granulosa cells
    (B) androstenedione to estrone by ovarian thecal cells
    (C) androstenedione to estrone by adipose tissue
    (D) estradiol to estrone by adipose tissue
    (E) testosterone to estradiol by adipose tissue

32. A 50-year-old woman presents to her health care provider complaining of hot flushes. Hot flushes are often the symptom in a perimenopausal woman that causes her to seek medical assistance. Hot flushes entail which of the following?

    (A) an average duration of about 30 minutes
    (B) peripheral redistribution of blood flow leading to sweating and elevated heart rate
    (C) peripheral vasodilatation reflecting an increase in core body temperature
    (D) peripheral vasodilatation resulting from a direct LH action on sympathetic neurons
    (E) subjective symptoms always accompanying objective signs of vasomotor instability

33. Prior to initiating estrogen replacement therapy (ERT), your patient is counseled regarding the long-term risks of estrogen deficiency associated with menopause. A major concern is osteoporosis. With osteoporosis, the accelerated bone loss occurring in the first 1 to 8 years after menopause is associated with which of the following?

    (A) an elevation in circulating parathyroid hormone levels
    (B) increased urinary loss of phosphorus and hydroxyproline
    (C) no influence on trabecular bone

    (D) primarily with affects on cortical bone
    (E) X-ray can diagnose early osteoporosis (osteopenia)

34. A postmenopausal patient is interested in hormone replacement therapy (HRT) with progesterone but is concerned about its dangers. Which of the following statements should be included in your discussion regarding the risks of HRT with combined therapy relative to no HRT?

    (A) Just as oral contraceptives may increase blood coagulability, HRT will also, due to high doses of hormone.
    (B) HRT may increase the risk of choleithiasis.
    (C) HRT may increase the risk of endometrial carcinoma.
    (D) HRT greatly increases the risk of breast carcinoma.
    (E) HRT may increase the risk of renal dysfunction.

DIRECTIONS (Questions 35 through 52): The following groups of questions are preceded by a list of lettered options. For each question, select the one lettered option that is most closely associated with it. Each lettered option may be used once, multiple times, or not at all.

## Questions 35 through 40

    (A) androstenedione
    (B) DHT
    (C) dehydroepiandrosterone sulfate (DHEAS)
    (D) estradiol
    (E) estrone
    (F) hCG
    (G) pregnenolone
    (H) testosterone
    (I) 17-hydroxyprogesterone

35. The birth of an infant that looks female (phenotype) but is genetically male will occur because of the lack of 5-alpha-reductase preventing the synthesis of due to an inability to make which hormone or enzyme.

36. Developing hirsutism in a 24-year-old woman prompts one to suspect an adult-onset 21-hydroxylase deficiency. The principal marker for such an enzyme deficiency is which of the above hormones or enzymes.

37. Principal androgen of adrenal origin.

38. Principal estrogen formed in a postmenopausal woman in peripheral tissue (e.g., adipose and muscle).

39. Hormone that can be used to simulate an LH surge and promote ovulation in an artificially stimulated cycle because it cross-reacts antigenically with LH.

40. Precursor for all hormonally active steroids.

**Questions 41 through 45: Match the chemical entity with its physiologic effect.**

(A) androstenedione
(B) arachidonic acid
(C) cholesterol
(D) DHEAS
(E) estradiol
(F) inhibin
(G) progesterone

41. Conversion of endometrium to secretory state that is necessary for successful implantation

42. Breast duct development in puberty

43. Substrate for aromatase by granulose cells to estrogen

44. Responsible for the increase in basal body temperature

45. Promotes proliferation of the functional endometrium

**Questions 46 through 49 refer to Figure 5–1:**

The following graph (Figure 5–1) demonstrates the relative hormonal changes during the normal menstrual cycle. Match the hormones with the graphic representation by letter.

46. FSH

47. LH

48. Estradiol

49. Progesterone

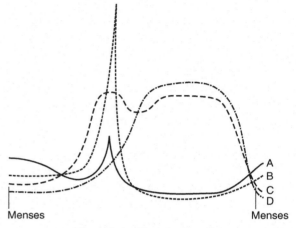

**Figure 5–1.** Menstrual cycle.

**Questions 50 through 52: Match the clinical situation with the associated hormonal state.**

(A) high circulating estradiol
(B) high circulating estrone
(C) high circulating FSH
(D) high circulating progesterone
(E) high circulating testosterone

50. Castrated young adult female

51. Obesity with Type II (BMI 35–39.9)

52. Presence of a dominant follicle

# Answers and Explanations

1. **(C)** Anterior pituitary hormones are regulated by hypothalamic hormones, which reach the pituitary via the portal hypophyseal vessels. The six hypothalamic hormones are: (1) TRH, which stimulates TSH; (2) GnRH, which stimulates FSH and LH; (3) CRH, which stimulates ACTH; (4) somatostatin inhibits GH; (5) growth hormone-releasing hormone (GHRH), which stimulates GH; and (6) prolactin-inhibitory factor (PIF), which inhibits PRL.

2. **(D)** Dopamine administration in vivo inhibits GnRH secretion. Serotonin and opiate peptides (produced under stressful conditions) also appear to inhibit GnRH release. Norepinephrine is produced in the mesencephalon and in the lower brain stem and stimulates GnRH secretion.

3. **(C)** Interruption of the hypophyseal portal circulation inhibits GnRH and dopamine delivery to the anterior pituitary causing a decline in circulating gonadotropin values and an increase in circulating PRL levels. AVP and oxytocin secretion from the posterior pituitary into the circulation is unaffected by interruption of the portal hypophyseal vessels (see Figure 5–2).

4. **(E)** PRL secretion is dominated by the inhibitory action of hypothalamic dopamine. Other mechanisms of PRL inhibition are GABA and histamine type II receptor activation. TRH is a potent stimulator of PRL and may induce galactorrhea under conditions of primary hypothyroidism, which should be checked for by measuring TSH.

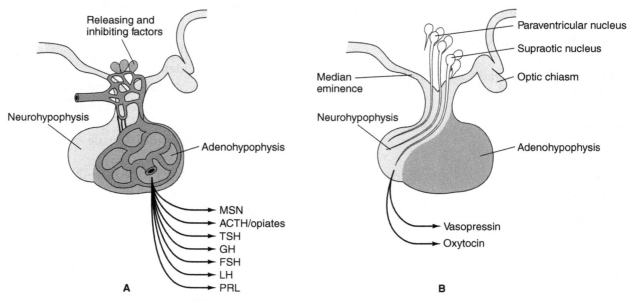

**Figure 5–2.** Diagram of (A) adenohypophysis and (B) neurohypophysis.

5. **(E)** Circulating PRL levels exhibit a diurnal variation with highest values occurring during sleep. High-protein meals (presumably mediated by ingestion of neurotransmitters) also cause a large increment in serum PRL levels, while carbohydrate meals have no such effect. Several stressful stimuli, including surgery, exercise, and hypoglycemia, cause an elevation in PRL secretion.

6. **(C)** Pituitary cells that secrete LH and FSH are called gonadotropes. GnRH action on LH secretion is enhanced by gonadotrope exposure to estrogen and diminished by gonadotrope exposure to testosterone. Pulsatile GnRH reduces a similar LH release pattern and stimulates LH synthesis, causing a greater amount of LH release during subsequent GnRH stimulation. The GnRH stimulation test used to diagnose the etiology of sexual precocity is based on this phenomenon. In contrast, exposure of gonadotropes to continuous GnRH reduces pituitary desensitization to GnRH, resulting in a decrease in LH release during subsequent continuous GnRH stimulation.

7. **(B)** Although DES is the only one of these compounds without a steroid configuration, it is strongly estrogenic. Before its ban as an antiabortifacient in 1971, the use of DES for miscarriage prevention was associated with Müllerian tract abnormalities and clear cell adenocarcinoma of the vagina in offspring exposed in utero. The most frequent Müllerian tract abnormality was a T-shaped uterus, with a small uterine cavity, accompanied by structural abnormalities of the cervix.

8. **(E)** The major breakthrough in steroid contraception occurred in 1938, when it was discovered that addition of an ethinyl group at the 17C position made estradiol active because of its reduced rate of hepatic degradation after oral ingestion. This stability with oral intake was necessary for hormonal contraception to be readily available to large numbers of women.

9. **(A)** Ethinyl estradiol is a potent estrogen and is prescribed in microgram doses (1 $\mu$g = 0.001 mg). The 0.625-mg dose of conjugated estrogens is roughly equivalent to 5 to 10 $\mu$g (i.e., 0.005–0.010 mg) ethinyl estradiol. Therefore, the most commonly used dosage of estrogen required for menopausal hormone replacement (0.625-mg conjugated estrogens) is less than that found in oral contraceptives, which contain approximately 30 $\mu$g ethinyl estradiol.

10. **(C)** The metabolic clearance rate (MCR) is defined as the volume of blood that is cleared of a substance per unit time. The circulating level of a substance is determined by its blood production rate (PR) divided by its MCR. With increased insulin resistance, insulin levels rise and inhibit hepatic production of SHBG. As most circulating testosterone is bound to SHBG, a decrease in SHBG will increase the amount of free testosterone and decrease the amount of free estrogen. The free testosterone and levels of estrone from peripheral conversion of androstenedione will keep FSH levels low. The underlying insulin resistance augments the stimulatory action of LH on the growth and androgen secretion of ovarian theca cells.

11. **(B)** Indomethacin is an inhibitor of PG synthesis and is used as a tocolytic agent. Inhibitors of PG synthesis may be prescribed for pain relief during menstruation (dysmenorrhea), since PGs also play a role in dysmenorrhea. Although progesterone may be a tocolytic agent it does not appear to be mediated primarily through the PG cascade.

12. **(E)** Fetal Leydig cells are the source of testosterone, which is produced in response to circulating hCG and fetal LH. Testosterone induces the mesonephric system (male internal genitalia) to undergo male sexual differentiation. DHT, which results from the peripheral conversion of testosterone, is responsible for formation of the external genitalia, including the prostate and Cowper's glands (from the urogenital sinus). DHT causes elongation of the genital tubercle into the phallus, forward migration of the urethral folds to create the penile shaft (corpus spongiosum), and caudal migration of the genital swellings to form the scrotum.

13. **(D)** With removal of the placenta at birth, the decline in circulating sex steroid levels causes loss of sex steroid negative feedback to the neonatal hypothalamus. A transient elevation in circulating gonadotropin levels temporarily stimulates gonadal steroidogenesis and disappears by 6 months of age in males and 1 to 2 years in females. During this time, circulating gonadotropins in infants may transiently induce formation of ovarian cysts, which results in estrogen stimulation of breast tissue.

14. **(D)** Sex steroid production during puberty stimulates development of secondary sex characteristics, growth of long bones (e.g., growth spurt), and changes in bone composition (maturation). The normal sequence of pubertal changes in the female is thelarche, maximal growth velocity, and menarche.

15. **(B)** The age at which menstruation begins has steadily decreased in the United States. The normal age range in which the first menstruation occurs is from 10 to 16 years, with an average of 12.8 years. It is unclear if this is due to increasing obesity among peripubertal females or overall better nutrition.

16. **(C)** During puberty, an increase in circulating gonadotropin levels stimulates gonadal steroidogenesis. The production of sex steroids induces secondary sex characteristics, endometrial proliferation (leading to menstruation), vaginal cornification, and growth of long bones. Between 6 and 9 years of age, an increase in adrenal function (adrenarche) is accompanied by an elevation in circulating DHEA and DHEAS levels, which induce pubic and axillary hair growth (pubarche).

17. **(B)** Puberty is delayed when secondary sex development fails to occur by 13 years of age in girls or 14 years in boys. Low circulating sex steroid levels delay epiphyseal closure, leading to prolonged growth of extremities. Delayed puberty results from the absence of either gonadal or hypothalamic–pituitary function. Absence of gonadal function due to defective gonadal development (gonadal dysgenesis) leads to a rise in circulating gonadotropin levels (hyper-gonadotropic hypogonadism) because negative feedback restraint is removed from the hypothalamus and pituitary. Moreover, absence of pulsatile GnRH due to hypothalamic suppression causes a decline in circulating gonadotropin levels (hypogonadotropic hypogonadism). Suppression of hypothalamic GnRH may reflect the presence of central nervous system (CNS) tumors and diseases, malnutrition, chronic illness, or stress. Kallmann syndrome refers to GnRH deficiency, combined with anosmia due to olfactory bulb agenesis. This syndrome may be due to a defect in migration of GnRH-containing neurons from the nasal placode to the hypothalamus.

18. **(C)** Precocious puberty refers to the onset of puberty prior to 8 years of age in girls or 9 years in boys. Premature onset of pubertal changes may reflect either early activation of the gonadostat (true precocious puberty) or exposure of target tissues to sex steroids without activation of the gonadostat (pseudoprecocious puberty). True precocious puberty occurs more commonly in females than males and leads to full reproductive function (e.g., ovulation or spermatogenesis). Ten percent of females with true precocious puberty have an underlying CNS abnormality (e.g., tumors, obstructions to cerebral spinal fluid outflow, granulomatous and infectious diseases, neurofibromatosis, and head trauma). Ninety percent of females have the idiopathic (constitutional) form of this disorder, in which no abnormality is detected.

19. **(D)** Opioid peptides are a group of peptides that bind to opiate receptors and demonstrate analgesic activity (like morphine). Opioid peptides inhibit gonadotropin secretion by suppressing hypothalamic GnRH release. The effect of opioid peptides on hypothalamic GnRH release is responsible for the low frequency of pulsatile LH secretion during the luteal phase. Melatonin, produced by the pineal gland (in response to environmental light and endogenous rhythm-generating mechanisms), suppresses GnRH release but has little apparent significance in humans. Norepinephrine stimulates GnRH release.

**20. (B)** FSH regulates ovarian steroidogenesis and stimulates folliculogenesis beyond the early preantral stage. The central principle of gonadotropin-dependent ovarian steroidogenesis is the "two-cell theory" of estrogen synthesis. This theory proposes that a developing follicle requires both granulosa cells and surrounding stromal cells (theca interna) for estrogen synthesis. Granulosa cells possess FSH receptors and respond to FSH by synthesizing aromatase and increasing FSH receptor sites. Thecal cells contain LH receptors and produce androgens in the presence of LH. Under these conditions, granulosa cells are able to convert androgens, produced locally by thecal cells, to estrogens and are the major source of circulating E2.

**21. (A)** Exposure of the hypothalamus and pituitary to a threshold E2 level (>200 pg/mL) for a critical interval (approximately 50 hours) induces a surge of circulating LH. This transient phenomenon is referred to as estrogen-positive feedback. As ovulation approaches, luteinized granulosa cells synthesize progesterone, which facilitates the E2-induced LH surge. Conversely, testosterone inhibits LH release by decreasing gonadotrope sensitivity to GnRH. Opioidergic mechanisms decrease LH secretion by diminishing the release of hypothalamic GnRH.

**22. (D)** The LH surge causes the primary oocyte to complete its first meiotic division, forming a secondary oocyte and first polar body. Each cell contains 23 double-structured chromosomes (haploid) with every chromosome consisting of two chromatids.

**23. (D)** The three principal hormones synthesized by the corpus luteum are progesterone, estrogen, and inhibin. These hormones are produced in greatest quantity 7 to 10 days after ovulation in anticipation and support of the implantation of the blastocyst. The corpus luteum also secretes relaxin, which rises in concentration 10 to 12 days after ovulation. There is no hormone called contractin.

**24. (D)** The development of secretory endometrium by progesterone action on an estrogen-primed endometrium is an indirect method of assessing whether ovulation has occurred. The changes are so characteristic that the histologic pattern can determine the postovulatory age of the endometrial tissue. This histologic analysis is called endometrial dating.

**25. (A)** Although the amounts vary with the menstrual cycle, 90% of cervical mucus consists of water and sodium chloride (NaCl). In the early follicular phase, a scant amount of cervical mucus containing leukocytes acts as a barrier to sperm and bacteria. During the late follicular phase, a rise in circulating estrogen levels alters vascular epithelial permeability and increases the water content of cervical secretions. The NaCl content of the mucus allows it to form a palm-leaf crystallization pattern on drying, a phenomenon referred to as ferning. Ferning is maximal when circulating estrogen levels are highest and is prevented by progesterone. The presence of progesterone that is present after ovulation is inhibitory to ferning since it causes the cervical mucous to thicken and become tenacious.

**26. (C)** Spinnbarkeit describes the elasticity of cervical mucus. High circulating estrogen levels cause the mucus to become profuse, thin, acellular, and clear, resulting in a high degree of stretchability (8–10 cm) when pulled from the cervix or stretched between a slide and a coverslip. Ferning will also occur at this time. These properties of estrogen-stimulated mucus promote formation of glycoprotein channels favoring sperm penetration. A high degree of spinnbarkeit in cervical mucus that ferns is clinically useful to time the postcoital test.

**27. (D)** Progesterone produced during the luteal phase inhibits GnRH pulsatility and shifts core body temperature upward from 0.6 to 1.0°F. Progesterone also produces secretory endometrium; induces thick, opaque cervical mucus (preventing passage of sperm and bacteria); and stimulates mammary alveolar development. Estrogen causes endometrial proliferation and mammary ductal development.

28. **(B)** The compact and spongy zones, collectively called the functional zone, are shed at menstruation. Endometrial shedding is facilitated by two types of arteries: the spiral arteries of the functional zone (which spasm from progesterone withdrawal) and the permanent arterioles of the basalis. There is no arteriole zone. The destruction of the basalis layer with scarring will prevent development of the functional zone and menses. This clinical situation is called Asherman's syndrome.

29. **(E)** Menstruation implies the sloughing of an estrogen- and progesterone-primed endometrium in response to the withdrawal of progesterone. Progesterone withdrawal induces spasm of the spiral arteries, leading to vascular collapse, endometrial necrosis, and sloughing.

30. **(C)** The endometrium contains a potent thromboplastin that initiates clotting. Activation of plasminogen causes lysis of blood clots typically prior to expulsion. If menstrual bleeding is excessive, some clotting will remain when the blood is expelled. The presence of clots supports her report of an increased rate of blood flow and the amount of blood loss is greater than usual. The "coagulum" usually represents a collection of mucoid material and red cells rather than a true clot during normal flow. Although heparin, von Willebrand, and sepsis with toxins may inhibit coagulation, this is not the cause for the usual menstrual flow. There is no such entity as organ hemophilia.

31. **(C)** The major circulating estrogen in postmenopausal women is estrone. Almost all of the estrone produced in postmenopausal women is derived from the peripheral conversion of androstenedione by fat, muscle, and other peripheral tissues. By definition of menopause, a patient does not have granulosa cells since there are no primary follicles. The theca cells are a source of androstenedione from LH stimulation, which is converted to estrone.

32. **(B)** The physiological changes accompanying the hot flush include peripheral vasodilation, sweating, elevated heart rate, and increased oxygen consumption. These events promote heat loss via redistribution of blood flow to the periphery and reflect a change in the set point of the hypothalamic thermoregulatory center. Peripheral blood flow increases approximately 1.5 minutes before and continues for several minutes beyond the subjective symptoms of the hot flush. Perspiration begins 2 to 3 minutes later and is followed by an increase in peripheral temperature, occurring several minutes after the initial rise in peripheral blood flow. At this time, core body temperature drops to $0.2°C$ and chills begin. The duration is typically a few minutes (1–5). Although in some women an increase in LH is associated with flushing, there is no causal relationship.

33. **(B)** Osteoporosis results when there is an imbalance between bone resorption and formation, with a chronic negative calcium balance causing mobilization of calcium from trabecular bone. Estrogen deficiency is a significant factor in the development of osteoporosis and has been associated with a transient increase in serum calcium, a compensatory decrease in serum parathyroid hormone levels, hypercalciuria (indicating negative calcium balance), and increased urinary loss of phosphorus and hydroxyproline. The rate of trabecular bone loss is 4% to 8% annually in the 5 to 8 years following menopause, and women lose 35% of their cortical bone and 50% of their trabecular bone through life. The bone loss can be slowed by ERT even though it had begun many years after menopause. Simple X-rays of vertebral column or hip do not detect early loss. The test of choice is a Dexa scan.

34. **(B)** The amounts of estrogen used for postmenopausal HRT are less than those found in oral contraceptives. Thus, they may theoretically, still slightly, increase the risk of thromboembolic disease but far less than oral contraceptive pills. However, the administration of estrogen by the transdermal patch, thereby avoiding the first pass through the liver, appears to have no effect on clotting factors. The use of exogenous estrogen unopposed by progesterone is associated with an increase in the incidence of endometrial carcinoma (four- to eightfold), but with the addition of progesterone,

the risk is less than half of the risk of using no replacement therapy at all. ERT may increase the risk of breast carcinoma, particularly after long-term therapy (>5 years), but this increase is small. Estrogen therapy also increases the risk of cholelithiasis. It does not increase the risk of renal dysfunction.

35. **(B)** DHT is the principal androgen formed in target tissues containing 5-alpha-reductase. This enzyme converts circulating testosterone to a more potent androgen, DHT. DHT is responsible for the development of the male external phenotype.

36. **(I)** The 21-hydroxylase enzyme is required to convert 17-hydroxyprogesterone (17-OHP) to 11-desoxycortisol. Its absence is associated with a marked elevation in circulating 17-OHP levels, which in turn become androgens. A deficiency of 21-hydroxylase is the cause of the most common form of congenital adrenal hyperplasia.

37. **(C)** DHEAS is produced almost entirely by the adrenal gland. The adrenal gland and ovary generally contribute about 50% each to androstenedione production. In females, approximately 50% of testosterone arises from peripheral conversion of androstenedione, while the adrenal gland and ovary contribute equal amounts (25%) to circulating testosterone levels. Any rapid or sudden development of hirsutism in a woman requires the determination of the source of the androgen.

38. **(E)** Estrone is the principal estrogen formed in peripheral tissue (e.g., adipose and muscle) by conversion of androstenedione. In obese women with chronic anovulation, circulating estrone levels may be elevated.

39. **(F)** The strong antigenic similarity between LH and hCG is useful in clinical practice. Administration of hCG in the presence of a dominant follicle will induce ovulation by mimicking an LH surge.

40. **(G)** Pregnenolone is the steroid precursor for all hormonally active steroids.

41. **(G)** Progesterone action on the endometrium increases glandular epithelial secretion, stimulates glycogen accumulation in stromal cell cytoplasm (decidualization), and promotes stromal vascularity (spiral arterioles) and edema. These changes vary daily throughout the luteal phase and are the basis of the histological analysis referred to as "endometrial dating."

42. **(E)** Estradiol induces mammary duct development, whereas progesterone induces mammary alveolar development.

43. **(A)** Theca interna cells of the ovary supply androstenedione to granulosa cells for aromatization to estradiol.

44. **(G)** Progesterone is thermogenic, causing a rise in basal body temperatures during the luteal phase of the menstrual cycle. A biphasic temperature usually confirms an ovulatory cycle, and persistence of the temperature elevation beyond 2 weeks suggests pregnancy.

45. **(E)** Estrogen stimulates the endometrium to proliferate during the follicular phase of the menstrual cycle. The endometrium increases in thickness during folliculogenesis, at which time mitotic figures are abundant throughout the glands and stroma.

46. **(A)** The small FSH midcycle peak is induced by the preovulatory rise in serum progesterone. Midcycle FSH production serves to free the oocyte from its follicular attachments (via hyaluronic acid), aid in follicular rupture (via plasminogen activator), and ensure sufficient LH receptor number for adequate luteal function. There is a rise of FSH at the very end and at the beginning of each cycle in response to the low estrogen levels. This recruits the next set of follicles.

47. **(B)** The LH surge is initiated by the positive feedback effect of unopposed estrogen. For purposes of ovulation induction, the LH surge can be mimicked by exogenous hCG administration.

48. **(C)** Circulating estradiol levels rise steadily during the follicular phase and have negative feedback on FSH release. Continued increase of estradiol levels is not due to increasing serum

FSH levels but because of the ability of the more dominant follicles to maintain an environment conducive to continued growth and production of estradiol.

49. **(D)** Although estrogen continues to be present during the luteal phase, circulating levels of progesterone (ng/mL) during the luteal phase are greater than those of estradiol (pg/mL). Progesterone withdrawal during luteolysis induces normal menses.

50. **(C)** With castration, loss of negative gonadal feedback (e.g., estrogen, progesterone, and inhibin) on FSH secretion causes a profound increase in circulating FSH levels.

51. **(B)** Peripheral aromatization of androstenedione to estrone accounts for the high circulating estrone levels associated with obesity. Since anovulation is common under these conditions, circulating estradiol levels remain in the early follicular range.

52. **(A)** Circulating estradiol is derived mostly from the dominant follicle and increases steadily in concentration to more than 200 pg/mL by the late follicular phase.

# CHAPTER 6

# Maternal Physiology During Pregnancy

## Questions

**DIRECTIONS (Questions 1 through 27): For each of the multiple choice questions in this section, select the lettered answer that is the one *best* response in each case.**

1. Most state-of-the-art serum pregnancy tests have a sensitivity for detection of $\beta$-human chorionic gonadotropin ($\beta$-hCG) of 25 mLU/mL. Such tests would diagnose pregnancy as early as which of the following?

    (A) 5 days after fertilization
    (B) 24 hours after implantation
    (C) day of the expected (missed) menses
    (D) 5 weeks' gestation age by menstrual dating
    (E) 6 weeks' gestation age by menstrual dating

2. A 35-year-old G5P4004 patient is found to have ASCUS on her Pap smear done at her new obstetrics (OB) visit. In your counseling of the patient as to what this result means, you note that the hormonal changes of pregnancy will cause changes in the cervix. Which of the following cervical changes may be found more frequently in the pregnant state than in the nonpregnant state?

    (A) atypical glandular hyperplasia
    (B) dysplasia
    (C) metaplasia
    (D) neoplasia
    (E) vaginal adenosis

3. A 16-year-old G1P0 patient is brought for an examination due to a probable pregnancy. The patient says that she became sexually active approximately 5 months ago. To estimate her gestational age, you palpate the abdomen. At approximately 20 weeks' estimated gestational age, which of the following best describes the uterus in a normal pregnancy?

    (A) not palpable abdominally
    (B) palpable at the level of the umbilicus
    (C) palpable at the level of the xiphoid
    (D) palpable just over the symphysis pubis
    (E) palpable midway between the umbilicus and the sternum

4. A 21-year-old G1 now P1 just delivered after a prolonged induction of labor due to being postdates. After the placental delivery she continues to bleed excessively. Your initial intervention to address this bleeding is to activate the normal physiologic mechanisms. Which of the following is the most important hemostatic mechanism in combating postpartum hemorrhage?

    (A) contraction of interlacing uterine muscle bundles
    (B) fibrinolysis inhibition
    (C) increased blood-clotting factors in pregnancy
    (D) intramyometrial vascular coagulation due to vasoconstriction
    (E) markedly decreased blood pressure in the uterine venules

5. The uterus must increase its volume over the course of a pregnancy from less than 20 cc to over 5 L. This is accomplished while still maintaining the ability for the uterine muscles to contract with enough force to expel the infant during labor. The uterine muscle mass enlarges during pregnancy primarily because of which of the following?

(A) atypical hyperplasia
(B) anaplasia
(C) hypertrophy and hyperplasia
(D) involution
(E) production of new myocytes

6. During a pelvic examination on a patient that is approximately 8 weeks' gestation by dates and pelvic examination, one adnexa is found to be slightly enlarged. This is most commonly due to which of the following?

(A) corpus luteum cyst
(B) ectopic pregnancy
(C) follicular cyst
(D) ovarian neoplasm
(E) parovarian cyst

7. A patient presents for her new obstetrical (OB) examination. She is 23 years of age and G1P0 at 10 weeks without problems. Her prepregnant body mass index (BMI) was 22. As part of her pregnancy-based education, you inform her that she should follow a balanced diet with a recommended weight gain of approximately how many pounds?

(A) 5–10
(B) 10–15
(C) 15–20
(D) 25–35
(E) 30–40

8. A patient presents for her routine prenatal visit at 34 weeks' estimated gestational age (EGA). She is complaining to the nurse of back pain. Her pulse and temperature are normal as well as her urine dip. After the examination you determine that it is due to exaggerate posture caused by her weight (BMI 35) and her pregnancy. Which of the following is a characteristic posture of pregnancy?

(A) hyperextension
(B) kyphosis
(C) lordoscoliosis
(D) lordosis
(E) scoliosis

9. A pregnant patient presents very concerned about some skin lesions/changes she is seeing that are just like her uncle's who has liver cirrhosis from hepatitis C. What lesions or changes are she likely referring to?

(A) hyperpigmentation and spider angiomata
(B) linea nigra and chloasma
(C) spider angiomata and palmar erythema
(D) striae and chloasma
(E) striae and linea nigra

10. The physiologic changes of pregnancy can alter many of the common laboratory tests. During the evaluation of a patient with tachycardia, hypertension, and headache you are considering both hyperthyroidism versus an atypical preeclampsia and draw the following laboratory tests. To correctly interpret the results, it is necessary to distinguish between normal versus abnormal changes during pregnancy. Which of the following would normally be expected to increase during pregnancy?

(A) alanine aminotransferase (ALT)
(B) aspartate aminotransferase (AST)
(C) hematocrit
(D) plasma creatinine
(E) thyroxine-binding globulin (TBG)

11. A patient presents complaining of a friable painful local buildup of her gums around the base of a number of teeth. This is starting to interfere with eating due to pain and bleeding. She has not seen a dentist for some time due to finances. The remainder of the pregnancy has been uncomplicated. These changes are likely due to which of the following?

(A) abscessed tooth
(B) decidualization

(C) epulis of pregnancy

(D) melasma

(E) spider hemangioma

**Questions 12 through 14 apply to the following patient:**

A patient at 19 weeks' EGA is evaluated for vague gastrointestinal/abdominal complaints, and there is concern for possible appendicitis. She notes diffuse abdominal pain, some nausea, and temperature of 37.3°C. She is not particularly hungry but lacks anorexia. She does have new onset nausea. She has positive bowel sounds. There is a negative psoas sign and only diffuse periumbilical tenderness without rebound. Her white blood cell (WBC) count is 11,000 and remainder of liver functions and pancreatic laboratories are within normal limits.

12. Considerations in the evaluation are sensitive to the changes in the gastrointestinal (GI) tract during pregnancy include which of the following?

(A) compression and downward displacement of the appendix by the uterus

(B) increased intestinal absorption helping to ensure weight gain

(C) increased intestinal tone and mobility

(D) more rapid gastric emptying

(E) physical elevation of the stomach

13. Given her presenting complaints and initial physical and laboratory testing, which one of the following represents an abnormal value?

(A) temperature 37.3°C

(B) only nausea without emesis

(C) negative psoas sign

(D) white blood cell (WBC) count of 11,000

(E) bowel sounds

14. It is determined that imaging is needed to evaluate the pain further. What is the best imaging test to order?

(A) abdominal/pelvic ultrasound

(B) KUB of the abdomen

(C) abdominal CT scan without contrast

(D) abdominal CT scan with contrast

(E) abdominal MRI

**Questions 15 and 16 apply to the following patient:**

A patient presents to OB triage unit with complaints of back pain and fever. She is 30 weeks' EGA. She had asymptomatic bacteria at her initial OB visit that was treated. Her temperature is 38.5°C and she has CVA tenderness. Because of changes in the urinary tract during pregnancy, patients are at greater risk for urinary tract infections.

15. Changes in the urinary tract during normal pregnancy include which of the following?

(A) decrease in renal plasma flow (RPF)

(B) increase in the amount of dead space in urinary tract

(C) increase in blood urea nitrogen (BUN) and creatinine

(D) increase in glomerular filtration rate (GFR)

(E) marked increase in both GFR and RPF when the patient is supine

16. On further questioning, a concern for renal stones possibly contributing to the infection is raised. It is decided to perform a one shot intravenous pyelogram (IVP) to evaluate for renal obstruction. If an IVP were performed in the third trimester, normal findings in pregnancy would include which of the following?

(A) kidneys appearing smaller than normal because of diaphragmatic compression

(B) obstruction of the right ureter secondary to the dextrorotation of the uterus

(C) sediment in the renal collecting system due to the stasis effect of progesterone

(D) ureteral dilation, probably secondary to progesterone effect, and compression of the lower urinary tract by the uterus

(E) vesicoureteral reflux secondary to stretching of the trigone by the enlarging uterus

17. At the initial OB visit your patients receive nutritional information. Iron supplementation is recommended in pregnancy in order to do which of the following?

    (A) maintain the maternal hemoglobin concentration
    (B) prevent iron deficiency in the fetus
    (C) prevent iron deficiency in the mother
    (D) prevent postpartum hemorrhage
    (E) raise the maternal hemoglobin concentration

18. A 22-year-old G3P2002 who had a hematocrit of 36% at her initial obstetrical examination at 12 weeks is found to have a hematocrit of 30% at 28 weeks when checked along with her 1 hour glucola. Based on the indices of the red blood cells on the CBC, you diagnose iron deficiency. She asks why that occurred since she has been taking her prenatal vitamins. As part of the explanation, you note that which of the following maternal measurements or findings is first decreased by the iron requirements of pregnancy?

    (A) bone marrow iron
    (B) hemoglobin
    (C) jejunal absorption of iron
    (D) red cell size
    (E) serum iron-binding capacity

19. During pregnancy the blood volume increases by 40%. The increase in blood volume in normal pregnancy is made up of which of the following?

    (A) erythrocytes
    (B) more erythrocytes than plasma
    (C) more plasma than erythrocytes
    (D) neither plasma nor erythrocytes
    (E) plasma only

20. In response to the increased vascular volume, the maternal cardiovascular system undergoes great change during pregnancy. During prenatal care, which of the following findings is part of the cardiovascular response to this increase in preload?

    (A) apical systolic murmurs are heard in approximately half of pregnant patients
    (B) arrhythmias are common
    (C) cardiac output is decreased by lying in the lateral position
    (D) the heart enlarges greatly, as can be demonstrated by standard chest X-rays
    (E) the stroke volume decreases

21. During pregnancy, the hormonal system of a woman is markedly altered since the fetus and placenta add their production to the maternal hormone production. This impacts maternal physiology and some of the findings of pregnancy. Estrogen is such a hormone that increases markedly. Most of this estrogen is produced by which of the following?

    (A) adrenals
    (B) fetus
    (C) ovaries
    (D) placenta
    (E) uterus

**Questions 22 and 23 apply to the following patient:**

A patient presents for preconceptive counseling. Her history is complicated by significant mitral stenosis. You tell her that this may be problematic at times of high cardiac output in pregnancy. Because of the fixed outflow, she could experience heart failure.

22. The time at which cardiac output is highest is during which phase of pregnancy?

    (A) in the first trimester
    (B) in the second trimester
    (C) in the third trimester
    (D) during labor
    (E) immediately postpartum (10–30 minutes)

23. Which of the following factors contribute to the increase in cardiac output in pregnancy?

    (A) decrease in blood volume
    (B) increase in ejection fraction
    (C) increase in heart rate

(D) increase in left ventricular stroke work index

(E) increase in systemic vascular resistance

**Questions 24 and 25 apply to the following patient:**

A 24-year-old nurse at 32 weeks' gestation complains of shortness of breath during her pregnancy, especially with physical exertion. She has no prior medical history. Her respiratory rate is 16; her lungs are clear to auscultation; and your office oxygen saturation monitor reveals her oxygen saturation to be 98% on room air.

24. You reassure her that this sensation is normal and explain which of the following?

(A) Airway conductance is decreased during pregnancy.

(B) Because of enlarging uterus pushing up on the diaphragm, her vital capacity is decreased by 20%.

(C) Maximal breathing capacity is not altered by pregnancy.

(D) Pulmonary resistance increases during pregnancy.

(E) Small amniotic fluid emboli are shed throughout pregnancy.

25. She urges you to perform pulmonary function tests. Assuming that your medical judgment is correct, these tests should show which of the following?

(A) diminished vital capacity

(B) increased functional residual capacity (FRC)

(C) increased reserve volume (RV)

(D) increased tidal volume

(E) unchanged expiratory reserve volume (ERV)

26. A 25-year-old G3P2 in her sixth week of pregnancy, by last menstrual period (LMP) calculation, has an endovaginal ultrasound examination because of vaginal bleeding. The ultrasound confirms an intrauterine pregnancy with fetal cardiac activity present and fetal pole length consistent with 6 weeks' gestation. Scan of the adnexae reveals a 5-cm simple cyst on the left ovary. Which of the following statements is true?

(A) This patient likely has both an intrauterine pregnancy and an ectopic pregnancy.

(B) This patient should be told that she will probably miscarry.

(C) The ovarian cyst should not be removed.

(D) First-trimester vaginal bleeding is uncommon and implies a poor pregnancy outcome.

(E) This patient has a blighted ovum.

27. Most obstetrical providers screen pregnant women for gestational diabetes around 28 weeks' gestation. The increased risk of developing diabetes in pregnancy is due to which of the following?

(A) decreased fetal glucose requirements

(B) decreased free fatty acids in maternal circulation

(C) increased maternal glucose requirements

(D) peripheral insulin resistance

(E) shorter insulin half life

# Answers and Explanations

1. **(C)** Circulating $\beta$-hCG in early pregnancy at a level of 25 mLU/mL is detected in most women by 12 to 13 days after the luteinizing hormone (LH) peak. Therefore, the test should be positive by the date of the expected menses.

2. **(C)** Metaplasia from hormonally induced changes in the squamocolumnar junction is common in pregnancy. Dysplasia or atypia is not common and needs to be evaluated. The cervix can be histologically evaluated for malignant change during pregnancy as well as during the nonpregnant state. Pap smears and colposcopy are both reliable. Dysplasia is probably best not treated until the postpartum period. However, CIS or microinvasive cervical cancer may be treated depending on the gestational age.

3. **(B)** This measurement is only a rough guide to the duration of gestation. It may be increased by twins, myomas, and hydramnios and decreased by oligohydramnios, intrauterine growth retardation, fetal death, and so on. Considerable individual variation is also common. One study found up to 3-cm difference, depending on whether the fundal height was measured with the gravida's bladder full or empty (see Figure 6–1).

4. **(A)** If uterine atony exists, the muscles do not provide the pressure on the endometrial vessels needed to occlude them. Methods such as massage and oxytocin administration will usually cause sufficient uterine contraction to inhibit such bleeding. Methergine, misoprostol, and prostaglandins (PGs) are also used as ther-

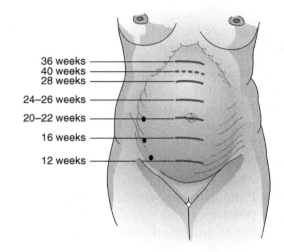

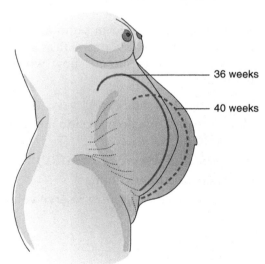

**Figure 6–1.** Fundal height in pregnancy. (Reproduced, with permission, from DeCherney AH, Nathan L. *Current Obstetric and Gynecologic Diagnosis and Treatment*, 9th ed. New York: McGraw-Hill, 2003.)

apeutic agents. Although pregnancy is a time of increased coagulation factors, those are not key to placental site hemostasis.

5. **(C)** During pregnancy, the enlargement of pre-existing myocyte cells is the primary source of growth. This is done by stretching and marked hypertrophy of the muscle cells. Also there is an accumulation of fibrous tissue in the muscle layers and a considerable increase in elastic tissues. These add strength to the uterus despite a thinning of the wall thickness. Involution occurs postpartum, when the uterus decreases from about 1,000 g to about 60 g. There are few new myocytes created during pregnancy. This increase is in a normal controlled fashion so there is no anaplasia or atypical.

6. **(A)** The corpus luteum normally decreases in its function after 8 weeks into the gestation. In midgestation, it is no longer needed to maintain the hormonal milieu of pregnancy (the placenta does that). Thus a slightly enlarged ovary and a positive pregnancy test signal normal pregnancy typically. If the uterus was not 8-week size and there was adnexal enlargement and tenderness the differential needs to include an ectopic pregnancy as well. Once the uterus is 8-week size this implies an intrauterine pregnancy since in a pregnancy not just hormonal change is necessary for uterine enlargement. A follicular cyst is uncommon after ovulation. An ovarian neoplasm is possible but less common unless markedly enlarged ovary (i.e., >6 cm). Ultrasound can be very helpful in differentiating between these.

7. **(D)** In 2009, the Institute of Medicine summarized studies and published guidelines for weight gain during pregnancy, which the American College of Obstetrics and Gynecology supports. It recommended a weight gain of 25 to 35 lb for normal-weight women to minimize low-birth-weight infants. The weight gain is accounted for by adding up the components that contribute to it, such as the fetus, placenta, increased blood volume, and increased maternal fat stores. More and more evidence is accumulating to show that low-weight gain when associated with inadequate diet is detrimental to the pregnancy. Women who are morbidly obese can gain less weight, but dieting to lose weight during pregnancy is never recommended. There continues to be controversy about the role of maternal weight gain to maternal obesity after pregnancy.

8. **(D)** The change in center of gravity caused by the enlarging uterus predisposes to a lordotic position and puts strain on paraspinal muscles and pelvic joints. Backache is a common complaint during pregnancy. Less commonly, the neck flexion and depressed shoulder girdle may cause median and ulnar nerve traction. Treatment is generally not effective and those complaints regress only after delivery. Use of heat, muscle relaxant, and exercise may help temporize these complaints.

9. **(C)** Hyperpigmentation in pregnancy includes the transformation of the linea alba to the linea nigra and the development of the "mask of pregnancy" or chloasma. Striae result from stretching of the skin under hormonal influences. The vascular changes occurring during states of high estrogen levels are common to both liver disease and normal pregnancy. These include the development of spider angiomata and palmar erythema.

10. **(E)** The mother and a rapidly growing infant use an increased amount of oxygen, resulting in an increased basal metabolic rate (BMR). When combined with elevated binding protein secondary to estrogen effect, one can be misled to diagnose hyperthyroidism when, in fact, these are normal pregnancy changes. For this reason, a thyroid evaluation in pregnancy will often use a free T4 level rather than total T4. Even mild hyperthyroidism probably does not merit treatment during pregnancy. AST and ALT are not elevated in normal pregnancy but may be elevated in patients with severe preeclampsia. Hematocrit will tend to drop because of plasma volume expansion. Creatinine also decreases because of increased glomerular filtration.

11. **(C)** This rather uncommon lesion tends to regress spontaneously with delivery. This is an extreme form of gingival hyperplasia that is common in pregnancy. There is no link to dental caries or permanent changes. It is often associated with poor dental hygiene and irritation of the gum line. Gums may bleed more easily in pregnancy. Melasma is the darkening of the skin over the cheeks and forehead. An abscess would be deeper in the gum line and not necessarily friable. Decidualization is glandular hyperplasia. A spider angioma is on the skin and is a vascular abnormality created by high estrogen levels.

12. **(E)** With prolonged gastric emptying time and an elevated stomach and progesterone acting to relax the sphincter mechanism of the stomach, the reflux of gastric contents into the esophagus becomes more frequent. These physiologic events are translated into the physical symptom of heartburn and/or gastroesophageal reflux disease (GERD), about which many patients complain. Appendicitis can be more difficult to diagnose because of the abnormal position of the appendix. It is elevated toward the right upper quadrant of the abdomen. The stomach is elevated and also somewhat compressed. Intestinal tone and mobility are slowed by progesterone effect. Intestinal absorbency remains the same, and for weight gain to take place, the gravida must increase caloric intake.

13. **(E)** The presentation of an acute abdomen in pregnancy is very difficult due to the anatomic and physiologic changes in pregnancy. Pregnant women often do not muster the inflammatory response due to an infectious process during pregnancy that a nonpregnant woman does. During pregnancy, C reactive protein and sedimentation rates are elevated as a baseline. WBC counts vary greatly during pregnancy from 5,000 to 12,000. Pregnant women also have a slightly elevated basal temperature. The elevation of the abdominal wall away from the intestines by the uterus may also decrease the findings of rebound, lack of bowel sounds, and anorexia. The positioning of the appendix in pregnancy appears to make the psoas sign less helpful. Given all these confounders, none of the findings in this woman make the diagnosis of appendicitis unlikely. The only abnormal value is the new onset of nausea even though there is no emesis. Given the serious ramifications of a ruptured appendicitis in pregnancy, one must be vigilant for this occurrence.

14. **(E)** Often imaging is needed to make diagnosis. Although an ultrasound has the least ionizing radiation impact and may identify other causes of pain such as ovarian mass or gallstones, by 20 weeks' EGA it is very hard to find little less compress the appendix. A KUB will be helpful only if there is free air under the diaphragm due to rupture. If a CT scan is to be done, oral contrast is safe and allows much better imaging for the diagnosis. The problem with CT scans is the ionizing radiation. MRI avoids the radiation and in expert hands has an excellent performance regarding sensitivity for appendicitis diagnosis. The problem is that it is very expensive, not always available 24/7 and expert readings may not be available 24/7. So although MRI is preferred often a CT scan is necessary if the cases are not clear enough to allow the surgeons to proceed to surgery without imaging.

15. **(D)** Renal function is generally enhanced during pregnancy partially due to vascular expansion, but is also dependent on position during pregnancy. This is largely due to the marked hemodynamic changes that occur in the upright and supine positions. There is also marked dilation up to twofold of the ureters, which is probably due to the effect of progesterone on smooth muscle. Serum BUN and creatinine are markedly decreased during pregnancy due to the increased GFR.

16. **(D)** The kidneys hypertrophy slightly in pregnancy. The effect of progesterone is dilatory on the collecting system. It does not dilate the ureterovesical junction and does not normally cause reflux. In rare cases, the enlarging uterus will cause ureteral obstruction, but this is not true in a majority of pregnancies.

17. **(C)** Because iron is actively transported to the fetus by the placenta against a high concentration gradient, fetal hemoglobin levels do not correlate with maternal levels. Further, the physiologic anemia of pregnancy occurs in both supplemented and nonsupplemented pregnant women because the increase in plasma volume exceeds the increase in RBC mass. Iron supplementation is to prevent iron deficiency in the mother. It has been estimated that women who are iron sufficient at the beginning of pregnancy and who are not iron supplemented need about 2 years after delivery to replenish their iron stores from dietary sources.

18. **(A)** Bone marrow iron will be depleted before the RBCs or binding are affected. Iron absorption would increase as the patient became anemic. Oral iron by diet or supplements can be used to prevent depletion of bone marrow stores.

19. **(C)** The erythrocytes increase approximately 33%, while total blood volume increases approximately 40% to 45%. This helps explain "physiologic" anemia. Again, adequate iron stores and intake will prevent iron depletion.

20. **(A)** The heart appears to enlarge on X-ray, but this is a function of position change. An electrocardiogram also reveals a left-axis shift. Systolic murmurs are common and often benign, but diastolic murmurs are pathologic. Because of the normal changes due to pregnancy, it can be very difficult to diagnose cardiac disease during gestation. Arrhythmia is not normal in pregnancy.

21. **(D)** Estriol is formed in large amounts by the placenta from maternal and fetal precursors. It has been used as an indicator of fetal well-being. Its production relies on interaction of fetus with the placenta and excretion into the maternal serum and urine. Problems with any of these decreases estriol in maternal serum.

22. **(E)** Cardiac output increases by 30% to 50% in pregnancy. In addition, it further increases as labor progresses to as much as 50% above baseline term pregnancy values. It reaches its maximum in the immediate postpartum period (10 to 30 minutes after delivery) with a further increase of 10% to 20%. At 1 hour postpartum, cardiac output returns to prelabor baseline values.

23. **(C)** Cardiac output is the product of stroke volume and heart rate (CO = SV × HR). Heart rate increases by approximately 15 to 20 beats per minute above the prepregnancy rate, and stroke volume increases largely as a result of increased blood volume. Under the influence of the smooth muscle-relaxing effects of elevated progesterone, systemic vascular resistance decreases. Normal pregnancy is not associated with a hyperdynamic left ventricular function, however.

24. **(C)** Vital capacity and maximal breathing capacity remain the same in normal pregnancy. The loss in lung volume due to elevation of the diaphragm is taken from the FRC and, therefore, does not affect the vital capacity. Pulmonary resistance decreases, making air conduction easier.

25. **(D)** In pregnancy, there is a 30% to 40% increase in tidal volume, which occurs at the expense of ERV. Owing to the elevation of the diaphragm, the RV is decreased approximately 20%. The FRC, comprising ERV and RV, is therefore also decreased. The vital capacity is unchanged and large airway function is unimpaired.

26. **(C)** Any woman in early pregnancy with unexplained vaginal bleeding should be evaluated for the possibility of an ectopic pregnancy. The risk of heterotopic pregnancy, that is, simultaneous intrauterine and ectopic pregnancy, is rare. Therefore, in general, confirming the presence of an intrauterine pregnancy by ultrasound effectively rules out ectopic pregnancy. First-trimester vaginal bleeding occurs in approximately 20% of intrauterine pregnancies that do not abort, and it is reported to be more common among multiparous women. A "blighted ovum" is defined as a gestational sac of 2.5 cm or more in which no fetus can be

identified on ultrasound. Such pregnancies are not viable. The corpus luteum of pregnancy produces progesterone to sustain pregnancy in its early weeks. Surgical removal before 7 weeks' gestation results in a rapid decline of maternal serum progesterone and ensuing spontaneous abortion.

27. **(D)** Pregnancy is often referred to as accelerated starvation since the metabolism is designed for the mother to utilize more free fatty acids as an energy source. Also, a relative insulin resistance will allow a higher level of glucose for fetal use since this is the preferred energy source for the fetus.

# Placental, Fetal, and Newborn Physiology

## Questions

1. Current research is placing the etiology of certain complications of pregnancy on the formation of a good placenta. To this end, the placental cotyledons are formed primarily by which of the following?

   (A) arterial pressure on the chorionic plate and decidua
   (B) fetal angiogenesis
   (C) folding of the yolk sac
   (D) maternal angiogenesis
   (E) mesenchymal differentiation secondary to unknown factors

2. Because the fetus is growing rapidly, its need for nutrients and energy exceeds the mother's on a gram-for-gram basis. Often, the placental transport will achieve a fetal concentration greater than maternal, but occasionally the converse occurs. Which of the following has a lower concentration in the fetus than in the mother?

   (A) amino acids
   (B) iron
   (C) oxygen
   (D) phosphate
   (E) vitamins

3. The placenta is supplied by two umbilical arteries that carry deoxygenated fetal blood. This blood flows into intervillous capillaries and back to the fetus in the single umbilical vein. The maternal circulation is designed to bathe the placental villi to optimize transport across the placenta of nutrients, oxygen, and metabolic wastes. Which of the following best describes the path of the maternal blood flow?

   (A) arteries to placental capillaries to veins
   (B) arteries to intravillous spaces to veins
   (C) intravillous spaces to arteries to veins
   (D) veins to intravillous spaces to arteries
   (E) veins to placental capillaries to arteries

4. The human placenta is a complex structure that serves as the interface between the fetus and maternal circulation to allow excretory, respiratory, and nutritional functions for the fetus. It does which of the following?

   (A) allows mainly small molecules and a few blood cells to pass
   (B) allows maternal blood to enter the fetal circulation but not vice versa
   (C) allows only large molecules to pass
   (D) allows total mixing of the maternal and fetal blood
   (E) maintains absolute separation between the maternal and fetal circulations

5. A chronic hypertensive patient presents with complaints of decreased fetal movement. Her prenatal care has been sporadic but it appears that she is at 37 weeks' gestation with an estimated fetal weight of 2,200 g. Concerns are raised regarding placental reserves for oxygenating the fetus. This can be most directly assessed by which of the following?

(A) biophysical profile
(B) a fetal ultrasound growth curve
(C) lecithin/sphingomyelin (L/S) ratio
(D) maternal alpha-fetoprotein
(E) maternal estriol production

6. Labor is induced at 38 weeks due to severe oligohydramnios. The infant is born with a congenital absence of the left hand. This is likely due to which of the following?

(A) amniotic bands
(B) chorioangioma
(C) genetic abnormalities
(D) maternal trauma
(E) true knots in the umbilical cord

7. A poorly controlled class D diabetic patient desired a repeat cesarean section. An amniocentesis to verify pulmonary maturity was done prior to scheduled surgery at 37 weeks' gestation. The L/S ratio was 2:1 and phosphatidylglycerol was absent. An infant was delivered who developed infant respiratory distress syndrome (IRDS). What was the most likely reason?

(A) Diabetic patients do not produce lecithin.
(B) Fetal lung maturation may be delayed in maternal diabetes.
(C) Foam test was not done.
(D) The L/S test was done on fetal urine.
(E) Maternal blood was present in the specimen.

8. A patient presents to labor and delivery complaining of regular uterine contractions. Upon reviewing her gestational dating criteria, the following is determined:

Last menstrual period (LMP) places her at 36 weeks' estimated gestational age (EGA).

Her clinical sizing at her initial obstetrical visit places her at 41 weeks.

Ultrasound done at 10 weeks places her at 38 weeks.

Ultrasound done at this presentation places her at 35 weeks.

Clinical size at presentation places her at 34 weeks.

You determine that she is how many weeks' EGA?

(A) 34 weeks' EGA
(B) 35 weeks' EGA
(C) 36 weeks' EGA
(D) 38 weeks' EGA
(E) 41 weeks' EGA

9. The fetal head is usually the largest part of the infant. Depending on the positioning of the head as it enters the pelvis, labor will progress normally or experience a dystocia due to cephalopelvic disproportion. The smallest circumference of the normal fetal head corresponds to the plane of which diameter?

(A) biparietal diameter
(B) bitemporal diameter
(C) occipitofrontal diameter
(D) occipitomental diameter
(E) suboccipitobregmatic diameter

10. A patient at her 34-week prenatal visit inquires as to the estimated fetal weight. When told it is likely 4 pounds she gets worried that with only a few more weeks that her fetus is too small and there is a problem. While reassuring her, she is told that most of the growth of an infant is in the last month or two of the pregnancy. During the last month of normal pregnancy, the fetus grows at a rate of approximately which of the following?

(A) 100 g/wk
(B) 250 g/wk
(C) 500 g/wk
(D) 759 g/ wk
(E) 1,000 g/wk

11. A patient is found to be blood type A negative during her first pregnancy. She receives antenatal RhoGAM at 28 weeks. At 32 weeks she develops severe preeclampsia and is induced, resulting in an uncomplicated vaginal delivery. The infant does well and is found to be A positive. The mother is found to have anti-D immunoglobulin at a titer of 1:1. Which of the following best describes how much RhoGAM the patient should receive?

(A) no RhoGAM since she is sensitized
(B) mini RhoGAM dose
(C) one dose of RhoGAM
(D) two doses of RhoGAM
(E) three doses of RhoGAM

12. A patient has an emergent cesarean section for an abruption. Because of a large anterior placenta, the placenta was entered during the surgery. The mother is Rh-negative. The infant appears anemic and is Rh-positive. To determine the amount of RhoGAM that needs to be given to prevent sensitization, an estimate of the amount of fetal red blood cells (RBCs) in the maternal circulation is necessary. Fetal RBCs can be distinguished from maternal RBCs by which of the following?

(A) lack of Rh factor
(B) lower amounts of hemoglobin
(C) nucleated RBCs
(D) resistance to acid elution
(E) shape

13. The oxygen dissociation curve of fetal blood lies to the left of the curve of maternal blood. Which of the following is implied?

(A) At any given $O_2$ tension, fetal hemoglobin (Hb F) binds less $O_2$ than adult hemoglobin (Hb A).
(B) At any given pH, Hb F binds less $O_2$ than Hb A.
(C) The fetus needs a greater $O_2$ tension than the mother.
(D) $O_2$ should transfer easily to the fetus.
(E) There is more Hb A than Hb F at delivery.

**Questions 14 through 17 apply to the following topic:**

In utero, the fetus exists in a "water"-filled environment. Oxygen is derived from the placenta. The fetal lungs are filled with amniotic fluid. Given the lower oxygen tension of the fetal blood, the circulation through the heart and lungs is altered to allow optimal oxygen delivery to the most critical structures. Yet this unique circulation must convert in minutes upon delivery to a typical adult circulatory flow.

14. Oxygenated blood from the umbilical vein enters the fetal circulation via which of the following?

(A) ductus arteriosus
(B) the inferior vena cava
(C) intrahepatic artery
(D) the lesser hepatic veins
(E) portal sinus and ductus venosus

15. In the fetus, the most well-oxygenated blood is allowed into the systemic circulation by which of the following?

(A) ductus arteriosus
(B) foramen ovale
(C) ligamentum teres
(D) ligamentum venosum
(E) right ventricle

16. In the fetal circulation, the highest oxygen content occurs in which of the following?

(A) aorta
(B) ductus arteriosus
(C) ductus venosus
(D) superior vena cava
(E) umbilical arteries

17. In systemic circulation of the fetus, the highest oxygen content occurs in which of the following?

(A) ascending aorta
(B) descending aorta
(C) ductus arteriosus
(D) left ventricle
(E) umbilical vein

18. A couple bring their newborn to the pediatrician with concerns regarding possible bruises on the infant's leg. There is no evidence of trauma or violence. The couple had an uncomplicated home birth. Concerns are raised regarding the infant's coagulation status. Which of the following best describes typical fetal coagulation at birth?

    (A) demonstrates a hypercoagulable state
    (B) depends solely on platelet activity until well into the first week of life when clotting factors are activated
    (C) differs significantly between male and female fetuses
    (D) is generally the same as in an adult
    (E) shows significantly less clotting capabilities than in the adult

19. The fetus can produce immune antibodies during development. Also there is some transport of immune antibodies across the placenta. In the fetal blood at birth (compared to maternal blood), there is/are generally which of the following?

    (A) more immunoglobulin G (IgG)
    (B) similar IgG levels
    (C) more immunoglobulin M (IgM)
    (D) more immunoglobulin A (IgA)
    (E) similar IgM levels

**Questions 20 through 22 apply to the following patient:**

A 21-year-old patient who is a G3P0111 at EGA of 33 weeks presents with preterm labor. She had a prior preterm infant at 28 weeks who still has pulmonary dysplasia, so she is very concerned about the pulmonary development of this fetus.

20. Lung surfactant is critical to pulmonary functioning by keeping surface tension in the alveoli low and thereby decreasing the occurrence of atelectasis and atrioventricular (AV) shunting. Surfactant is formed in which of the following?

    (A) epithelium of the respiratory bronchi
    (B) hilum of the lung
    (C) placental syncytiotrophoblasts
    (D) type I pneumocytes of the lung alveoli
    (E) type II pneumocytes of the lung alveoli

21. The presence of which of the following substances is most reassuring that fetal lungs will be mature?

    (A) phosphatidylinositol
    (B) phosphatidylethanolamine
    (C) phosphatidylglycerol (PG)
    (D) phosphatidylcholine
    (E) phosphatidylinositol deacylase

22. Fetal breathing movements can be an indicator of fetal well-being in utero and should occur in what interval of time?

    (A) every 30–60 seconds
    (B) every 30–60 minutes
    (C) 8 breathing movements in 2 hours
    (D) every 24 hours with a diurnal pattern
    (E) every 24 hours associated with fetal movement

23. A patient presents for her routine prenatal visit at 32 weeks' EGA. Her pregnancy up to now has been uncomplicated. Her BMI is 25. Her laboratory testing is normal including a 1-hour glucose screen. An anatomic ultrasound done at 22 weeks was normal and confirmed her dating. Her fundal height is 37 cm today. A brief bedside ultrasound reveals an amniotic fluid index (AFI) of 30 cm. Which of the following situations is most likely to be the etiology of polyhydramnios?

    (A) duodenal atresia
    (B) renal atresia
    (C) pulmonary hypoplasia
    (D) gestational diabetes
    (E) anencephale

24. A fetus has an infection that is causing acute hemolysis. At birth, the infant is not jaundiced though the liver is enlarged. The lack of fetal jaundice is because of which of the following?

(A) Fetus has a great capacity for conjugating bilirubin.

(B) Fetus produces biliverdin.

(C) Liver has high levels of uridine diphosphoglucose dehydrogenase.

(D) Liver plays no part in fetal blood production.

(E) Unconjugated bilirubin is cleared by the maternal liver.

25. Which of the following ratios best describes the serum insulin and glucose levels in the newborn infant of a poorly controlled diabetic mother in comparison to the newborn infant of a euglycemic mother?

|  | Insulin | Glucose |
|---|---|---|
| (A) | Higher | lower |
| (B) | Same | same |
| (C) | Lower | lower |
| (D) | Higher | higher |
| (E) | Lower | higher |

26. Which of the following best describes the fetal kidneys?

(A) They are first capable of producing highly concentrated urine at 3 months.

(B) They are first capable of producing highly concentrated urine at 6 months.

(C) They are not affected by urinary tract obstruction in utero.

(D) If absent, they are associated with pulmonary hypoplasia.

(E) They produce only normotonic urine.

27. A woman presents for her new obstetrical visit at 12 weeks' EGA. Her medical history is complicated by Graves thyroiditis that has been treated with radioactive iodine a few years prior. The patient is currently being maintained on thyroid replacement. She is worried that this will compromise the fetus. She is told that the interaction between maternal and fetal physiology relative to thyroid function is complex. Which of the following is an accurate description of this interaction?

(A) Maternal thyroid hormones (T4 and T3) readily cross the placenta.

(B) Maternal thyrotropin easily crosses the placenta.

(C) The athyroid fetus is growth retarded at birth.

(D) The fetal thyroid concentrates iodide.

(E) The placenta serves as a barrier to maternal iodine crossing to the fetus.

28. A fetus has genotype 46,XY. Early in embryogenesis, the right testis does not form (dysgenesis). What will be the resulting developments?

(A) development of the right mesonephric duct

(B) development of a right ovary

(C) development of the right paramesonephric duct

(D) female phenotype

(E) true hermaphrodite

29. A female fetus has partial fusion of the two Müllerian ducts and complete failure of septal resorption. What is the resulting uterine anomaly called?

(A) didelphys uterus

(B) Müllerian agenesis

(C) septate uterus

(D) unicornuate uterus

(E) vaginal septum

# Answers and Explanations

1. **(A)** About 6 weeks after conception, the trophoblast has 12 to 15 major arteries invading deeply into the myometrium and 20 or more lesser arteries. The pressure generated by these major vessels forces the chorionic plate away from the decidua and forms 12 to 20 cotyledons. Fetal angiogenesis is partly contributory to cotyledon formation as well.

2. **(C)** Although much of placental transport is passive, a large number of necessary metabolic products are actively transported against a concentration gradient. This accounts for many instances of nutritional sparing of the fetus even though maternal nutrition is poor. Fetal $PO_2$, however, is significantly less than maternal. This is why Hb F is needed to facilitate transport of the decreased oxygen to the fetal tissue. The average oxygen saturation of intervillous blood is estimated to be 65% to 75% with a partial pressure ($PO_2$) of 30 to 35 mm Hg. The oxygen saturation of umbilical vein blood is similar but with a lower oxygen partial pressure.

3. **(B)** Oxygenated maternal arterial blood flows into the intervillous spaces, exchanging oxygen with the fetal blood across the placental tissues. It is then collected in maternal veins and reenters the maternal vascular system. The fetal and maternal vascular systems do not normally mix maternal and fetal blood. The human placenta is a hemochorial placenta.

4. **(A)** The placenta allows a few maternal and a few fetal cells to cross. There may be as much as 0.1 to 3.0 mL of fetal blood in the maternal circulation normally; however, there is no free passage. The systems should be separate and to the degree to which they are not, maternal sensitization may occur.

5. **(A)** This is a series of assessments utilizing ultrasound evaluation and a nonstress test. It is the only immediate and direct measure of placental respiratory function and fetal activity listed. Estriol changes can be delayed as can a fall-off in fetal growth. L/S ratio is a test for lung maturity of the fetus, not the placental reserve. Maternal serum alpha-fetoprotein (MSAFP) is a prenatal screen for neural tube defects. Although asymmetric intrauterine growth retardation can result from a decreased reserve and be detected by ultrasound, this is not an immediate assessment of status.

6. **(A)** Amniotic bands can cause severe fetal deformities and even amputations by constricting fetal parts. They are thought to result when small areas of amnion tear and form tough bands from the resultant scarring with healing. The phenomenon is also associated with oligohydramnios. Placental abnormalities have also been noted with a full-blown amniotic band syndrome.

7. **(B)** In diabetic patients, the L/S ratio alone may not be adequate to predict the onset of IRDS, hence the recommendation to assess for the presence of PG as a better indicator of lung maturity. Fetal urine would not have a high L/S ratio. Maternal blood would lower the L/S ratio in most cases, as it has an L/S ratio of about 1.4. Fetal lung biochemical measurements are

less reliable predictors of fetal lung maturity in poorly controlled pregnant diabetic patients.

8. **(D)** Dating a pregnancy is critical to determining the best management. Traditionally, the first day of the LMP is used. However, with the advent of ultrasound, which allows measurement of the fetus, dating has become more accurate. The first ultrasound done during a pregnancy should be compared with the dating from the LMP. If dating based on the LMP is within the error of the ultrasound, LMP dating is used. The error of the ultrasound is roughly +1 week for the first trimester, +2 weeks for the second trimester, and +3 weeks for the third trimester. Since the initial ultrasound was done in the first trimester and was 2 weeks different from the LMP, the ultrasound dating is used. Later ultrasounds are not used to change the due date but can be used for estimating the fetal growth rate. Given that the ultrasound and clinical sizing is smaller than the EGA of 38 weeks determined by the initial ultrasound, concerns of growth restrictions or a constitutionally small fetus can be raised.

9. **(E)** A vertex presentation offers the smallest circumference of the fetal head to the pelvic passage. The circumference at this point is about 32 cm. At the greatest point of the circumference (the occipitofrontal diameter), it is about 34 cm. In addition to the circumference, the ability of the fetus to negotiate the pelvic curve is very much dependent on the position of the presenting vertex, with a well-flexed head in the occiput anterior (OA) position being optimal.

10. **(B)** A good rule of thumb is that the fetus gains one-half pound a week during the last few weeks of gestation. Of course, if placental insufficiency exists, such weight gain does not occur. In uncontrolled diabetes mellitus, classes A, B, and C, growth during this period is accelerated. More severe forms of diabetes (e.g., F, R, or H) may have small-vessel disease with resulting placental insufficiency.

11. **(C)** RhoGAM consists of anti-D immunoglobin. Since she received RhoGAM only a month ear-

lier, there would still be some detected during the "RhoGAM" workup postpartum. She should still receive 1 ampule of RhoGAM unless testing determines a large fetal–maternal bleed, which is not likely in an uncomplicated vaginal delivery.

12. **(D)** Small numbers of fetal red cells can be detected in the maternal circulation by the Kleihauer–Betke test, which uses the fetal cells resistant to acid elution for identification. Fetal red cells can exist and function at lower pH values than adult RBCs. Fetal RBCs have less than two-thirds the life span of adult RBCs. Fetal RBCs may also be nucleated. The nucleation helps identify fetal RBCs on a smear. This nucleation disappears early in normal pregnancy. Fetal cells then closely resemble reticulocytes.

13. **(D)** The pH of the fetus is slightly lower than the maternal pH. The difference in $O_2$ affinity is very small in vivo. The fetus lives at a lower $O_2$ concentration with an oxygen-loving hemoglobin (Hb F), which allows oxygen transport to fetal tissues despite very low maternal oxygen tension. Although Hb A starts being produced in the third trimester, the Hb F is still the dominant form at delivery.

14. **(E)** The umbilical vein comes directly from the placenta and distributes highly oxygenated blood to the liver, the portal system, and the inferior vena cava. The umbilical vein enters the fetus and divides immediately into the portal sinus (carrying blood to the hepatic veins) and the ductus venosus (carrying blood to the vena cava). The ductus arteriosus connects the fetal pulmonary vasculature with the fetal aorta (see Figure 7–1).

15. **(B)** The foramen ovale lets oxygenated blood into the left side of the heart. The ligaments mentioned are found after birth and represent occluded vessels from the fetal circulation. Before birth; however, they serve as the shunting mechanism that makes fetal oxygenation possible. The ductus arteriosus allows the flow from the right ventricle to enter the systemic circulation after the aortic arch.

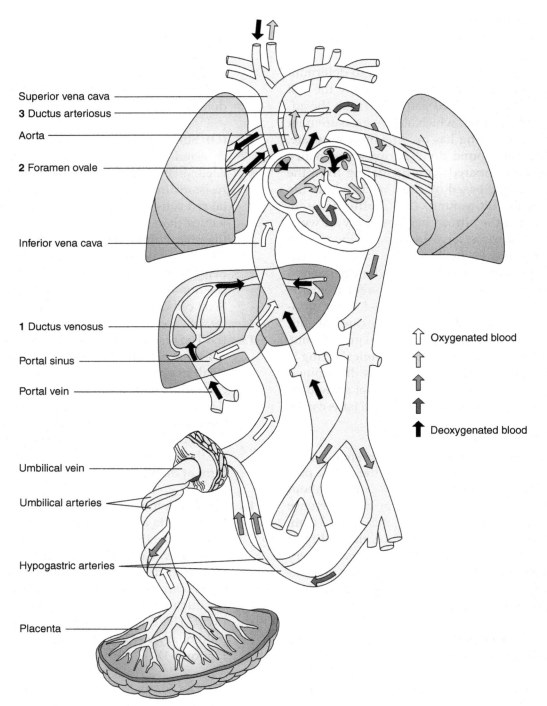

Superior vena cava

**3** Ductus arteriosus

Aorta

**2** Foramen ovale

Inferior vena cava

**1** Ductus venosus

Portal sinus

Portal vein

Umbilical vein

Umbilical arteries

Hypogastric arteries

Placenta

⇧ Oxygenated blood

⬆ Deoxygenated blood

**Figure 7–1.** The fetal circulation.
(Reproduced, with permission, from Cunningham FG, Levenoe KJ, Bloom S, Hauth JC, Rouse DJ,
Spong C. *Williams Obstetrics*, 23rd ed. New York: McGraw-Hill, 2001.)

**16. (C)** The fetal venous blood from the placenta has the highest oxygen content. This is true because fetal venous blood in the ductus venosus has most recently received oxygenation. Pulmonary fetal oxygenation does not occur until the infant's first breath. The superior vena cava has oxygen-deficit blood. The ductus arteriosus and aorta have mixed blood that eventually goes to umbilical arteries.

17. **(E)** The umbilical vein always has the highest oxygen concentration. The next highest oxygen concentration in the systemic circulation is in the ascending aorta prior to the insertion of the ductus arteriosus. The arteries supplying the fetal brain branch off that part of the ascending aorta allowing the blood with the highest systemic oxygen levels to be preferentially shunted to the brain. The left ventricle is not part of the systemic circulation.

18. **(E)** Fetal and early neonatal blood clotting may be compromised because the fetus is low in factors II, VII, IX, X, XI, XII, and XIII and fibrinogen. These do not cross the placenta from the mother. Levels are generally 50% of adult levels. Vitamin K-dependent coagulation factors decrease further in the first few days after birth. This decrease is amplified in breast-fed infants. Newborn infants are given vitamin K to stimulate the lipid-soluble coagulation factors. It is the mother who is in a hypercoagulable state.

19. **(B)** IgG crosses the placenta easily from 16 weeks' gestation onward. At birth, fetal and maternal IgG levels are equal since most of the IgG present is from maternal diffusion. IgM cannot cross, and a normal fetus (noninfected) produces very little IgM. Thus an elevated IgM level represents a fetal infectious insult such as with rubella, CMV, or toxoplasmosis. IgA is not produced and later will be absorbed through the fetal gut from the colostrum in small-to-moderate amounts. Even these small amounts are able to provide mucosal protection against enteric infections. The fetus normally has lower levels of IgM and IgA than the mother.

20. **(E)** There are more than 40 cell types in the fetal lung. Surfactant is specific to the type II pneumocytes of the alveoli. Surfactant is produced in the lamellar bodies of these cells. The presence of air-to-tissue interface as the infant takes its first breath allows the surfactant to "uncoil" from the lamellar bodies and line the alveolus, thus preventing alveolar collapse. It is the capacity of the lungs to produce surfactant and not the actual laying down of it in utero that establishes lung maturity before birth.

21. **(C)** The first four are all components of mature surfactant. Fifty percent of surfactant is composed of phosphatidylcholine, but the presence of PG seems to play a crucial role in the prevention of infant respiratory distress. Its presence is nearly a guarantee of fetal lung maturity.

22. **(B)** Fetal breathing movements can be seen episodically in the normal human fetus. They occur about every 30 to 60 minutes. Asphyxia appears to reduce the frequency of fetal breathing movements. Eight to ten fetal movements in 2 hours are referring to the fetal kick count pattern, which is felt to be reassuring.

23. **(A)** The sudden development of polyhydramnios raises the possibility of a number of pathologies although the most common is idiopathic. Given a normal diabetes screen and anatomy ultrasound, the presence of diabetes and major anatomical issues such as anencephaly is very rare. Renal atresia would cause oligohydramnios with the development of pulmonary hypoplasia if it happens early enough in the pregnancy. This is the common presentation for duodenal atresia with the obstruction preventing absorption of the fluid and excretion across the placenta.

24. **(E)** Because of a relative lack of enzymes, the liver conjugates bilirubin poorly. Some is excreted into the bowel where it is oxidized to biliverdin and colors the meconium. However, the unconjugated bilirubin is transported across the placenta and cleared by the maternal liver. This prevents fetal jaundice. Neonatal jaundice will appear hours to days after birth due to the poor ability of the newborn liver to conjugate bilirubin and excrete it through the intestines. The fetal liver is active in blood production early in pregnancy, hence the liver enlargement in this case. Uridine diphosphoglucose dehydrogenase plays only a minor role in intermediary metabolism. Fetal levels of glycogen are two to three times that of adult levels.

25. **(A)** Insulin levels are elevated in the infants of diabetic mothers. In fact, high insulin levels may cause a precipitous drop in newborn serum

glucose, causing the baby to be metabolically unstable. This is why all babies of diabetic mothers and macrosomic infants (potentially undiagnosed diabetic mothers) are screened quickly after birth and for the first few hours for hypoglycemia.

26. **(D)** The number and function of glomeruli can be used as a rough index of fetal maturity. Creatinine concentration in the amniotic fluid mirrors renal function. Maximum fetal urine production is about 650 mL/d of hypotonic solution. Fetal urine production is often decreased in infants with growth retardation. The fetal kidneys cannot significantly concentrate the urine until after delivery. Intrauterine obstruction of the fetal urinary tract can cause severe damage to the fetal kidneys. Absence of fetal kidneys will result in severe oligohydramnios and pulmonary hypoplasia and is incompatible with life. Many of these infants have a specific syndrome called Potter's syndrome.

27. **(D)** Generally, the placenta serves as a barrier to maternal thyrotropin and thyroid hormones. The fetus concentrates iodide very effectively, hence the need to avoid radioactive iodine and high iodide-containing medications. There is limited action of the thyroid hormone during fetal life. The athyroid fetus will appear normally grown at birth. This is why all newborns are screened in the first week of life for thyroid function.

28. **(C)** The Müllerian-inhibiting substance (MIS) is active only in the immediate area. Thus, the lack of a testis on the right will mean there is no MIS, the Müllerian ducts (paramesonephric) will develop, and the Wolffian duct will regress. Because 5 alpha-dihydrotestosterone is present from the left testis, the external genitalia will be male. Thus, the newborn will have a male phenotype. Since there was gonadal dysgenesis, there will not be a right ovary.

29. **(A)** The formation of a normal internal female reproductive system requires the fusion of the two Müllerian tubes and then reabsorption of the resulting septum to a single uterine cavity and cervix. Vaginal agenesis is a failure of the Müllerian ducts to elongate to the level of the urogenital sinus. A vaginal septum is formed when there is a septal reabsorption defect. A septate uterus has successful Müllerian fusion but incomplete reabsorption of the septum. A unicornuate uterus results when there is agenesis of one Müllerian duct. A uterine didelphys results when there is partial fusion and complete septal resorption defect. This results in two uterine cavities and two cervices.

# CHAPTER 8

# Prenatal Care

## Questions

**DIRECTIONS (Questions 1 through 38): For each of the multiple choice questions in this section, select the lettered answer that is the one *best* response in each case.**

1. Worldwide, which of the following is the most common problem during pregnancy?

    (A) diabetes

    (B) preeclampsia

    (C) heart disease

    (D) urinary tract infection (UTI)

    (E) iron-deficiency anemia

2. In the United States, it appears that maternal mortality is increasing after years of decline. To address this increase, efforts must be directed toward the leading causes. Which of the following choices lists those leading causes?

    (A) infection, cardiomyopathy, and stroke

    (B) motor vehicle accidents, homicide, and suicide

    (C) embolism, hypertension, and ectopic pregnancy

    (D) complications related to abortion and anesthesia

    (E) human immunodeficiency virus (HIV) and infections related to immunodeficiency

3. A patient presents with a positive pregnancy test, the exact date of the start of her last normal menses, and the date of her luteinizing hormone (LH) surge from a urine kit. Her expected date of delivery can most correctly be calculated by which of the following?

    (A) adding 254 to the date of the start of the last menstrual period (LMP)

    (B) counting 10 lunar months from the time of ovulation

    (C) counting 280 from the first day of the LMP

    (D) counting 40 weeks from the last day of the LMP

    (E) adding 256 to the date of the elevated urinary LH when detected by home testing

4. A friend mentions to you she just had a positive pregnancy test and wonders if you can tell her when she is likely due. The LMP was June 30. Her expected date of confinement (EDC) is approximately which of the following?

    (A) March 23

    (B) April 7

    (C) March 28

    (D) April 23

    (E) March 7

5. A patient presents to your clinic complaining of nausea and vomiting. She is currently ingesting combined oral contraceptive pills (OCP) and has used them for over a year. When you tell her she has a positive pregnancy test, she reports that her last bleeding on the OCPs was 8 weeks ago. In such a situation, determination of the most accurate estimated date of delivery can then be made by which of the following?

   (A) eliciting when breast tenderness or morning sickness began

   (B) assessing uterine size by physical examination

   (C) counting 280 days from the first positive serum pregnancy test

   (D) asking the patient when she first felt pregnant

   (E) obtaining fetal biometry by ultrasound prior to 20 weeks' gestation

6. A 24-year-old patient who has signs and symptoms of renal lithiasis is to have an intravenous pyelogram (IVP) as part of a urologic investigation. Before proceeding with the study, which of the following should you determine?

   (A) whether she is using contraception

   (B) whether she is in the follicular phase of a menstrual cycle

   (C) whether she is sexually active

   (D) whether she has a history of children with birth defects

   (E) whether she may be pregnant

7. A 20-year-old primigravida, who is 24 weeks pregnant, expresses concern about the normality of her fetus after learning that a close friend has just delivered an infant with hydrocephalus. Which of the following details about hydrocephalus should be included in her counseling?

   (A) occurs spontaneously in 1 in 500 pregnancies

   (B) has a multifactorial etiology

   (C) is usually an isolated defect

   (D) can be cured by intrauterine placement of shunts

   (E) can be identified as early as 10 weeks' gestation

8. Fundal height, part of the obstetric examination, is taken from the top of the symphysis pubis to the top of the fundus. How is it measured?

   (A) by calipers, approximating the week of gestation

   (B) in inches, approximating the lunar month of gestation

   (C) in centimeters and divided by 3.5, approximating the lunar months of gestation

   (D) in centimeters, approximating the weeks of gestation beyond 22 weeks

   (E) by calipers in centimeters, prognosticating the fetal weight

9. Using your knowledge of normal maternal physiology, which of the following would you employ if a patient at 38 weeks became faint while lying supine on your examination table?

   (A) aromatic ammonia spirit (smelling salts)

   (B) turning the patient on her side

   (C) oxygen by face mask

   (D) intravenous (IV) drugs to increase blood pressure

   (E) IV saline solution

10. A woman in early pregnancy is worried because of some recent discomfort in her left breast. On examination, her skin appears normal, she has no axillary or clavicular adenopathy, but you palpate a smooth, nontender, 2-cm mass. Your immediate management should be which of the following?

   (A) breast ultrasound

   (B) needle aspiration of the mass

   (C) excisional biopsies of the mass

   (D) mammography

   (E) warm compresses and antibiotics

11. The management of vaginal bleeding in a first-trimester pregnancy requires a trending of human chorionic gonadotropin (hCG) levels. Because urine pregnancy tests can typically be less expensive and results are more rapidly available, it is important to know their sensitivity. Immunologic tests for pregnancy can detect hCG in the urine in which of the following concentrations?

(A) 2 IU/L
(B) 20 IU/L
(C) 100 IU/L
(D) 200 IU/L
(E) 1,000 IU/L

12. The new obstetrical visit typically includes a general well woman assessment as well as pregnancy evaluation. Which of the following is true about Pap smears taken from the uterine cervix during a normal pregnancy?

(A) They should be part of routine obstetric care, if needed, based on pap frequency for the individual patient.
(B) They are indicated only in patients with clinically assessed risks.
(C) They are difficult to interpret because of gestational changes.
(D) They are a cost-effective replacement for cultures for sexually transmitted diseases (STDs).
(E) They are likely to induce uterine irritability.

13. Prenatal care is a structured approach to obstetric care to assess for increase risk of complications or the actual development of problems. Which of the following would most predispose the patient to obstetrical complications?

(A) maternal age 39
(B) maternal age 17, with menarche at age 13
(C) history of four normal deliveries
(D) history of ovarian dermoid cyst removed 4 years ago
(E) a clinically measured pelvic diagonal conjugate of 12 cm

14. A pregnant woman at 4 weeks' gestation had an upper gastrointestinal (GI) series and is worried about possible fetal effects from radiation. You inform her that the risk for mental retardation to the fetus is greatest during which phase of pregnancy?

(A) implantation stage from 0 to 9 days
(B) 1st to 8th week of gestation
(C) 8th through 15th week of gestation
(D) 15th through 25th week of gestation
(E) last trimester

15. Advising a 34-year-old woman at 12 weeks' gestation about the risk of chromosomal defects in the fetus, you can correctly state which of the following?

(A) There is little worry regarding Down syndrome before the age of 35.
(B) Paternal age is very important in the etiology of Down syndrome.
(C) Maternal serum alpha-fetoprotein (MSAFP) is a very specific test for Down syndrome.
(D) Screening for Down syndrome can be improved by checking amniotic fluid for acetylcholinesterase level.
(E) Efficacy of screening for Down syndrome is improved by adding estriol, inhibin A, and hCG concentration to the MSAFP (quadruple screen).

16. The most worrisome sign or symptom of potentially serious pathology in late pregnancy is which of the following?

(A) swollen ankles
(B) constipation
(C) visual changes
(D) nocturia
(E) heartburn

17. During late pregnancy, which of the following implies urinary tract disease?

    (A) decreased serum creatinine
    (B) failure to excrete concentrated urine after 18 hours without fluids
    (C) glucosuria
    (D) dilation of the ureters
    (E) decreased creatinine clearance

18. Because treatment of HIV during pregnancy and labor can significantly decrease fetal transmission as well as maternal morbidity, which of the following is the standard of care regarding HIV testing in pregnancy?

    (A) It should not be offered to patients in low-risk populations.
    (B) Universal screening is required by law.
    (C) It is performed routinely without patient consent in federal facilities serving high-risk populations.
    (D) Testing is done only at the request of the patient.
    (E) Universal screening using an *opt-out* approach is recommended.

19. Routine screening procedures at her first prenatal care visit for a 35-year-old primigravida with an estimated gestational age (EGA) of 8 weeks should include which of the following?

    (A) quadruple test
    (B) 1-hour glucose challenge
    (C) family history
    (D) toxoplasma titer
    (E) ultrasound

20. Many fetal anomalies found on ultrasound are associated with other anomalies that the sonographer must assess. Which of the following abnormal ultrasound findings of the fetus are usually found in isolation and not as part of a collection of abnormalities or a syndrome?

    (A) omphalocele
    (B) gastroschisis
    (C) diaphragmatic hernia

    (D) duodenal atresia
    (E) posturethral value

21. An abnormal biophysical profile (BPP) predicts which of the following?

    (A) higher risk for antepartum death within 1 week
    (B) a baby that will be small for gestational age (SGA)
    (C) maternal preeclampsia
    (D) meconium staining
    (E) placental abruption

22. A pregnant woman not previously known to be diabetic, who is at 26 weeks' gestation, had a routine 50-g (GTT) with a 1-hour blood glucose value of 144 mg/dL. A follow-up 100-g, 3-hour oral GTT revealed plasma values of fasting blood sugar of 102; 1 hour, 180; 2 hours, 162; and 3 hours, 144. You should do which of the following?

    (A) begin American Diabetes Association (ADA) diet and daily glucose monitoring
    (B) repeat the GTT in early or mid-third trimester
    (C) start oral hypoglycemic agents in the diet
    (D) perform an immediate Contraction Stress Test (CST)
    (E) treat the patient as one with normal gestation

23. A patient is measuring size larger than dates at her initial obstetric visit at 24 weeks' EGA. She is worried about twins since they "run" in the family. The best method to safely and reliably diagnose twins is by which of the following?

    (A) ultrasonography
    (B) Leopold's maneuvers
    (C) auscultation
    (D) X-rays
    (E) computed tomography (CT) scan

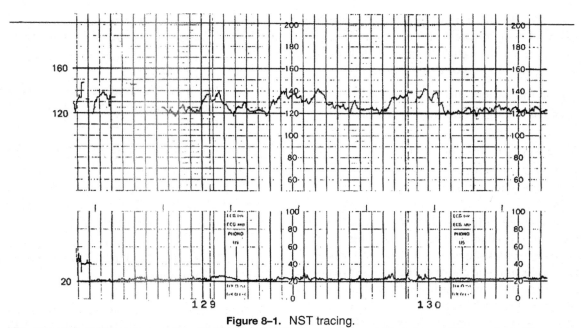

**Figure 8–1.** NST tracing.
(Reproduced, with permission, from DeCherney AH, Nathan L. *Current Obstetric and Gynecologic Diagnosis and Treatment*, 9th ed. New York: McGraw-Hill, 2003.)

**24.** A 24-year-old G1P0 at 38 weeks' EGA presents to labor and delivery for a complaint of decreased fetal movement. The nonstress test (NST) results are shown in Figure 8–1. What is the interpretation of this NST?

(A) The tracing does not meet the criteria for reactivity.

(B) A fetus with this pattern is at risk for fetal death in utero within the next week.

(C) The pattern demonstrates short-term but not long-term variability.

(D) The pattern is common during the sleep cycle of the fetus.

(E) This is a reactive NST, indicating that the fetus is not likely to be acidotic.

**25.** Of the following evaluations done during routine prenatal care in a normal pregnancy, which of the following is most important in the initial clinic visit?

(A) routine measurement of the fundus

(B) determination of the gestational age

(C) determination of maternal blood pressure

(D) maternal urinalysis

(E) maternal weight

**26.** There is good evidence that a woman who gave birth to an infant with a neural tube defect (NTD) can substantially reduce the risk of recurrence by taking periconceptional folic acid supplementation. What is the recommended dose?

(A) 0.4 mg

(B) 0.8 mg

(C) 1.0 mg

(D) 4 mg

(E) 8 mg

**27.** Which of the following is the most prominent cause of pregnancy loss?

(A) contraception

(B) stillbirths

(C) neonatal mortality

(D) fetal deaths in utero

(E) abortion

28. A 32-year-old G2P1 female presents for routine prenatal visit at 36 weeks' EGA. You note a 7-lb weight gain in the last 2 weeks? Which of the following should be your first priority?

    (A) give the patient diuretics
    (B) assess for signs and symptoms of preeclampsia
    (C) markedly restrict her diet
    (D) encourage vigorous exercise
    (E) place her on bed rest

29. An 18-year-old single, sedentary, obese female (gravida 1, para 0) is first seen by you for prenatal care at 16 weeks' gestation. Her history is unremarkable, and she claims to be in good health. Her dietary history includes high carbohydrate intake with no fresh vegetables. Physical examination is within normal limits except that she is somewhat pale. Suggested nutritional counseling should include which of the following?

    (A) a strict diet to maintain her current weight
    (B) 25–30 g of protein in the diet everyday
    (C) intake of 1,200 calories a day
    (D) folic acid supplementation
    (E) at least 1 hour of vigorous aerobic exercise daily

30. A 19-year-old primigravida with unsure LMP presents to initiate prenatal care. You attempt to estimate gestational age. The uterine fundus is palpable at the level of the pubic symphysis, and fetal heart tones are audible by electronic Doppler. On the basis of this information, what is the approximate gestational age?

    (A) 8 weeks
    (B) 12 weeks
    (C) 16 weeks
    (D) 20 weeks
    (E) 24 weeks

31. A 28-year-old (gravida 3, para 1, abortus 1) at 30 weeks' gestation reports some recent intermittent contractions. Which of the following correlates with the greatest risk for preterm labor?

    (A) patient is a smoker (half pack per day)
    (B) prior 32-week delivery

    (C) history of colposcopy
    (D) history of *Chlamydia trachomatis*
    (E) prior 8-week spontaneous abortion

32. A 32-year-old (gravida 2, para 1) initiates care at 8 weeks' gestation. Which of the following is most worrisome for poor obstetric outcome?

    (A) trace proteinuria on urine dipstick
    (B) blood pressure of 144/92 mm Hg
    (C) inaudible fetal heart tone by electronic Doppler
    (D) maternal height of 4 ft 10 in.
    (E) the presence of curd-like discharge consistent with *Candida* on speculum examination

33. Between obesity, irregular menses, erratic use of contraception and unknown LMP ultrasound is commonly used to determine the EDC. How many weeks after LMP is ultrasound most accurate in dating a pregnancy?

    (A) between 2 and 4 weeks after LMP
    (B) between 7 and 9 weeks after LMP
    (C) between 12 and 14 weeks after LMP
    (D) between 19 and 21 weeks after LMP
    (E) between 30 and 32 weeks after LMP

34. How many weeks after LMP is ultrasound most useful in evaluating fetal anatomy?

    (A) between 2 and 4 weeks after LMP
    (B) between 7 and 9 weeks after LMP
    (C) between 12 and 14 weeks after LMP
    (D) between 19 and 21 weeks after LMP
    (E) between 30 and 32 weeks after LMP

35. Which of the following nutrients is most likely to be deficient during pregnancy?

    (A) iron
    (B) vitamin D
    (C) vitamin A
    (D) calcium
    (E) folic acid

36. A 32-year-old woman has a twin pregnancy at 8 weeks' gestation. During her initial prenatal care visit, you review risks for multifetal pregnancies. Which of the following statements reflects the most frequent risks in twin pregnancies?

   (A) Pregnancy-induced hypertension occurs at a higher rate than in singletons.
   (B) Cesarean delivery is necessary in greater than 90% of twin deliveries.
   (C) Shoulder dystocia occurs more in the aftercoming vertex twin , as compared to a singleton.
   (D) Perinatal death rate is less than that of singletons.
   (E) Congenital anomalies occur at the same rate as in singletons.

37. Periconceptional dietary adjustments have been shown to have a profound impact on which of the following diseases or malformations?

   (A) Tay-Sachs disease
   (B) preeclampsia
   (C) clubfoot (talipes equinovarus)
   (D) diabetes mellitus
   (E) cystic fibrosis

38. Which of the following should be prescribed for the average pregnant woman?

   (A) an increase of no more than 15–20 lb in pregnancy
   (B) iron supplementation, in addition to prenatal vitamins
   (C) continuation of moderate exercise
   (D) 4-mg folic acid supplementation
   (E) vinegar–water douches in the third trimester

**DIRECTIONS (Questions 39 through 51): The following groups of questions are preceded by a list of lettered options. For each question, select the one lettered option that is most closely associated with it. Each lettered option may be used once, multiple times, or not at all.**

### Questions 39 through 43

Match the specific ultrasound findings with the commonly associated abnormality.

   (A) interventricular cardiac defect
   (B) NTD
   (C) duodenal atresia
   (D) Potter's syndrome
   (E) thalassemia

39. Absent kidneys

40. Banana sign

41. Lemon sign

42. Double bubble sign

43. Hydrops fetalis

**Questions 44 through 51**

Match the potential abnormality or complication associated with the medications below.

    (A) craniofacial abnormalities

    (B) Ebstein's anomaly

    (C) spina bifida

    (D) scalp defects

    (E) abortion

    (F) stillbirth

    (G) none of the above

**44.** Fluoxetine

**45.** Podophyllin resin

**46.** Tetracycline

**47.** Captopril

**48.** Valproic acid

**49.** Isotretinoin

**50.** Methimazole

**51.** Misoprostol

**DIRECTIONS (Question 52): For the following multiple choice question, select the lettered answer that is the one *best* response.**

**52.** Pregnancy should be avoided within 1 month of receiving which of the following vaccinations?

    (A) measles, mumps, rubella (MMR)

    (B) influenza

    (C) hepatitis B

    (D) tetanus

    (E) pneumococcus

# Answers and Explanations

1. **(E)** The National Institutes of Health estimates that 50% of all pregnant women worldwide are iron deficient. In the United States, the average woman has iron stores of less than 1 g. This amount is needed for the increased maternal blood volume and fetal growth during pregnancy. Poorly nourished women have an even greater deficiency. The National Academy of Sciences recommends 27-mg iron supplementation—the amount found in most prenatal vitamins. All women should be routinely screened for iron-deficiency anemia during early pregnancy and be given additional supplementation as needed.

   Preeclampsia, diabetes, UTIs, and heart disease do complicate pregnancies but to a lesser extent overall, as compared with iron-deficiency anemia.

2. **(C)** Maternal death is the demise of any woman from any pregnancy-related cause while pregnant or within 42 days after termination of pregnancy. A direct maternal death is the result of obstetric complications of pregnancy, labor, or the puerperium. An indirect maternal death is not directly due to obstetric causes but may be aggravated by the physiologic changes of pregnancy. Studies vary in reporting the most frequent causes of maternal death, but collectively embolism, hypertension, and ectopic pregnancy represent nearly 50% of direct maternal deaths. Maternal mortality, along with other statistics of pregnancy outcome, is a measure of the effectiveness of obstetrical care.

3. **(C)** To determine the EDC, add 280 days to the LMP. If the patient has an altered cycle length, the EDC may be different from that calculated earlier. Ultrasound is a useful adjunct for the determination of EDC.

4. **(B)** Nägele's rule allows rapid estimation of the expected date of delivery. From the LMP, add 7 days, subtract 3 months, and add 1 year. It works for the patient with regular monthly cycles and a sure LMP.

5. **(E)** A certain, documented LMP in a woman with normal, regular menstrual cycles is an excellent means to determine gestational age and estimated date of delivery. Without this, we must rely on other clinical information to date the pregnancy. The most accurate means is an early ultrasound, preferably in the first trimester (crown-to-rump length), or, at the latest, biometry done before 20 weeks' gestation. Assessment of uterine size—if done in the first trimester by an experienced obstetrical clinician—can also provide an accurate estimate, but objective early ultrasound measurements are preferable.

6. **(E)** One should always determine whether the patient is pregnant before ordering diagnostic X-rays on any menstrual-age woman. Although mutagenic radiation is unlikely from low doses, cumulative effects may be more damaging. The other answers are immaterial to the type or timing of imaging studies.

7. **(B)** Hydrocephalus occurs in approximately 1 per 2,000 births and may be due to neoplasm, infections (such as toxoplasmosis) or genetic inheritance, frequently by the mechanisms of aqueductal stenosis. It is usually found in

conjunction with other neurologic or systemic anomalies. Ultrasound has greatly facilitated our ability to diagnose hydrocephalus in utero by using either the absolute size of greater than 10 mm of the lateral ventricular atrium or a ratio of greater than 50% of the lateral ventricular width to the hemispheric width of the brain. Although surgery has been tried, results have been discouraging.

8. **(D)** Measurement of fundal height is a routine component of prenatal care. The repetitive, consistent measurements may allow the obstetrician to detect the SGA fetus or a fetus with accelerated growth, as may occur in the setting of maternal diabetes. After 22 weeks, uterine fundal height in centimeters coincides with weeks of gestation. Unfortunately increasing incidence of obesity in the pregnant population makes this technique less accurate. However, interval growth between visits should be consistent with the number of interval weeks. Precise knowledge of the age of the fetus is essential for appropriate obstetric management.

9. **(B)** In the third trimester, the supine position facilitates the large pregnant uterus to compress the venous system that returns blood from the lower half of the body. This results in potentially decreased cardiac filling and cardiac output. In about 10% of women, this causes significant arterial hypotension, sometimes referred to as the supine hypotensive syndrome. Altering material position is usually sufficient to remedy this compression and alleviate the hypotension. Administration of fluids or pressors is rarely necessary.

10. **(A)** Breast cancer is one of the most common malignancies diagnosed during pregnancy, although the actual incidence is still quite low: 1 in 3,000 pregnancies). The differential of a breast mass in the pregnant or lactating woman includes malignancy, fibroadenoma, adenoma, cysts, abscess, and hyperplasia. The evaluation of any breast mass should include a thorough history and physical examination. In pregnancy, breast ultrasound is typically the first imaging modality to determine the characteristics of the mass. Depending on this result, additional

imaging such as MRI or mammography may be used. On the basis of these results coupled with the physical examination, biopsies, either core or fine needle may be needed.

11. **(B)** The lower range of detectable hCG has dropped dramatically in recent years. Because of this sensitivity, one can use pregnancy tests to detect low hCG levels. More sensitive tests have greatly improved the ability to diagnose pregnancy. The tests are now inexpensive, specific, sensitive, and highly accurate.

12. **(A)** According to the December 2009 American College of Obstetricians and Gynecologists (ACOG) Practice Bulletin, cervical cancer screening should begin at age 21 and be repeated every 2 years, if normal. Once a woman turns 30, paps should be performed every 3 years, if three prior consecutive paps are normal. More frequent paps may be indicated in patients with HIV, immunosuppressed, Diethylstilbestrol (DES) exposed, and prior treatment for CIN 2, CIN 3, or cancer. There are no special considerations for women who are pregnant, therefore they follow the same recommendations. Paps are just as valid during pregnancy. A Pap smear does not assess for STDs. Additional testing may be done on the fluid sample left after a liquid-based pap for gonorrhea and chlamydia. There may be a slightly higher incidence of nonsignificant spotting with the pap during pregnancy.

13. **(A)** Older women have an increased risk during pregnancy for chromosomal abnormalities, mostly due to nondisjunction. They also have an increased number of abnormalities associated with advancing age, such as hypertension, gestational diabetes, and need for cesarean delivery. Extremely young women are also at a greater risk for problems during pregnancy. This is particularly true under the age of 16 and particularly if menarche occurs less than 2 years before the pregnancy. Normal deliveries are not a problem, but a history of prior abnormal deliveries, such as preterm delivery and cesarean section, is concerning. The presence of an ovarian cyst that is treated adequately is of little concern regarding current pregnancy risk. The diagonal conjugate of 12 cm is normal.

14. **(C)** Data derived from the survivors of the atomic bomb place the greatest risk for mental retardation from radiation when the fetus is exposed at 8 to 15 weeks' gestation and virtually no risk with small (i.e., <5 rads) doses before 8 or after 25 weeks' gestation. If a woman is exposed in the preimplantation time period, 0 to 9 days, an "all or none" phenomenon occurs with either the loss of the pregnancy or a fetus that is unaffected. An Upper GI series exposes the uterus/embryo to 0.56 mrad. Single exposures much higher than this would be necessary to affect the fetus.

15. **(E)** Although the risk of Down syndrome increases with maternal age, most Down infants are born to women younger than 35 years, because there are a greater number of pregnancies in this age group. Therefore, a good test to detect it is important. Paternal age does not have much effect on the incidence of Down syndrome, although it is important in autosomal dominant genetic disease. Amniotic fluid acetylcholinesterase is valuable for detecting NTDs but not for Down syndrome. Screening for Down syndrome can be performed in first trimester, when indicated, by chorionic villous sampling. MSAFP is a reasonably good test for NTDs when elevated, and a low serum value of AFP is useful, particularly when combined with maternal age to detect Down syndrome. Still, most women who have a low MSAFP will not have children with Down syndrome. The efficacy of screening can be improved by adding estriol, hCG, and inhibin A. This is the so-called quadruple screen and is performed between 16 and 20 weeks' gestation. Many centers now have the ability to offer an "integrated" first and second trimester screen, which includes the following: ultrasound between 11 and 13 weeks to assess fetal nuchal translucency, serum levels for free beta-hCG and PAPP-A between 11 and 13 weeks, combined with the quadruple screen in the second trimester. This integrated approach detects 95% of babies with Down syndrome with only a 1.2% false-negative rate.

16. **(C)** Cerebral visual disturbances such as scotomata can occur in preeclamptic patients, and such women require further evaluation. The other listed choices are common nuisances related to the physiologic changes of pregnancy.

17. **(E)** Because of increased glomerular filtration rate (GFR), serum creatinine is usually low during pregnancy and creatinine clearance is increased. Decreased creatinine clearance may be seen in a variety of conditions such as preeclampsia and renal insufficiency. The increased GFR is also responsible for glucosuria in gravidas with normal glucose levels. The kidneys often excrete excess extracellular fluid after a period of recumbency, so the urine may not be concentrated after decreased oral intake of fluid, and urine is often the least concentrated in the morning. There is usually normal dilation of the collecting system on IVP during pregnancy.

18. **(E)** Universal HIV testing with patient notification was recommended by the Institute of Medicine in an effort to reduce the rate of perinatal HIV transmission in the United States. By 2008, the American Academy of Pediatrics, United States Preventive Services Task Force, the Centers for Disease Control and Prevention, and the ACOG supported recommendation for universal screening using an *opt-out* approach. The use of patient notification allows the woman to decline to be tested. No signed consent is required.

19. **(C)** All women are counseled regarding chromosomal risks, not just women older than 35 years. All women should be informed of all available testing including an ultrasound between 11 and 13 weeks for nuchal translucency. The quadruple test is performed in the second trimester. A 1-hour glucose challenge test is done routinely in the second trimester (24–28 weeks) to predict gestational diabetes in an otherwise asymptomatic woman without risk factors such as obesity, history of macrosomia, history of gestational diabetes or a family member with diabetes, or an unexplained stillbirth. A family history to evaluate familial retardation or birth defects, as well as different ethnic origins, is important for screening purposes and needs to be done at the first visit to guide subsequent recommendations. A Toxoplasma titer is not beneficial as the incidence in the

United States is very low, and the treatment options are not good. It may be done in selected cases in a preconceptual testing program but as yet is not routine in the United States. Ultrasound at 8 weeks' gestation may be used to date a pregnancy if LMP is uncertain, but it need not be performed routinely.

20. **(E)** Omphalocele (abdominal contents of the fetus covered only by a two-layered sac of amnion and peritoneum), diaphragmatic hernia, and duodenal atresia are associated approximately 50% of the time with other congenital anomalies. Gastroschisis, a defect in the anterior abdominal wall, is associated with other anomalies approximately 30% of the time. Other stenotic areas of the GI tract do not usually indicate chromosomal abnormalities. Posterior urethral valves may cause significant dilation of the urinary collecting system. It is usually not associated with other abnormalities. It is amenable to surgical correction with a good outcome.

21. **(A)** The BPP measures amniotic fluid volume (requiring a fluid pocket of 2 cm), the results of the NST, an episode of fetal breathing that lasts at least 30 seconds, three discrete limb movements of the fetus, and at least one episode of extension with return to flexion by a fetal limb or trunk. Each of these factors is given two points. A normal score is 8 or 10, indicating fetal well-being. Progressive perinatal mortality rate correlates with decreasing BPP score. A normal BPP has a false-negative rate, as defined by antepartum death, of 1 per 1,000. The other conditions are not predicted by the antepartum assessment of fetal well-being.

22. **(A)** Many authorities advise universal screening of pregnant woman with a GTT because at least one-third of women with gestational diabetes will be missed when only women who have risk factors for diabetes are screened. Based on the Fifth International Workshop-Conference on Gestational Diabetes, a diagnosis of gestational diabetes is made if two or more of the four values meet or exceed the following:

Fasting serum glucose concentration >95 mg/dL (5.3 mmol/L)

One-hour serum glucose concentration >180 mg/dL (10 mmol/L)
Two-hour serum glucose concentration >155 mg/dL (8.6 mmol/L)
Three-hour serum glucose concentration >140 mg/dL (7.8 mmol/L)

Since the fasting and all three other levels meet or exceed these values, this patient has gestational diabetes and would therefore be recommended to start an ADA diet (under the counseling of a diabetic nutritionist), monitor fasting, and postprandial sugars daily. If values consistently exceed 90 and 140 (1-hour postprandial), medications would be instituted.

23. **(A)** Leopold's maneuvers are used to assess fetal lie, presentation, and engagement by palpation of the gravid abdomen. They are not intended as a means to diagnose twins. Auscultation of two fetal heartbeats may help in diagnosing twins, but the diagnosis may be uncertain and is generally confirmed by ultrasound. The three radiologic methods listed can all diagnose twins, but the use of ultrasound can reliably make the diagnosis early and safely in pregnancy.

24. **(E)** Fetal heart rate tracings are a common method for assessing fetal well-being. Nonstress testing is done by recording fetal heart rates during a 20-minute period. The test requires at least two accelerations of the fetal heart rate of at least 15 beats and lasting for at least 15 seconds. A reactive tracing demonstrates both short-term (instantaneous change in heart rate from one heartbeat to the next) and long-term (changes occurring in the course of 1 minute in a cycle of 3–5 waves per minute) variability. With a reactive NST, the probability of fetal demise is less than 3 per 1,000 within the next week. Reactivity, such as seen in the tracing in Figure 8–1, is unlikely during a fetal sleep cycle. If a reactive pattern is not seen within the first 20 minutes, attempts to stimulate the fetus may be done because a nonreactive pattern is often due to a sleep cycle and will become reactive within the following 20 minutes.

25. **(B)** The early determination of the gestational age allows informed decision making if any

pregnancy complication demands treatment that depends on knowledge of the gestational age. Although it is true that all of the evaluations listed are important, the accurate assessment and recording of gestational age is generally deemed most important in otherwise clinically normal pregnancies.

26. **(D)** In a randomized prospective trial of women with a previously affected child, the recurrence risk of NTDs was lowered by 72% in women taking 4-mg folic acid daily. For women without a previously affected child, ACOG recommends at least is 0.4 mg daily immediately prior to conception and during the early weeks of neural tube closure.

27. **(E)** Contraception that prevents pregnancy is not pregnancy wastage. Abortion, which is the loss of pregnancy before 500 g or approximately 20 weeks, exceeds all other causes of loss of pregnancy. Ten to twenty percent of known pregnancies will end in spontaneous abortion. In addition, over 1 million voluntary abortions are performed yearly in the United States. Stillbirth and intrauterine fetal demise are basically the same and have a rate of 6–7 per 10,000. Neonatal deaths have a rate of 5–6 per 10,000.

28. **(B)** Diuretics are rarely indicated in pregnancy. A well-balanced, protein-rich diet with adequate rest in a lateral recumbent position is better treatment for edema than diuretics. Rapid weight gain secondary to fluid retention may be a sign of impending preeclampsia. Other signs and symptoms include nausea, vomiting headache, visual disturbance, and Right Upper Quadrant (RUQ) pain. Physical findings could include hypertension, tenderness in RUQ, and hyperreflexia. As preeclampsia is a serious, potentially life-threatening entity, every effort must be made to determine if this is the reason for the weight gain.

29. **(D)** Overweight women should limit weight gain to 15 to 25 lb in pregnancy. Most weight gain occurs in the second half of pregnancy. Folic acid requirements are increased during pregnancy, and an individual with this dietary history is apt to be severely deficient in folic acid as well as having deficiencies of iron, protein, and many other nutrients. She needs 70 g of protein a day, plus other nutrients. Her diet should be supplemented in any area of deficiency: calories, constituents, or minerals. While aerobic exercise is recommended and would be of benefit to her, it is inadvisable to initiate a vigorous program in a previously sedentary woman during pregnancy. Regular mild to moderate exercise, such as walking, three to five times per week should be advised.

30. **(B)** Fetal heart tones can be documented by 10 weeks' gestation by Doppler devices. Before 12 to 14 weeks' gestation, uterine size can give a fairly accurate estimate of gestational age. At about 12 weeks' gestation, the uterus has reached the pubic symphysis. And at about 20 weeks' gestation the uterus is at the umbilicus. Moreover, at 16 weeks' gestation the uterus is half way between the umbilicus and symphysis.

31. **(B)** Prior preterm delivery is the single most significant risk factor associated with preterm birth. Preterm birth is also associated with smoking, but the association is not as strong. Other risk factors include maternal genital tract infection, reduced cervical competence, low socioeconomic status, and uterine malformations. Colposcopy alone would not increase a woman's risk for cervical incompetence, but depending on the amount of tissue removed, cervical conization/Loop Electroexcision Procedure (LEEP) may. First-trimester spontaneous abortion is common, and it is not associated with preterm delivery in subsequent pregnancies.

32. **(B)** Minimal protein loss of 100 to 300 mg per 24 hours is normal in nonpregnant women and in pregnancy. Fetal heart tones are not consistently audible by Doppler until about 10 weeks' gestation. Candidiasis, a common cause of vaginitis, is common in pregnancy and can be safely treated with topical agents. Short stature in itself does not portend a poor prognosis for pregnancy. Gravidas with chronic hypertension (BP >140/90 before 20 weeks' gestation), however, are more likely to develop superimposed preeclampsia, one of the leading causes of maternal morbidity and mortality.

33. **(B)** Ultrasound measurement of crown-to-rump length in the first trimester will provide accurate estimation of gestational age to within a few days. Because of variation in growth among fetuses, ultrasound is much less accurate for dating pregnancies beyond the second trimester. In women with normal cycles, conception should occur approximately 2 weeks after LMP. At 4 weeks, the conceptus is implanting within the uterus and is not yet visible by ultrasound.

34. **(D)** The best time to thoroughly evaluate fetal anatomy is between 16 and 20 weeks' gestation. Often, a complete evaluation of the fetal heart is more easily accomplished a few weeks later in gestation.

35. **(A)** Dietary allowances for most substances increase during pregnancy, including vitamin D, calcium, and folic acid. The most significant deficiency, however, is for iron. Few women have sufficient iron stores or dietary iron intake to supply the amount needed for the growing fetus and placenta. Unlike the others, vitamin A is not required in greater amounts in pregnancy since it is felt to be stored adequately.

36. **(A)** Twin pregnancies are high-risk pregnancies, accounting for a disproportionately large share of adverse pregnancy outcomes. Pregnancy-induced hypertension and hypertensive disorders in general occur with more frequency in multiple gestations. The incidence is up to 20% for twin pregnancies. Twin (and higher-order) pregnancies carry a higher risk of preterm delivery, low birth weight, and resultant perinatal death. Congenital anomalies are more common: 2% for major malformations and 4% for minor malformations. Because of a variety of reasons, such as malpresentation, fetal distress in labor, pregnancy-induced hypertension, congenital anomalies, cesarean sections are also more common for twin gestations. Approximately 60% of twins will be delivered via cesarean section. Shoulder dystocia rates appear to be lower than those for singletons.

37. **(D)** There is evidence that periconceptional glycemic control in diabetic women has been shown to decrease the risk of congenital malformations in their offspring. Specifically, a $HbA_{1c}$ of 8 or greater is linked to increased risk of spontaneous abortion and congenital malformations. Ideally, the $HbA_{1c}$ is <6.

38. **(C)** For the average woman, a weight gain of 25 to 35 lb is optimal in pregnancy. Moderate exercise should be encouraged in the normal pregnancy, but fatigue should be avoided. Additional iron supplementation is only recommended to improve iron stores in women with anemia, as evidenced by their hematocrit in the first trimester. For the average woman, the Centers for Disease Control and Prevention and the U.S. Public Health Service recommend 0.4-mg folic acid as a daily supplement for women of reproductive age and during pregnancy. For women with a history of a prior pregnancy affected by a NTD or who is on an anticonvulsant medication, 4 mg is the recommended supplement dose. Douching is not recommended for the pregnant or nonpregnant woman.

39–43. **(39-D, 40-B, 41-B, 42-C, 43-E)** Bilateral renal agenesis will result in severe oligohydramnios because of no urine production. The infant develops pulmonary hypoplasia and atypical facies and has frequent cardiac anomalies. This is Potter's syndrome. The banana sign is found frequently in infants with open spina bifida. It is due to a flattening of the cerebral hemispheres with an obliteration of the cisterna magna, which results in a centrally curved banana-like appearance on ultrasound. The lemon sign is also associated with NTDs and may occur with spina bifida. It is a scalloping of the frontal bones to give a lemon-shaped appearance of the head and usually disappears after 24 weeks. One should be suspicious of an open spina bifida if there is a small head, lemon and banana signs, enlarged ventricles, and absence or obliteration of the cisterna magna. The double bubble sign is found with duodenal atresia. Homozygous alpha-thalassemia results in the formation of tetramers of beta chains known as Bart's hemoglobin. This hemoglobinopathy can result in hydrops fetalis.

44. **(G)** For any drug to be prescribed during pregnancy, its benefits must outweigh its risks.

According to the Food and Drug Administration classification, fluoxetine is category C; that is, animal studies have shown that the drug exerts teratogenic or embryocidal effects, and there are no adequate, well-controlled studies in pregnant women. However, no malformations or congenital effects have been documented. Several neonatal effects have been reported, including difficulty in environmental adaptation.

45. **(F)** Podophyllin resin, a common treatment for condyloma acuminata, has been associated with stillbirth. It causes local vascular spasm, ischemia, and necrosis of tissue. During pregnancy the lesions are profuse and vascular, predisposing to systemic absorption. This is a category X drug.

46. **(G)** Tetracycline causes yellow-brown discoloration of deciduous teeth or be deposited in fetal long bones when used after 25 weeks.

47. **(G)** Captopril is an angiotensin-converting enzyme (ACE) inhibitor. ACE inhibitors are category C/D. Category D means that fetal risk has been identified, but use in pregnancy may be indicated if benefits outweigh the risks. Its use in pregnancy has been associated with severe oligohydramnios, pulmonary hypoplasia, and neonatal anemia. In general, there is reduction in uteroplacental perfusion, which can be fatal. Patients who use this drug and then become pregnant must seek alternative antihypertensive medications.

48. **(C)** Valproic acid, a drug used in the treatment of seizure disorders, has been associated with a 1% to 2% risk of spina bifida. It is category D.

49. **(A)** Isotretinoin (Accutane) is a vitamin A isomer marketed for treatment of severe cystic acne. It is a category X drug. Use of this drug in pregnancy poses a significant risk of both structural anomalies and mental retardation. Malformed infants have a characteristic pattern of craniofacial, cardiac, thymic, and central nervous system (CNS) anomalies.

50. **(D)** Methimazole is used for treatment of hyperthyroidism. A small number of cases of unusual scalp defects, aplasia cutis, have occurred in infants born to mothers taking the drug. Like propylthiouracil, it is a category D drug.

51. **(E)** Misoprostol is a synthetic prostaglandin E1 that induces uterine contractions. In obstetrics, it is effective in ripening the cervix for labor induction. In the first trimester, it is used in conjunction with mifepristone or methotrexate to produce a medical abortion.

52. **(A)** MMR is a live attenuated viral vaccine and should be avoided immediately before and during pregnancy, according to the Centers for Disease Control and Prevention. All other immunizations listed are safe in pregnancy. Influenza vaccine is highly recommended to all pregnant women.

# CHAPTER 9

# Diseases Complicating Pregnancy

## Questions

**DIRECTIONS (Questions 1 through 77): For each of the multiple choice questions in this section, select the lettered answer that is the one *best* response in each case.**

**Questions 1 through 5 apply to the following patient:**

A 28-year-old G2P0 at 39 weeks is in early labor. She is 2 cm dilated and 90% effaced, with contractions every 4 to 5 minutes. The fetal heart tones are reassuring. Her nurse steps out for a moment and returns to find her having a seizure.

1. The nurse administers a 4-g magnesium bolus. The seizure stops. The fetal heart tone variability is flat, but there are no decelerations. What would your next therapies be aimed at?

   (A) reducing edema with diuretics
   (B) giving hypotensive agents until the blood pressure is 110/70 mm Hg
   (C) giving 3 g of magnesium sulfate every 3 hours
   (D) prepare for immediate delivery by cesarean section
   (E) keeping the patient free of convulsions, coma, and acidosis

2. Which of the following would be the most common warning sign/symptom of her eclamptic seizure?

   (A) proteinuria
   (B) severe headache
   (C) facial edema
   (D) increased blood pressure >160/120 mm Hg
   (E) epigastric pain

3. This patient is most at risk for mortality from which of the following complications?

   (A) infection
   (B) uremia
   (C) congestive heart failure
   (D) fever
   (E) cerebral hemorrhage

4. This patient and other women with severe preeclampsia, when compared with pregnant women without preeclampsia, will have a decrease in which of the following?

   (A) response to pressor amines
   (B) plasma volume
   (C) total body sodium
   (D) uric acid
   (E) serum liver functions

5. If this patient were to have a renal biopsy, what would the most likely pathologic finding be?

   (A) glomerular endothelial swelling
   (B) pyelonephritis
   (C) hydroureter
   (D) cortical necrosis
   (E) acute tubular necrosis

**Questions 6 and 7 apply to the following patient:**

A 19-year-old woman without prenatal care (gravida 1, para 0) in the third trimester of pregnancy arrives in the emergency department. She has presented because of headache and visual change. While being examined, she had a convulsion.

6. You should do which of the following while waiting for the magnesium sulfate bolus to arrive from the labor and delivery department?

   (A) obtain an ultrasound to rule out molar pregnancy
   (B) prepare to perform an emergency cesarean delivery
   (C) give intravenous (IV) phenytoin
   (D) protect the patient from self-harm
   (E) obtain a chest film

7. After she awakes from her seizure and the postictal state, she complains of blurry vision. What is the most likely finding upon fundoscopic examination?

   (A) exudates and hemorrhage
   (B) loss of corneal curvature
   (C) retinal edema
   (D) arteriolar spasm
   (E) macular degeneration

8. A patient and her husband are extremely anxious about your suggestion that she be given magnesium sulfate for seizure prophylaxis. In assuring her about the safety of the drug, you can emphasize which of the following?

   (A) The drug is rapidly excreted via the kidney.
   (B) It is a mild smooth-muscle constrictor and thus safe for the infusion.
   (C) The drug has a narrow margin of safety so that we start off with a lower dose in preeclamptics, and administer it by an IV pump.

(D) As a central nervous system (CNS) stimulant it should not deprive her of the awareness of her delivery, unlike barbiturates.
(E) The drug does not cross the placenta and thus should not affect her fetus/infant.

9. In eclampsia, which of the following is one of several unfavorable prognostic signs?

   (A) tachycardia
   (B) 2+ proteinuria
   (C) urine output greater than 100 cc/h
   (D) more than one but less than three convulsions
   (E) swelling of the tongue

10. A 24-year-old woman (gravida 1, para 0) at 37 weeks' gestation was noted to have a 6-lb weight gain and an increase in blood pressure from 100/60 to 130/80 mm Hg in the past week. She also has 1+ proteinuria. The examination was repeated 6 hours later and the same results were obtained. Which of the following is the best diagnosis?

   (A) normal pregnancy
   (B) preeclampsia
   (C) eclampsia
   (D) pregnancy-induced hypertension
   (E) transient hypertension of pregnancy

11. What is the most common association with heart disease in pregnancy?

   (A) rheumatic fever
   (B) previous myocardial infarction
   (C) hypertension
   (D) thyroid disease
   (E) congenital heart disease (CHD)

12. A 22-year-old primiparous woman presents for her first prenatal evaluation. On physical examination you hear a grade 3/6 holosystolic murmur. Which is the most common CHD in pregnancy that would cause that type of murmur?

(A) ventricular septal defect (VSD)

(B) patent ductus arteriosus (PDA)

(C) pulmonary stenosis

(D) atrial septal defect (ASD)

(E) aortic stenosis

13. You are seeing for the first prenatal visit a 19-year-old woman with an artificial porcine valve placed 6 months ago for CHD. She is 10 weeks pregnant, tired, and does not sleep particularly well. The fetus is size-date appropriate. Of the following choices, which is the best first step in management?

(A) evaluate for valve replacement due to assumed cardiac enlargement

(B) anticoagulate with aspirin and a platelet inhibitor

(C) recommend termination of the pregnancy as she had not postponed conception for the mandatory 24 months after valve replacement

(D) anticoagulate with heparin

(E) keep on low-dose oral antibiotics

14. A 16-year-old woman with CHD is referred at 8 weeks' gestation by her cardiologist. She has peripheral cyanosis, a hematocrit of 65%, and is 95 lb and 5 ft. 4 in tall. You counsel her that the most likely fetal outcome is which of the following?

(A) not affected

(B) marked prematurity

(C) intrauterine growth restriction

(D) spontaneous abortion or fetal death

(E) postmaturity

15. A 33-year-old Type 1 diabetic patient (gravida 1, para 0) is scheduled for induction of labor at 37 weeks' gestation. Which of the following should her insulin dosage should be?

(A) maintained at her preinduction level

(B) increased by 10–15%

(C) decreased by half

(D) put on a sliding scale with q3–4h blood glucose measurements

(E) put on an IV insulin infusion

16. Which of the following histories might lead you to suspect the existence of diabetes in a patient now pregnant for the third time?

(A) Spontaneous rupture of the membranes occurred during the second trimester in both preceding pregnancies.

(B) Jaundice appeared in the last trimester of her second pregnancy.

(C) Both preceding infants were premature.

(D) Unexplained intrauterine death occurred at 38 weeks' gestation in her last pregnancy.

(E) Abruptio placentae occurred in the second pregnancy.

17. A complete blood cell count is typically obtained at the initiation of prenatal care. This test is important as an indicator of general nutritional status. In the pregnant population, anemia can best be defined as which of the following?

(A) high total iron binding capacity

(B) a genetic defect in ferritin synthesis

(C) low folic acid

(D) a hemoglobin below 11 g/dL

(E) low plasma volume

18. The most common type of anemia in pregnancy is due to which of the following?

(A) iron deficiency

(B) sickle cell disease

(C) folate deficiency

(D) thalassemia

(E) vitamin $B_{12}$ deficiency

19. Your patient has microcytic anemia with a hemoglobin of 9 and normal iron stores. What is the most likely diagnosis?

(A) folate deficiency

(B) vitamin $B_{12}$ deficiency

(C) thalassemia

(D) vitamin $B_6$ deficiency

(E) acute blood loss

**Questions 20 through 22 apply to the following patient:**

An African American couple presents for prenatal care. They are interested in complete screening as indicated for genetic diseases. They are unaware of their sickle cell status regarding the presence of trait or not.

20. What is the percentage of African Americans with sickle cell anemia disease?

 (A) less than 1
 (B) 5
 (C) 10
 (D) 25
 (E) 50

21. The mother is found to have sickle trait. If the father has trait, what percentage of their children will be born with sickle disease?

 (A) 0
 (B) 25
 (C) 50
 (D) 75
 (E) 100

22. Since sulfa drugs are commonly prescribed for urinary tract infections (UTIs) during pregnancy, you include as part of counseling that G6PD homozygous deficiency is present in what percentage of African American women?

 (A) less than 1
 (B) 2
 (C) 5
 (D) 10
 (E) 33

**Questions 23 and 24 apply to the following patient:**

A 22-year-old patient presents with a hematocrit of 31% at 28 weeks' gestation. Her mean corpuscular volume (MCV) is 105, her mean corpuscular hemoglobin (MCH) is 33, and her mean corpuscular hemoglobin concentration (MCHC) is 36. Serum iron is 100 mg/dL. There is no evidence of abnormal bleeding.

23. Which of the following is the best diagnosis?

 (A) normocytic, normochromic anemia
 (B) normal
 (C) macrocytic anemia
 (D) microcytic anemia
 (E) hemolysis

24. The most likely cause of anemia in this patient is which of the following?

 (A) gastrointestinal (GI) bleeding
 (B) G6PD deficiency
 (C) iron deficiency
 (D) folic acid deficiency
 (E) pernicious anemia

25. You are seeing a 28-year-old woman (gravida 3, para 2) with suspected UTI. To obtain a urine specimen, which of the following should you order?

 (A) clean-void midstream urine
 (B) catheterization
 (C) suprapubic tap
 (D) 24-hour urine
 (E) first morning void

26. Because of concerns of a maternal renal stone, a renal ultrasound is ordered in a 35-year-old G4P3003 at 34 weeks' estimated gestational age (EGA). Renal imaging during the eighth month of gestation normally reveals what?

 (A) mild to moderate ureteral reflux
 (B) the same findings as those of a normal, nonpregnant woman
 (C) hydroureter bilaterally
 (D) ureteral spasm above the pelvic brim
 (E) nephroptosis

27. You are called by the radiologist who was performing an obstetric ultrasound. He has found extensive hydroureter in a woman who is 26 weeks pregnant. She has mild right-sided pain that bothers her during the day but does not wake her from sleep. What is the best treatment at this point?

(A) intermittent bladder catheterization to keep the bladder as empty as possible

(B) ureteral stent on the right

(C) bed rest on her left side

(D) increased fluid intake

(E) no treatment

**Questions 28 and 29 apply to the following patient:**

A 16-year-old patient (gravida 1) is seen for the first time when 16 weeks pregnant. History and examination are entirely normal except for a large solid mass in the posterior pelvis. It is slightly lobulated, immobile, and smooth and cannot be completely palpated. There is some question as to whether or not it will obstruct labor.

28. Which of the following procedures should be carried out?

(A) "one shot" intravenous pyelogram (IVP)

(B) barium enema

(C) exploratory laparotomy

(D) abortion

(E) pelvic/abdominal ultrasound

29. Which of the following is the most likely diagnosis?

(A) anterior meningomyelocele

(B) pelvic kidney

(C) carcinoma of the bowel

(D) sacculated uterus

(E) idiopathic retroperitoneal fibrosis

**Questions 30 through 32 apply to the following patient:**

A 34-year-old woman (gravida 3, para 2) at 35 weeks' gestation complains of sharp, excruciating pain in the right flank radiating into her groin. No chills or fever have been noted. The pain resolved shortly after the patient was seen. Urinary analysis reveals numerous red blood cells (RBCs), some WBCs, and no bacteria. WBC and hematocrit are normal.

30. Which of the following options is the most likely diagnosis?

(A) appendicitis

(B) pyelonephritis

(C) round ligament pain

(D) ureteral lithiasis

(E) Meckel's diverticulum

31. Which of the following laboratory tests should be performed?

(A) serum iron

(B) serum glutamic oxaloacetic transaminase (SGOT)

(C) tine test

(D) bilirubin

(E) serum calcium

32. Ureteral stones during pregnancy are rare. Which of the following best characterizes them?

(A) They are more likely to produce pain during pregnancy than in the nonpregnant state.

(B) They are usually discovered during workup for vague abdominal pain.

(C) They are associated with hyperparathyroidism.

(D) They are frequently a cause of acute obstruction.

(E) A prophylactic ureteral filter may need to be placed.

33. A 14-year-old girl is seen for her first prenatal visit at 34 weeks' gestation by menstrual history. On examination her BP is 148/96 mm Hg and her fundus measures 33 cm. Her urine dipstick is 1+ positive for protein. Which of the following is the most likely diagnosis?

(A) hypertensive disease with superimposed preeclampsia

(B) mild eclampsia

(C) third-trimester pregnancy

(D) preeclampsia

(E) chronic hypertension

34. If the patient has hyperparathyroidism, which of the following will the infant possibly be at increased risk for postpartum?

    (A) hyaline membrane disease
    (B) tetany
    (C) coma
    (D) hyperglycemia
    (E) malabsorption syndrome

35. A healthy mother delivers a term infant with microcephaly. The mother's urine was found to contain cells with inclusion bodies. Which of the following is the most likely diagnosis?

    (A) chromosomal abnormality
    (B) cytomegalovirus disease
    (C) syphilis
    (D) poliomyelitis
    (E) granuloma inguinale

36. A patient is seen in the early third trimester of pregnancy with acute onset of chills and fever, nausea, and backache. Her temperature is 102°F. The urinary sediment reveals many bacteria and WBCs. Which of the following is the most likely diagnosis?

    (A) acute appendicitis
    (B) ruptured uterus
    (C) pyelonephritis
    (D) abruptio placentae
    (E) labor

37. A 19-year-old G1P0 at 27 weeks' gestation is found to have a fetus with mildly dilated ventricles, calcifications in the brain and liver (fetal) during her ultrasound. Her toxoplasmosis immunoglobulin M (IgM) titer is 1:256 and her immunoglobulin G (IgG) is 1:1024. What is the most likely mode of transmission?

    (A) ascending passage of a virus
    (B) delivery through the infected tissue
    (C) transplacental passage of the protozoa
    (D) sexual intercourse by the mother during pregnancy
    (E) hematogenesis spread of the bacteria

38. An asymptomatic pregnant woman consults you because she has been sexually active with a partner who has been diagnosed with gonorrhea. What should be your next step?

    (A) reassure her and await symptoms
    (B) culture her endocervix and treat on the basis of a positive culture
    (C) treat when she is past 12 weeks (the first trimester) pregnant
    (D) treat her with 2.4 million units of oral penicillin over 10 days
    (E) treat her with ceftriaxone 250-mg intramuscular (IM)

39. Which of the following is a major complication of maternal gonorrhea in the third trimester?

    (A) gonorrheal ophthalmia of the newborn
    (B) gonococcal arthritis
    (C) miscarriage in subsequent pregnancies
    (D) infection of the patient's sexual partner
    (E) tubo-ovarian abscess

**Questions 40 through 42 apply to the following patient:**

A 24-year-old married white woman was exposed to rubella at 7 to 8 weeks' gestation. Several days later she developed a red macular rash and had a rubella antibody titer of 1:160 when seen by you at 11 weeks' gestation.

40. What is the approximate risk of the fetus having serious congenital abnormalities?

    (A) 0%
    (B) 1–24%
    (C) 25–50%
    (D) 50–75%
    (E) 100%

41. Which of the following may be anticipated in an infant born to this mother?

    (A) rhagades
    (B) hepatosplenomegaly
    (C) trisomy 21
    (D) Hutchinson's incisors
    (E) cri du chat syndrome

42. The mother was not interested in therapeutic abortion. After spontaneous labor with epidural anesthesia, she delivered a fetus with a marked purpuric rash. This was most likely due to which of the following?

    (A) ulcerations from rubella
    (B) marked thrombocytopenia causing the purpura
    (C) placental heparinase
    (D) an allergic reaction to the anesthetic agent
    (E) Group strep infection

**Questions 43 through 47 apply to the following patient:**

A 24-year-old patient now 17 weeks' pregnant is found to have a positive VDRL (Venereal Disease Research Laboratory) of 1:16 titer. She gives no history of syphilis. A fluorescent treponemal antibody test (FTA) is drawn but will require 1 to 2 weeks to be returned. Cerebrospinal fluid (CSF) tests are negative. The patient denies allergies.

43. Serologic tests for syphilis will usually be positive first in which of the following periods of time after contact with the disease?

    (A) 1–2 days
    (B) 6–8 hours
    (C) 18–20 days
    (D) 4–6 weeks
    (E) 4–6 months

44. What is the most appropriate course of action?

    (A) wait until the FTA results are known
    (B) treat with 4.8 million units of procaine penicillin
    (C) treat with 2.4 million units of benzathine penicillin IM
    (D) treat with 3.5 g ampicillin PO
    (E) redraw the VDRL

45. After adequate treatment, the maternal VDRL titer slowly decreases but is still positive. At the time of delivery, the fetus appears normal but the cord VDRL is also positive. Which of the following is the most likely explanation?

    (A) The baby has a biologic false positive.
    (B) The baby has congenital syphilis.
    (C) The baby has levels of maternal antibody.
    (D) The baby has been treated but its antibody level is still elevated.
    (E) The mother was treated but the baby was not and has reinfected the mother.

46. To distinguish whether or not the infant is infected, you should do which of the following?

    (A) biopsies
    (B) serial VDRLs
    (C) serial Frei's tests
    (D) dark-field examinations
    (E) an X-ray of long bones

47. Which of the following is recommended as treatment for early syphilis diagnosed by a positive VDRL, and fluorescent treponemal antibody–antibody absorption test (FTA–ABS) during pregnancy who reports being penicillin allergic?

    (A) doxycycline PO
    (B) desensitization and procaine penicillin IM stat with probenecid
    (C) desensitization and benzathine penicillin IM stat
    (D) ceftriaxone IM
    (E) erythromycin PO

**Questions 48 and 49 apply to the following patient:**

An agitated patient is seen during the first trimester of pregnancy with an enlarged thyroid, a BP of 110/70 mm Hg, a resting pulse of 110, and an increased RBC uptake of triiodothyronine T3.

48. What should be your first step?

    (A) measure thyroid-stimulating hormone (TSH)
    (B) obtain an iodine 131 ($I^{131}$) uptake by the thyroid
    (C) obtain a basal metabolic rate (BMR)
    (D) evaluate free thyroxine (T4)
    (E) evaluate thyroid-binding globulin

49. Among other tests, the free thyroxine is elevated. Your initial treatment should be to do which of the following?

    (A) treat with $I^{131}$
    (B) give propylthiouracil (PTU)
    (C) give PTU and propranolol
    (D) give PTU and low-dose thyroid hormone
    (E) advise subtotal thyroidectomy in the second trimester

50. A 35-year-old patient at 31 weeks' gestation complains of a firm lump in her left breast. On examination, a 2 cm × 3 cm × 3 cm firm nodule surrounded by some erythema is discovered in the upper outer quadrant. There is no skin retraction, and the nodule is somewhat mobile. Which is the most appropriate plan of management?

    (A) to reassure the patient, see her regularly, and evaluate the mass at 6 weeks' postpartum
    (B) mastectomy
    (C) hot packs on the breast and antibiotics for mastitis
    (D) mammogram
    (E) ultrasound directed biopsy

51. One of your more demanding patients is worried about having a Pap smear. She has read on the Internet the procedure can cause miscarriage during pregnancy. She is a 27-year-old G1P0 at 12 weeks' EGA and her last Pap smear was over 3 years prior. What should you advise her about her Pap smears?

    (A) contraindicated in the third trimester
    (B) consistently overread and to be judged with caution
    (C) normally return as atypical or abnormal squamous cells of unknown significance (ASCUS)
    (D) of poor diagnostic importance
    (E) part of the normal workup if she is due for screening

52. A patient 8 weeks pregnant is found to have Stage III carcinoma of the cervix. In regard to the malignancy, you discuss the various options and their risks. She has a chance to ask questions. Her husband asks what is the safest and "recommended" choice for her. How should you respond?

    (A) deliver by cesarean section at 34 weeks and irradiate
    (B) deliver vaginally at term and irradiate
    (C) perform hysterotomy now and irradiate
    (D) perform radical hysterectomy and pelvic lymphadenectomy now
    (E) irradiate now

**Questions 53 and 54 apply to the following patient:**

A 17-year-old single female (gravida 1, para 0), last menstrual period (LMP) 32 weeks ago, menstrual formula (MF) 12/28/4–5, with occasional cramps and no history of contraception, comes for her first OB clinic visit and routine care. The patient admits to a 40-lb weight gain during pregnancy with ankle swelling for the past 4 weeks. Rings on her fingers are tight. Otherwise, she feels well. She has been staying with a cousin who is on welfare. She has had no prior prenatal care and no iron or vitamin supplementation.

*History:* Noncontributory except for appendectomy; age 14. Generally in good health.

*Social history:* High school dropout; parents divorced.

*Family history:* No history of renal disease, diabetes, cancer, hypertension, congenital anomalies, or twins.

*Physical findings:* BP, 135/85; P, 84; T, 37; R, 20. BMI 35. Head ears eyes nose throat (HEENT): Fundi not examined.

*Neck:* Thyroid, 1 to 1½ times enlarged; chest, clear; breasts, full, slightly tender; heart, grade 11/VI, systolic murmur at the left sternal border (LSB).

*Abdomen:* Uterus, 42 cm; fetal heart tones (FHTs), 136 and 156 taken simultaneously; extremities, 2+ edema, 3+ reflexes. Brief ultrasound confirms twins in breech presentation.

*Pelvis:* Normal measurements; cervix, one-half effaced, soft, and not dilated, station +1. The above findings were all confirmed 6 hours later.

*Laboratory tests:* Urinalysis (UA), color cloudy yellow; specific gravity, 1.013; protein, 2+; RBCs, rare; WBC, 2 to 5; bacteria, 0; WBC, 9800; Rh, VDRL, rubella titer, and Pap smear were obtained but not yet returned.

53. What is the most likely diagnosis?

    (A) abruption
    (B) accreta
    (C) acute fatty necrosis of the liver
    (D) abortion
    (E) Crohn's disease
    (F) preeclampsia
    (G) chronic hypertension
    (H) renal disease

54. Given the history of this patient, several more laboratory and diagnostic tests are obtained. She is stable and the fetuses have reassuring heart rate tracings. Which of the following do you expect to see in the test results?

    (A) chest X-ray to show decreased pulmonary vascular markings
    (B) urine to show infection
    (C) creatinine clearance to be increased above normal pregnancy levels
    (D) serum uric acid to be increased
    (E) a decreased hematocrit

55. An unconscious obstetric patient is admitted to the emergency department in the eighth month of pregnancy with a BP of 60/20 mm Hg and a pulse of 120 per minute. If there has been no vaginal bleeding, which diagnosis may be excluded?

    (A) abruptio placentae
    (B) placenta previa
    (C) premature rupture of membranes with septic shock
    (D) eclampsia
    (E) amniotic fluid embolism

56. A 23-year-old patient, amenorrheic for 16 weeks, had vaginal spotting. She was found to have a uterus enlarged to 20 weeks' size and no FHTs audible with the Doppler or fetoscope. Human chorionic gonadotropin (hCG) serum levels were approximately 150 IU/mL. Which of the following tests is most appropriate at this time?

    (A) human chorionic somatomammotropin (hCS)
    (B) pelvic ultrasound
    (C) serial hCGs
    (D) Apt test on vaginal blood
    (E) serial clotting function studies

57. Which clinical scenario is most associated with metastatic gestational trophoblastic disease?

    (A) after spontaneous abortion of a chromosomally abnormal embryo
    (B) spontaneously during the childbearing years
    (C) after hydatidiform mole
    (D) after normal pregnancy
    (E) after a second trimester pregnancy termination

**Questions 58 and 59 apply to the following patient:**

A 28-year-old woman noted loss of fetal motion at 36 weeks' gestation by dates. FHTs were not heard at 40 weeks by dates, when the patient was next seen. The uterus measured 30 cm from symphysis to fundus.

58. Which of the following tests would be valuable to perform at this time?

   (A) maternal serum estriol
   (B) clotting screen
   (C) lecithin/sphingomyelin (L/S) ratio
   (D) karyotype of amniotic cells
   (E) amniotic fluid creatinine

59. Which of the following is the most well-recognized maternal complication that may occur in this case?

   (A) uterine rupture
   (B) coagulation defect
   (C) amniotic fluid embolus
   (D) thrombophlebitis
   (E) endometritis

60. Massive hydramnios (>3,000 mL) is associated with congenital malformation in what percentage of cases?

   (A) less than 1
   (B) 5–10%
   (C) 20–30%
   (D) 50–60%
   (E) 90–100%

61. In women with polyhydramnios, what is the most common cause?

   (A) maternal hypertension
   (B) fetal urinary tract anomalies
   (C) maternal diabetes
   (D) postmature pregnancy
   (E) twins
   (F) fetal intestinal obstruction

   (G) fetal aneuploidy
   (H) fetal muscular disease inhibiting swallowing
   (I) idiopathic

62. Hydramnios is characterized by which of the following?

   (A) amniotic fluid volumes greater than 2,000 cc
   (B) negligible increase in perinatal morbidity
   (C) a lack of symptoms, depending on rapidity of onset
   (D) marked increase in intrauterine pressure
   (E) an increase in endometritis

**Questions 63 and 64 apply to the following patient:**

A 23-year-old woman (gravida 1) at about 12 weeks' gestation develops persistent nausea and vomiting that progresses from an occasional episode to a constant retching. She has no fever or diarrhea but lost 5 lb in 1 week and appears dehydrated.

63. What is your diagnosis?

   (A) anorexia nervosa
   (B) morning sickness
   (C) ptyalism
   (D) hyperemesis gravidarum
   (E) gastroenteritis

64. Which of the following is the best choice of therapy for this patient?

   (A) phenothiazines
   (B) hypnosis
   (C) IV hydration
   (D) psychiatric referral
   (E) outpatient antiemetic therapy

**Questions 65 and 66 apply to the following patient:**

A patient at 34 weeks' gestation develops marked pruritus especially on her palms and soles, and mildly elevated liver function tests and elevated bile acids.

65. Which of the following diagnostic possibilities is most consistent with the clinical presentation?

    (A) pancreatitis
    (B) hyperthyroidism
    (C) diabetes insipidus
    (D) cholestasis of pregnancy
    (E) progesterone allergy

66. Under which of the following conditions are the pruritus and jaundice from the previous patient likely to recur?

    (A) menopause
    (B) after discontinuation of breast-feeding
    (C) poor diet
    (D) with another pregnancy
    (E) with the use of antihypertensive medication

67. You are seeing a 25-year-old woman (gravida 1, para 0) with sickle cell disease at 12 weeks' gestation for her first prenatal visit. Suggestions for her care should include which of the following?

    (A) folic acid
    (B) transfusions of fresh hemoglobin for hematocrit less than 25%
    (C) antibiotic prophylaxis to prevent UTI
    (D) oral iron in double the usual dosage (650 mg tid)
    (E) delivery at 36 weeks after documentation of fetal lung maturity

68. You are seeing a patient for preconception counseling. She has complex cardiovascular problems for which she will be seeing the cardiologist next week. She is concerned that her cardiac disease may lead to cyanosis. Which cardiac diagnosis exempts her from that complication?

    (A) VSD
    (B) PDA

    (C) tetralogy of Fallot
    (D) Ebstein's anomaly
    (E) Marfan's syndrome

69. During pregnancy, blood tests for diabetes are more apt to be abnormal than in the nonpregnant state. Also nondiabetic women may develop gestational diabetes during the last half of the pregnancy. This is due in part to which of the following?

    (A) decreased insulin production
    (B) increased food absorption from the GI tract
    (C) increased placental lactogen
    (D) decreased hepatic secretion of insulin-binding globulin
    (E) hemoconcentration

70. A 26-year-old Caucasian woman presents for her first prenatal visit. She is 14 weeks' pregnant and has had a history of a deep vein thrombosis in her left leg when she had taken birth control pills 3 years ago. She was tested and found to be homozygous for Factor V Leiden. What should you advise the patient?

    (A) During pregnancy she is not at increased risk for a deep venous thrombosis (DVT) as long as she is not on bed rest.
    (B) Low dose (81 mg) of aspirin should be taken during pregnancy and postpartum.
    (C) She should be placed on prophylactic warfarin therapy since she is past the first trimester.
    (D) She would benefit from prophylactic doses of low-molecular-weight heparin twice a day until 6 weeks postpartum.
    (E) Since she has already had one DVT, she should be on therapeutic doses of subcutaneous heparin until after delivery when estrogen levels will fall.

71. A patient is found to be Rh negative with a negative antibody screen. Anti-D immune globulin should be given for which of the following situations?

    (A) after an abortion, spontaneous or therapeutic, prior to 6 weeks' gestation in an Rh-negative female
    (B) a Du positive mother who has an Rh-positive baby
    (C) an Rh-negative female infant with an Rh-positive mother
    (D) postpartum to Rh-positive females with Rh-negative husbands
    (E) after a motor vehicle accident to an Rh-negative mother

72. A woman with Class II cardiac disease is pregnant. She has no other health problems. What should be included in the management plans for her pregnancy?

    (A) a 2200 cal ADA diet to obtain adequate weight gain and prophylaxis against gestational diabetes
    (B) limit weight gain to 20–25 lb
    (C) prophylactic low-dose aspirin (81 mg)
    (D) vaginal delivery unless obstetric indications for C-section
    (E) deliver at the verification of lung maturity around 37 weeks

73. A 34-year-old woman with long-standing systemic lupus erythematosus (SLE) is pregnant for the first time. You are seeing her at 10 weeks' gestation. Special testing will be required for her during pregnancy because of marginal renal function secondary to the severity of her disease. Recommendations for management include which of the following?

    (A) serial ANA titers to follow the course of her disease
    (B) modified bed rest to decrease the risks of developing superimposed preeclampsia
    (C) serial complete blood cell counts to evaluate platelet counts
    (D) regular ultrasounds for fetal growth
    (E) C-reactive protein levels at each trimester

74. A patient with suspected cholestasis of pregnancy develops a slight hyperbilirubinemia and slight elevation of SGOT. You obtain serum bile salts that are positive, confirming the diagnosis. Relief of the pruritus may be obtained by which of the following?

    (A) amitriptyline
    (B) bland diet
    (C) oral $H_2$ blockers
    (D) cholestyramine
    (E) mild diuretic therapy

75. In developed countries (western societies) what is the most common cause of direct maternal mortality?

    (A) hemorrhage
    (B) congenital cardiac disease
    (C) infection
    (D) hypertension
    (E) amniotic fluid embolism

76. What is the most common cause of nonmaternal or indirect mortality?

    (A) domestic violence
    (B) amniotic fluid emboli
    (C) motor vehicle accidents
    (D) heart disease
    (E) asthma

77. On her first prenatal visit, a 17-year-old single woman (gravida 1, para 0), 32 weeks by good dates, is found to have vital signs as follows: BP, 135/85; P, 84; T, 98.6°F; and R, 20. She also has ankle and hand edema and a uterine fundus measuring 42 cm with breech concordant twins on ultrasound. She has normal pelvic measurements and the cervix is closed and soft, with the presenting part at station −1. Her UA revealed no WBCs or bacteria with 2+ protein. Her hematocrit is 38, and her WBC count is 9800. The next step in care of this patient should include which of the following?

    (A) trial of home bed rest for 24 hours, with repeat evaluation at that time
    (B) hospitalization with bed rest and frequent vital signs

(C)  oxytocin induction of labor

(D)  antihypertensive drugs

(E)  cesarean section because of the twins

**DIRECTIONS (Questions 78 through 92): The following group of questions is preceded by a list of lettered options. For each question, select the one lettered option that is *most* closely associated with it. Each lettered option may be used once, multiple times, or not at all.**

## Questions 78 through 83

Match the effects of the following medications during pregnancy with the appropriate medication.

(A)  tetracycline

(B)  nitrofurantoin

(C)  sulfas

(D)  streptomycin

(E)  chloramphenicol

(F)  PTU

(G)  acetaminophen

(H)  ibuprofen

(I)  warfarin

78.  Is excreted after binding, utilizing glucuronyl transferase

79.  May cause aplastic anemia in the neonate

80.  Ototoxic

81.  Discolors decidual teeth

82.  Agranulocytosis in the mother

83.  Oligohydramnios

## Questions 84 through 88

(A)  mild preeclampsia

(B)  severe preeclampsia

(C)  chronic hypertensive disease

(D)  eclampsia

(E)  chronic renal disease

(F)  lupus nephritis

84.  A 30-year-old woman at 16 weeks' gestation with a BP of 144/95, no edema, no proteinuria, FHT 140

85.  A 19-year-old woman at 36 weeks' gestation with a BP of 150/100, 2+ edema, and 2+ proteinuria with no other symptoms

86.  A 21-year-old woman in early labor at 39 weeks' gestation who has just convulsed

87.  A 16-year-old woman at 37 weeks' gestation with a BP of 145/105, 2+ proteinuria, and pulmonary edema

88.  A 35-year-old woman (gravida 5, para 4) now at 32 weeks' gestation with a BP of 180/120, no proteinuria or edema, but retinal exudates and hemorrhage, as well as a history of hypertension for 8 years

## Questions 89 and 90

Match the following disease entities with the most applicable statement.

(A)  SLE

(B)  carcinoma of the breast

(C)  herpes gestationis

(D)  melanoma

(E)  influenza

89.  Appears to affect pregnant women much more severely than nonpregnant women

90.  May be exacerbated in the postpartum period

## Questions 91 and 92

(A)  *Listeria monocytogenes*

(B)  multiple sclerosis

(C)  hiatal hernia

(D)  polyostotic fibrous dysplasia (McCune–Albright syndrome)

(E)  influenza

91.  Associated with fetal demise

92.  Is often worse postpartum than antepartum

# Answers and Explanations

1. **(E)** Diuretics are contraindicated in eclampsia, and a rapid decrease in blood pressure may not allow adequate tissue perfusion. Magnesium sulfate should be titrated to keep reflexes 1+. As soon as the patient is stabilized, delivery should be attempted. Given how the fetus tolerates these events, eventually a C-section may be indicated but only after stabilization of the mother.

2. **(B)** Although all of the signs and symptoms may occur prior to a seizure, the most common symptom immediately preceding a seizure is a severe headache. Patients often describe it as the worst headache they have ever had.

3. **(E)** Prevention of eclampsia is one of the concerns in the treatment of preeclampsia. Both fetal and maternal mortality rates rise if the disease becomes complicated because of convulsions. There may be a severe compromise of cardiac function, gastric content aspiration, and pulmonary edema. Of the choices listed, the most frequent cause of death is cerebral hemorrhage.

4. **(B)** Severely preeclamptic or eclamptic patients have marked hemoconcentration due to a decrease in plasma volume. The hematocrit is uniformly high. Albumin is low in spite of the hemoconcentration. The plasma volume may decrease by as much as 30%. She will have an increased response to pressors. Because of the decreased plasma volume preeclamptic or eclamptic patients do not tolerate excess blood loss and need to be carefully monitored and replaced with fluid or blood products.

5. **(A)** This lesion is transient and will usually regress rapidly after delivery. This is often associated with subendothelial deposition of proteinaceous material. The process has been called *glomerular capillary endotheliosis*.

6. **(D)** In such an emergency situation, the immediate concern is to protect the patient from self-inflicted injury and to stop the convulsion. Magnesium sulfate is still the best first line of therapy. Morphine, magnesium sulfate, barbiturates, and diazepam have all been used acutely to decrease convulsions and relax the patient. Care must be exercised not to depress respiration.

7. **(D)** Exudates and hemorrhages are usually found in chronic hypertensive states and not in preeclampsia. The arteriolar spasm is representative of the generalized vasospasm that occurs in preeclampsia. Retinal hemorrhage or detachment may occur. It is usually unilateral and seldom causes total visual loss.

8. **(A)** Magnesium sulfate ($MgSO_4$) is excreted by the kidney. Therefore, if kidney function is decreased, the amount of $MgSO_4$ given must also be decreased. Because of its smooth muscle-relaxing properties, blood vessels relax slightly and blood supply to the uterus may be increased. This agent is thought to have a wide margin of safety.

9. **(A)** Prolonged coma, more than 10 convulsions, and high proteinuria are other poor diagnostic signs. Given these problems, maternal and fetal mortality are high.

10. **(B)** Criteria for mild preeclampsia are met—namely, a rise in systolic BP of 30 mm Hg and in diastolic BP of more than 15 mm Hg, along with proteinuria. These signs and symptoms were observed on two occasions, 6 hours apart. The patient should be treated in an appropriate manner.

11. **(E)** As the incidence of rheumatic fever decreased, CHD gained importance. More of the congenital defects are repaired and rheumatic fever decreased secondary to good antibiotic therapy. CHD has now become the most common heart defect.

12. **(A)** Combined data show that VSD is much more common than the other forms of congenital heart defects. The physiologic effects of VSD are related to its size. Large unrepaired defects result in pulmonary hypertension and risk of bacterial endocarditis.

13. **(D)** Anticoagulation is recommended to prevent embolic phenomena. Heparin and low-molecular-weight heparin do not cross the placenta and will not harm the fetus, but dicumarol does cross the placenta and may cause fetal bleeding and other abnormalities. Aspirin and platelet inhibitors are ineffective; however, heparin is not as protective as dicumarol for the mother and has been associated with an increased risk of maternal mortality unless levels are monitored carefully. When monitored, anticoagulation with heparin or low-molecular-weight heparin is the treatment of choice. Patients with three artificial heart valves have had successful pregnancies. Antibiotics are necessary at the time of operative procedures. If a patient truly has a metal mechanical valve, anticoagulation is critical and this is one of the few situation where Coumadin would be considered indicated despite the fetal risks.

14. **(D)** Such patients should not become pregnant if possible. Their own life expectancy is markedly diminished. Maternal concerns must be considered first in such situations. The fetus will almost always be lost.

15. **(E)** Induction of labor usually is intense and long in a primiparous woman. Insulin infusion is most commonly the optimal form of management for these patients.

16. **(D)** Alertness to several clinical and historical signs may allow one to diagnose diabetes early in pregnancy and by proper care decrease the fetal mortality associated with the disease. However, approximately one-half of the pregnant patients with gestational diabetes will be missed if only high-risk factors are used for diagnosis.

17. **(D)** Anemia is a common finding in pregnancy. A fairly standard definition of anemia is important. In pregnancy, a hemoglobin below 10 g/dL is considered to reflect an anemic state. The anemia may be partly "physiologic," from the normal vascular volume increase with a great expansion of plasma volume than RBC mass, but it should and can be treated in most cases.

18. **(A)** Many women have small iron stores secondary to blood loss during menses, childbirth, and inadequate intake. Their intake should be increased to make up for the lack of bone marrow iron. The poor tolerance to iron and poor intestinal absorption also add to the problem.

19. **(C)** Thalassemia is a disease of defective production of either the alpha- or beta-globin that make up the hemoglobin molecule. Deficient production may lead to microcytic anemia. Acute blood loss does not manifest as a change in the red-cell indices.

20. **(A)** Sickle cell disease is found in less than 1 in 500 African Americans. Sickle cell trait is found in approximately 8% of African Americans.

21. **(B)** Sickle cell disease is autosomal recessive. Thus, the children must have both copies of the abnormal gene to have the disease. Each child will have a 50% chance of receiving an abnormal gene from the parent who has sickle cell trait. Thus 50% or a 25% chance of disease. This also explains the 1/500 rate of sickle cell disease with $1/12 \times 1/12 \times 1/4 = 1/576$.

22. **(B)** G6PD deficiency is a disease found in 2% of African American women. The enzyme deficiency may lead to anemia when a woman is exposed to certain drugs with sulfa drugs being particularly problematic.

23. **(C)** The MCV is greater than normal with a lower than normal hematocrit.

24. **(D)** Folic acid deficiency is the most common cause in a young person of macrocytic anemia. $B_{12}$ deficiency also may cause macrocytic anemia but is rare in this age group.

25. **(A)** A clean-void urine specimen is best for routine cultures, provided meticulous care is taken during collection. Other methods that avoid contamination of the specimen—namely, catheterization and suprapubic aspiration—may be used, but both invade the bladder, and catheterization is known to predispose to UTIs.

26. **(C)** X-rays of the lower abdomen should not be done routinely during pregnancy because of the radiation exposure to both mother and fetus. However, one should be aware of the physiologic hydroureters present during pregnancy. This finding may be misinterpreted as obstruction.

27. **(E)** As this is a normal physiologic finding, it does not require any treatment. Total obstruction is unlikely. Stenting is unnecessary.

28. **(E)** Pelvic kidney must always be considered in the presence of a large, firm, posterior pelvic mass. In pregnancy, ultrasound is an even better study than an IVP, which gives a low dose of radiation.

29. **(B)** A single pelvic kidney is susceptible to trauma at the time of delivery and to infection during pregnancy. However, if it is functioning properly, there is no need to terminate the pregnancy. Transplant patients deliver vaginally with few problems.

30. **(D)** Stones can be passed during pregnancy. The possibility of long-standing renal calculi must be kept in mind, in which case low-grade chronic infection is likely to be present. Symptomatic treatment is provided with surgical removal, if necessary.

31. **(E)** Hyperparathyroidism during pregnancy is a rare disease, usually caused by an adenoma or hyperplasia of the parathyroids. However, the presence of renal stones in young women should make one think of this disease. Other tests, such as urine cultures and serum calcium and phosphorus, should also be done. The urine can be strained for other stones.

32. **(C)** Because of the rarity (<0.01%) of ureteral stones in the normal age group of pregnant women and the large ureters secondary to pregnancy hormones, one should look for predisposing factors such as hyperparathyroidism if renal stones are discovered. The diagnosis, evaluation, and therapy are similar as in the nonpregnant patient, except lithotripsy is contraindicated. Pain caused is usually excruciating. There is no such thing as a ureteral filter.

33. **(D)** Eclampsia requires the presence of convulsions and/or coma. Preeclampsia is the only diagnosis that can be substantiated. At age 14 chronic hypertension is very unlikely, especially given fundal size equally EGA.

34. **(B)** During intrauterine life, the infant of a hyperparathyroid mother is exposed to high serum calcium levels, which may result in tetany when no longer present. Such symptoms in the newborn may be the first indication of the maternal disease.

35. **(B)** Fortunately, cytomegalic disease is almost never recurrent and often does not affect the infant even if the asymptomatic mother excretes the virus. Up to 1% of all newborns excrete the virus at birth. Only 5% to 10% of these infants are symptomatic. Cells with inclusion bodies are most likely seen with cytomegalovirus.

36. **(C)** Generally, the signs and symptoms of pyelonephritis are clear-cut. Women with prior asymptomatic bacteriuria are at greater risk of developing pyelonephritis than women without

bacteriuria. Up to 2% of pregnancies are complicated by pyelonephritis.

37. **(C)** The mother may contract the protozoa from exposure to cat feces or by eating undercooked meat. Most women are asymptomatic. Many of the newborns will be infected. Fetal infection with toxoplasmosis may be devastating.

38. **(E)** Because of the large number of asymptomatic carriers of gonorrhea (both male and female), the decreasing sensitivity of the organism, and the inability to culture the gonococci adequately from the female, this patient should be treated with ceftriaxone 250 mg IM if she is not allergic. She should be recultured in 2 weeks. Her partner should also be treated. She should also be evaluated and/or treated for chlamydia, as the probability of simultaneous exposure is high.

39. **(A)** Most pregnant patients should have a gonococcal culture taken. Any disease so discovered should be treated promptly. Prevention is the best means to avoid poor neonatal outcome. Given the seriousness of gonococcal ophthalmia, all newborns receive prophylactic eye drops.

40. **(C)** During the second month of pregnancy, maternal rubella results in an 80% fetal infection, with a 25% to 50% incidence of major abnormalities. With rubella, during the first month, the incidence of anomalies is even higher. The anomalies can be and usually are multiple.

41. **(B)** Several major anomalies are also known to occur following rubella. These include eye and heart lesions, intrauterine growth retardation, and chromosomal abnormalities. Most common is congenital hearing loss.

42. **(B)** Purpura is a recognized abnormality occurring in infants with congenital rubella. It is due to thrombocytopenia. Anemia is also possible.

43. **(D)** Obtaining a VDRL only at the time of contact or within a few days may lead one to a sense of false security. However, the serologic tests for syphilis will almost always be positive within 4 to 6 weeks after exposure.

44. **(C)** If syphilis in pregnancy can be treated early, it is less likely to cross the placenta and infect the fetus. Treatment beyond 18 weeks often leaves the fetus with serious sequelae. A titer of 1:16 is unlikely to be a biologic false positive. Any patient with a positive test for syphilis should be screened for HIV.

45. **(C)** There is a slim chance that the mother was reinfected, but it is far more likely that the baby has maternal antibody. The VDRL should become negative without therapy.

46. **(B)** If the baby has the disease, the VDRL titer will increase. If it simply has passive maternal antibody, the titer will disappear within 3 months. Positive IgM levels provide a useful, though not specific, indication of infection. If there is any doubt, it is better to treat the infant. Darkfield examinations will help if lesions are present; otherwise, there is no place from which to obtain specimens.

47. **(C)** Short-acting penicillin may cure incubating syphilis but is not adequate for the established disease. Late syphilis requires higher doses. If duration is greater than 1 year or if neurosyphilis is suspected, spinal fluid must be obtained for analysis. Even though the patient is penicillin allergic, no other antibiotic adequately crosses the placenta to treat the infant. Therefore the patient must be desensitized and treated with a long-acting penicillin. This is one example of how the placental barrier impacts selection of medications for mother.

48. **(D)** BMR, protein-bound iodine (PBI), and binding globulin will all be elevated during pregnancy. $I^{131}$ uptake determination is contraindicated during pregnancy. The T3 uptake is normally decreased in pregnancy because the increased serum-binding globulin competes with the RBCs added for the test for uptake of labeled T3. To diagnose hyperthyroidism, measurements of unbound or free T4 can be done. PBI, BMR, and assays other than TSH, T4, and T3 resin (or RBC) uptake are seldom done.

**49. (B)** I$^{131}$ treatment is contraindicated in pregnancy and thyroidectomy may not be necessary. Some arguments exist as to the best medical regimen. However, initial treatment is thyroid suppression with PTU.

**50. (E)** Carcinoma of the breast can arise at any time, and nodules should be worked up in spite of pregnancy. Mistaking a cancer for a mastitis is not unusual. Delay in evaluation or treatment only decreases the chance of long-term survival.

**51. (E)** Many women see a physician for the first time in years when they are pregnant. Pap smears should be done routinely as indicated. Pregnancy does not alter cytologic findings significantly enough to alter the reading of Pap smears in pregnancy.

**52. (E)** In general, the best results are achieved if one disregards the pregnancy and treats the cancer. Irradiation will soon result in abortion. Radical surgery has no place in Stage III disease, and hysterotomy is not necessary so early in gestation. The patient, of course, may desire another course of action after all the possibilities have been explained.

**53. (F)** The most likely diagnosis is preeclampsia. Patients with multiple gestation are more likely to develop preeclampsia, and at younger gestational ages.

**54. (D)** Increased uric acid levels are probably from microangiopathic cell destruction and endothelial damage.

**55. (B)** Septic shock, as well as coma, postictal state, or pulmonary hypertension, could cause such symptoms. The absence of vaginal bleeding virtually rules out placenta previa as a diagnosis for a state of shock. Abruptio placentae can have hidden bleeding. Eclampsia usually has associated hypertension. Amniotic embolism usually occurs during labor.

**56. (B)** If the patient had a hydatidiform mole, which is certainly a strong possibility from the history, you would anticipate a very high level of hCG. Serial hCG would be elevated well beyond normal levels. Ultrasound will show classic signs of molar tissue and is the test of choice. The Apt test is to detect fetal hemoglobin, of which there is none in complete molar pregnancies. Serial clotting function will not help in the immediate diagnosis.

**57. (C)** Those occurring after gestation seem to be related to poor nutrition and an advanced maternal age. Spontaneous occurrence is extremely rare. Asian patients are at the highest risk. The most common time is after hydatidiform mole.

**58. (B)** In the presence of long-standing fetal death, tests to determine fetal viability are fruitless. The mother, however, may develop a consumptive coagulopathy. This is rare before 1 month after fetal death.

**59. (B)** A dead fetus that is retained in utero beyond 5 weeks is likely to cause hypofibrinogenemia; therefore, maternal clotting ability should be evaluated. Delivery is indicated.

**60. (C)** Defects that inhibit fetal swallowing appear to be most common. The importance of recognizing the association of poor fetal outcome with severe degrees of hydramnios is greater than the importance of knowing the absolute percentages. Most fetuses will not have anomalies, and the cause of hydramnios is usually not found. Amniotic fluid index, calculated by adding the vertical depth of the largest pocket of amniotic fluid in each of four quadrants, has been used as a measure.

**61. (I)** The distention of the uterus will tend to cause preterm labor. Fetal urinary tract anomalies are associated with a decreased volume of amniotic fluid because urine makes up a lot of the amniotic fluid. Hypertension is generally not related to hydramnios, although often it is related to oligohydramnios. Diabetes in the mother will cause an osmotic diuresis in the infant, resulting in increased fluid, and neurologic deficits may compromise swallowing; both can increase amniotic fluid. However, the most common cause is idiopathic in >40% of cases.

62. **(A)** The pressure within the amnion is not elevated in the majority of cases but may be increased in the presence of uterine contractions. Hydramnios implies greater than 2,000 mL of fluid, with severe hydramnios being more than 3,000 mL. Hydramnios is associated with a variety of fetal abnormalities. The uterus is often overdistended and may contract very poorly.

63. **(D)** The duration and intensity place this episode beyond the realm of usual nausea and vomiting of pregnancy. Ptyalism is excessive salivation. Flu is possible but less likely without associated intestinal symptoms.

64. **(C)** If the patient is acutely dehydrated and unable to retain ingested food, she should be treated with fluids and electrolytes. Often, hydration with a dilute glucose solution will relieve the vomiting.

65. **(D)** Cholestatic hepatosis or cholestasis of pregnancy is characterized by mild icterus and pruritus. This entity may be associated with adverse fetal outcome.

66. **(D)** High estrogen levels appear to be etiologically implicated in the syndrome of cholestatic hepatosis. Why they predispose to cholestasis is unclear. This may also recur with the use of birth control pills.

67. **(A)** Sickle cell anemia is not managed with iron supplementation because the patient has high iron stores. Transfusions are with the packed cells, not with hemoglobin. Early delivery is not otherwise indicated.

68. **(E)** In Ebstein's anomaly, there is downward displacement of an abnormal tricuspid valve into the right ventricle. Cyanosis is due to right-to-left shunting through the foramen ovale. Tetralogy of Fallot is a combination of VSD, right ventricular hypertrophy, and an overriding aorta with cyanosis. Cyanosis gets worse during pregnancy when peripheral resistance decreases and the shunt increases. PDA also allows right-to-left shunting when systemic pressure falls. VSD will allow right-to-left shunting when

pulmonary hypertension develops. Marfan's syndrome is an inherited weakness of connective tissue that commonly leads to aortic dilation and dissecting aneurysm.

69. **(C)** Human placental lactogen acts to inhibit insulin activity.

70. **(D)** Women with a previous DVT and a thrombophilia, such as Factor V Leiden, are at an increased risk or recurrent DVT in pregnancy and for 6 weeks postpartum. Low-molecular-weight heparin is the treatment of choice, and warfarin may be used after delivery since it does not cross into breast milk.

71. **(E)** Anti-D immune globulin is given after an event such as trauma, amniocentesis, or delivery, which may lead to exposure of maternal Rh-negative blood to the Rh antigen. Women who are DU positive do not need RhoGAM.

72. **(D)** Class II disease is usually asymptomatic in pregnancy. Patient should be closely monitored to detect early signs of congestive heart failure (CHF). Decreasing vital capacity is an early sign of CHF. If CHF occurs, rapid medical treatment with digitalis, oxygen, and diuretics is indicated. Patients with CHF do best with vaginal delivery.

73. **(D)** Most often in pregnancies complicated by SLE, the worst complications will be renal. Declining function with exacerbation or onset of hypertensive disease are the manifestations. Renal function must be monitored throughout pregnancy. While blood urea nitrogen (BUN) and creatinine levels are specifically used to monitor current renal function, sharply declining C3 and C4 levels are predictors of exacerbations of this disease. Many authorities recommend monthly monitoring of these serum complement levels. Serial antinuclear antibodies (ANA) titers will not help monitor disease. Growth restriction is common, and ultrasounds will be helpful in monitoring fetal growth

74. **(D)** The signs and symptoms of obstetric hepatosis disappear after delivery. Antihistamines and cholestyramine have been reported to be

helpful. Monitoring for fetal well-being is important since there is a risk of sudden infant death due to cholestasis.

75. **(D)** The three most common causes of maternal mortality are hemorrhage, hypertension, and pulmonary embolism. Of these, the hypertensive disorders are the most common. Anesthesia, heart disease, collagen diseases, and asthma are also causes of maternal death, but they are not among the top three as recorded in current maternal death statistics. Maternal mortality is steadily declining, and causes are changing in relative incidence.

76. **(A)** Nonmaternal deaths are due to factors that have nothing to do with the pregnancy, such as gunshot wounds or motor vehicle accidents. Domestic violence is, sadly, the most common cause.

77. **(B)** The patient should be stabilized before any attempt at induction. One must be sure that the fetuses are mature. If the mother and fetuses are not in danger, there is no great urgency for delivery. Antihypertensives are not used at this level of blood pressure.

78. **(C)** Sulfas compete with bilirubin for an excretory pathway. This may result in increased bilirubin in the fetus and may require therapy.

79. **(E)** Aplastic anemia from chloramphenicol is a rare occurrence and one that can be avoided. Usually, many other effective drugs are available that do not have so serious a side effect. However, it remains the first choice for treatment of typhoid fever.

80. **(D)** Streptomycin is not a drug of choice for the usual infections, as the range of bacterial coverage is not great and there is risk of toxicity. Many broad-spectrum aminoglycosides are now available that can be used in place of streptomycin.

81. **(A)** High concentrations of tetracycline will develop in patients with decreased renal function, as excretion will be impaired. Therefore, dosage should be decreased if renal function is impaired. It can cause staining of deciduous teeth and has been associated with acute fatty liver.

82. **(F)** An uncommon side effect of PTU therapy is agranulocytosis

83. **(H)** Ibuprofen and other nonsteroidal anti-inflammatory agents may induce decreased renal blood flow in the fetus resulting in decreased amniotic fluid.

84. **(C)** In this instance, the BP elevation was discovered before 20 weeks' gestation, and there was no evidence of hydatidiform mole. Therefore, the most likely diagnosis is chronic hypertensive disease. Preeclampsia is usually a disease of the third trimester.

85. **(A)** This patient does not have any of the signs or symptoms required to make the diagnosis of severe preeclampsia. These signs are somewhat arbitrary and constitute a continuum.

86. **(D)** The presence of convulsions or coma, or both, in late pregnancy must be considered eclampsia until proved otherwise. Epilepsy, brain tumors, or hepatic disease may be at fault, but the most likely diagnosis is eclampsia. Primary seizure disorders may present in pregnancy, but pregnancy-related seizures are more likely.

87. **(B)** The presence of pulmonary edema or cyanosis is sufficient to make the diagnosis of severe preeclampsia. Pulmonary complications are one of the major causes of death from preeclampsia. They are treated best by delivery and supportive measures.

88. **(C)** The long history of increased BP with the retinal changes makes chronic hypertensive disease the most likely diagnosis. However, this patient must be observed closely for superimposed toxemia.

89. **(E)** Pneumonia, as a complication of epidemic influenza, is very serious in the pregnant woman. Children, pregnant women, and the aged appear to be at the greatest risk from this

disease. Vaccination for influenza during pregnancy is safe and recommended.

90. **(A)** Many autoimmune diseases become more severe or "flare" after delivery. For unknown reasons, perhaps due to a depressed immune response with a rebound during postpartum, multiple sclerosis often flares postpartum

91. **(A)** *Listeria* has been found in abortuses although the exact association with abortion in humans is unclear. It can cause fetal infection, with a high fetal mortality rate.

92. **(C)** Hiatal hernia is quite common during pregnancy, perhaps from reflux of gastric acid into the esophagus, causing the symptom of heartburn. This is common because of increased intra-abdominal pressure. Antacids are the best treatment. The symptom of heartburn can be mistaken for the epigastric pain of preeclampsia and vice versa.

# CHAPTER 10

# Normal Labor and Delivery

## Questions

**DIRECTIONS (Questions 1 through 34): For each of the multiple choice questions in this section, select the lettered answer that is the one *best* response in each case.**

1. At term, the ligaments of the pelvis change. This may result in which of the following to aid fetal passage?

   (A) a slight increase in the rotation of the femoral shaft

   (B) transient degeneration of pelvic ground substance

   (C) inferior placed angle to the iliosacral ligament

   (D) mild enlargement of the pelvic cavity

   (E) posterior rotation of the levator muscles allowing improved fetal passage

**Questions 2 and 3 apply to the following patient:**

A 4 ft 11 in Southeast Asian woman has an estimated fetal weight by ultrasound of 4,000 g. To estimate the pelvic capacity, you perform clinical pelvimetry.

2. Which of the following does this procedure measure?

   (A) true conjugate

   (B) transverse diameter of the inlet

   (C) shape of the pubic arch

   (D) flare of the iliac crests

   (E) elasticity of the levator muscles

3. You estimate that the pelvic outlet is adequate, but there may be a problem in the midpelvis. The interspinous diameter of a normal pelvis should be at least how many centimeters?

   (A) 5

   (B) 6–8

   (C) 9–11

   (D) 12

   (E) The interspinous diameter is not a clinically important assessment

4. To appreciate how different positioning of the presenting part can impact the second stage of labor, one needs to understand the pelvic axis. During the delivery, the fetal head follows the pelvic axis. What is the best way to describe this axis?

   (A) a straight line in parallel to the vaginal canal

   (B) a curve first directed anteriorly and then caudad

   (C) a curve first directed posteriorly and then caudad

   (D) a curve first directed posteriorly and then cephalad

   (E) a straight line perpendicular to the vaginal canal

**5.** The position of fetal presentation has a large impact on the success of the second stage of labor. The diagram in Figure 10–1 depicts which position of the fetus in the female pelvis?

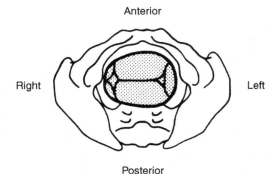

Anterior

Right                                                        Left

Posterior

**Figure 10–1.**

(A) right occipitoposterior (ROP)

(B) left mentotransverse (LMT)

(C) left occipitoanterior (LOA)

(D) left sacrotransverse (LST)

(E) left occiput transverse (LOT)

**Questions 6 and 7 apply to the following patient:**

You are counseling an extremely anxious 37-year-old primigravida who admits that she is "into control." She has researched analgesia in labor and has a few more questions about pudendal nerves.

**6.** The pudendal nerve can be easily blocked by local anesthetics. What does the neurological effect of the pudendal nerve block affect?

(A) the levator ani muscle

(B) the obturator internus muscle

(C) sensation to the uterus

(D) motor innervation of the bladder

(E) sensory innervation of the perineum

**7.** A pudendal anesthetic blockade accomplishes its effects through which of the following nerves?

(A) autonomic motor pathways

(B) autonomic sensory pathways

(C) T11, 12

(D) L2, 3, 4

(E) S2, 3, 4

**8.** When repairing a perineal laceration, what is the optimal suture to use because of healing time and least pain and inflammation produced?

(A) Dexon (polycaprolate)

(B) plain catgut

(C) chromic catgut

(D) monocryl (poliglecaprone)

(E) polydioxanone (PDS)

**9.** Which of the following is the major problem associated with the administration of barbiturates during labor?

(A) sudden fetal death

(B) fetal depression after birth

(C) lack of maternal cooperation during the birth process because of narcosis

(D) the likelihood of maternal aspiration causing pneumonitis

(E) their effect is not better than placebo

**10.** It is important to be able to estimate the blood loss at a delivery to determine if more aggressive management of uterine bleeding is indicated. Average blood loss during normal deliveries is how many milliliters?

(A) 700

(B) 500

(C) 250

(D) 100

(E) 50

**11.** During an obstructive labor, a retraction ring can form on the uterus that can compound the lack of progress in labor. Where does the physiologic retraction ring occur?

(A) internal os

(B) external os

(C) level of the round ligament insertion

(D) junction of the upper and lower uterine segments

(E) at the level of the tubal ostia

**12.** In a cephalic presentation, the position is determined by the relationship of what fetal part to the mother's pelvis?

(A) mentum

(B) sacrum

(C) acromion

(D) occiput

(E) sinciput

**13.** The relation of the fetal parts to one another determines which of the following?

(A) presentation of the fetus

(B) lie of the fetus

(C) attitude of the fetus

(D) position of the fetus

(E) intention of the fetus

**14.** A primigravid patient has been having a long prodromal labor but has finally entered active phase of Stage 1. She is excited and wants to know what she should expect as a typical labor course. Average durations of active labor without epidural analgesia are best expressed by which of the following?

(A) first stage, 750 minutes; second stage, 80 minutes; third stage, 30 minutes

(B) first stage, 80 minutes; second stage, 20 minutes; third stage, 5 minutes

(C) first stage, 120 minutes; second stage, 80 minutes; third stage, 5 minutes

(D) first stage, 80 minutes; second stage, 20 minutes; third stage, 20 minutes

(E) first stage, 750 minutes; second stage, 80 minutes; third stage, 5 minutes

**15.** A patient has failed to have any further dilation after achieving 6 cm. As possible reasons for this secondary arrest of dilation are explored, you place an intrauterine catheter to calculate the intensity of her contractions which are measured in Montevideo units. Which of the following is a Montevideo unit?

(A) number of contractions in 10 minutes

(B) number of contractions per minute times their intensity

(C) intensity of any 10 contractions times the time it took for them to occur

(D) number of contractions over 50 mm Hg in 10 minutes

(E) number of contractions in 10 minutes times their average intensity

**16.** In the normal labor, the pressure produced by uterine contractions is greatest at which of the following times?

(A) latent phase

(B) active phase

(C) second stage

(D) third stage

(E) when Braxton Hicks' sign is evident

**17.** At 39 weeks during a pelvic examination, due to Braxton Hicks contractions, the patient is found to be 2 cm dilated. She asks if anything can be done to promote labor since she is exhausted from days of B H contractions. A sweeping (stripping) of the membranes is done based on the idea that this disrupts the lysosomes in the lower decidual. Which of the following, when released from lysosomes, may initiate labor?

(A) arachidonic acid

(B) phosphatidylinositol

(C) phospholipase A

(D) thromboxane

(E) phosphatidylglycerol

**18.** Engagement is best defined as which of the following?

(A) when the presenting part goes through the pelvic inlet

(B) when the presenting part is level with the ischial spines

(C) when the greatest biparietal diameter of the fetal head passes the pelvic inlet

(D) when the greatest biparietal diameter of the head is level with the ischial spines

(E) when the greatest diameter of the fetal presenting part passes through the narrowest and lowest part of the maternal pelvis

19. A patient is experiencing an arrest of decent. During the evaluation one can feel that it is a vertex presentation with the sagittal suture transverse or oblique but closer to the symphysis than the promontory. What is this specific condition called?

    (A) posterior asynclitism
    (B) internal rotation
    (C) anterior asynclitism
    (D) extension
    (E) restitution

20. When educating a patient about the possible signs of labor you mention "bloody show." This is which of the following?

    (A) a result of small placental abruptions
    (B) not seen in breech presentations
    (C) a consequence of effacement and dilatation of the cervix
    (D) associated with the passage of meconium
    (E) problematic in Rh-negative mothers if not given RhoGAM within 72 hours

21. A patient is being evaluated for excessive postpartum vaginal bleeding after a successful VBAC (vaginal birth after C-section) of a 3,500-g infant. One concern is retained placental tissue. Placental separation is facilitated by which of the following?

    (A) deep placental growth into the myometrium
    (B) presence of a layer of decidua
    (C) decreased uterine muscle contractibility
    (D) the changing configuration of the uterus after fetal delivery
    (E) bleeding into the uterus

22. Eight minutes after a normal delivery under pudendal anesthesia, the patient has not completed the third stage of labor. The uterus is discoid and firm; no bleeding is evident. What should you do?

    (A) pull steadily but with greater traction on the cord
    (B) perform Crede's maneuver

    (C) augment the contractions with intramuscular (IM) methergine
    (D) manually remove the placenta
    (E) gently massage the uterus and wait

23. A 20-year-old G1P0 patient is having a protracted active phase with irregular contractins that appear to be of inadequate intensity. It is determined that the patient would benefit from oxytocin (pitocin) augmentation. The patient is very nervous about this and asks a number of questions about the drug. Which of the following is a characteristic of oxytocin?

    (A) half-life of about 8 minutes
    (B) prolonged effect
    (C) immediate hypertensive effect if given intravenously
    (D) inactivated by oxytocinase
    (E) inhibited by nonsteroidal anti-inflammatory agents

24. A 21-year-old primiparous patient arrives in Labor and Delivery with poor prenatal care, her last visit being 8 weeks ago. She is 41 weeks by dates, and states she ruptured membranes approximately 12 hours ago. On examination, estimated weight is 9 lb. She has thick meconium. Her cervix is 3 cm, dilated, and the presenting part is at −2 station. The presenting part is a face. The fetal heart tones are excellent; she is not contracting. What is the best management?

    (A) oxytocin induction with group B strep prophylaxis
    (B) Misoprostol 25 $\mu$g, group B strep prophylaxis
    (C) expectant management with group B strep prophylaxis
    (D) epidural anesthesia to relax the pelvis, group B strep prophylaxis, and then oxytocin
    (E) cesarean section

**Questions 25 and 26 apply to the following patient:**

A 21-year-old primigravida at 39 weeks' gestation presents to labor and delivery with complaints of uterine contractions since 5 AM that day. She is seen for a routine clinic visit at 3 PM and her cervix is found to be 2 cm dilated, 50% effaced, midposition, and moderate in consistency, with the fetal vertex at 0 station. Reexamination on labor and delivery at 7 PM shows no significant cervical change. Fetal heart tones are reassuring. She begs you to admit and augment her because she is tired of being pregnant. You explain that she and the fetus are doing well and that her Bishop's score predicts the likelihood of a successful labor augmentation.

25. What is this gravida's Bishop score?

    (A) 8, cervix unripe

    (B) 4, cervix unripe

    (C) 2, cervix ripening

    (D) 6, cervix ripening

    (E) 9, cervix ripe

26. What would be the optimal obstetrical management at that time?

    (A) labor augmentation with a high dose of oxytocin

    (B) performance of primary cesarean section for prolonged labor with presumed cephalopelvic disproportion

    (C) reassurance and rest, offering narcotics to aid relaxation and sleep

    (D) artificial rupture of the membranes

    (E) cervical ripening with misoprostol

**Questions 27 and 28 apply to the following patient:**

A 32-year-old woman (gravida 3, para 1, abortus 1) at term is admitted in labor with an initial cervical examination of 6-cm dilatation, complete effacement, and the vertex at −1 station. Estimated fetal weight is 8 lb, and her first pregnancy resulted in an uncomplicated vaginal delivery of an 8-lb infant. After 2 hours, there is no cervical change. An intrauterine pressure catheter is placed. This shows three contractions in a 10-minute period, each with a strength of 40 mm Hg.

27. What is this abnormality of labor termed?

    (A) prolonged latent phase

    (B) active-phase arrest

    (C) failure of descent

    (D) arrest of latent phase

    (E) protraction of descent

28. What is the best course of action at this time?

    (A) wait 2 more hours and repeat the cervical examination

    (B) start oxytocin augmentation

    (C) perform a cesarean section

    (D) discharge the patient, instructing her to return when contractions become stronger

    (E) therapeutic rest with analgesia and short-acting anti-anxiety medication

29. The routine use of midline episiotomy during delivery has been shown to do which of the following?

    (A) prevent urinary stress incontinence in the fourth decade of life

    (B) decrease the incidence of fetal cranial molding

    (C) decrease maternal blood loss

    (D) increase the incidence of third- and fourth-degree lacerations

    (E) prevent the development of a rectocele and uterine prolapsed postmenopausal

30. Normal labor is dependent on the unique aspects of the uterine smooth muscle. Which statement characterizes uterine muscle cells during normal labor?

    (A) The muscle regains full strength between contractions.

    (B) The entire uterus contracts simultaneously.

    (C) Muscle cells rely on placental transfer for generation of adenosine triphosphate (ATP).

    (D) They demonstrate a contractile sensitivity to oxytocin.

    (E) Muscle cells return to the original length after contraction.

31. Which of the following statements most accurately describes postpartum hemorrhage?

    (A) It is prevented primarily by the increased concentration of clotting factors in maternal blood.
    (B) Grand multiparity is a risk factor.
    (C) Women with severe pre-eclampsia are more tolerant of heavy blood loss.
    (D) Changes in pulse and blood pressure are good early indicators of excessive blood loss.
    (E) Placenta accreta is the most frequent cause.

32. A relative contraindication for induction of labor includes which of the following?

    (A) prolonged pregnancy
    (B) severe pre-eclampsia
    (C) intrauterine growth restriction
    (D) previous myomectomy entering the uterine cavity at the fundus
    (E) prolonged rupture of membranes without labor

**Questions 33 and 34 apply to the following patient:**

A 19-year-old primigravida at term presents to labor and delivery reporting irregular contractions and rupture of membranes 21 hours prior to arrival. She has not received prenatal care but reports that her pregnancy was uncomplicated. She is afebrile, and electronic fetal monitoring is reactive with occasional mild variable decelerations.

33. Which method is the most sensitive test to confirm rupture of membranes?

    (A) nitrazine test
    (B) vaginal pooling
    (C) pelvic examination
    (D) ferning
    (E) Coombs' test

34. Cervical examination reveals a dilatation of 3 cm, 50% effacement, −1 station, vertex presentation. Spontaneous rupture of membranes is confirmed. What is the best course of action at this time?

    (A) perform an immediate low transverse cesarean section
    (B) start intravenous (IV) antibiotics for group B streptococcal (GBS) prophylaxis
    (C) begin an amnioinfusion
    (D) conduct a contraction stress test
    (E) ambulate the patient

**DIRECTIONS (Questions 35 through 42): The following group of questions is preceded by a list of lettered options. For each question, select the one lettered option that is *most* closely associated with it. Each lettered option may be used once, multiple times, or not at all.**

**Questions 35 through 38**

    (A) first stage of labor
    (B) second stage of labor
    (C) third stage of labor
    (D) effacement
    (E) lightening
    (F) fourth stage of labor
    (G) postpartum period
    (H) engagement

35. Dropping of the fetal head into the pelvis

36. Ends with complete dilation of the cervix

37. Begins with the delivery of the baby

38. Ends with the delivery of the baby

**Questions 39 through 42**

    (A) McRoberts maneuver
    (B) Mauriceau–Smellie–Veit maneuver
    (C) external cephalic version
    (D) Ritgen maneuver
    (E) Leopold's maneuvers
    (F) Ferguson's maneuver
    (G) Crede maneuver
    (H) Wood's corkscrew maneuver

39. At 39 weeks' gestation, a woman is admitted to labor and delivery. Her cervix is long and closed. The fetus is found to be a vertex presentation by palpation.

40. Gentle constant abdominal pressure is applied to cause the fetal vertex to rotate out of the fundal area and into the lower uterine segment.

41. The vertex delivers, but gentle downward traction fails to effect delivery of the anterior shoulder.

42. A rapid labor with a vertex presentation has taken place, and the infant is crowning. Mother is in poor control so attempts are made to slow the delivery of the vertex to avoid perineal/vaginal lacerations.

**DIRECTIONS (Questions 43 through 45): For each of the multiple choice questions in this section, select the lettered answer that is the one *best* response in each case.**

**Questions 43 through 45 apply to the following patient:**

A 24-year-old G3P0 Ab 2 presents in early labor at 39 weeks. She has a prepregnancy BMI of 48. Her 1 hour 50 g glucose screen was 138 mg%. No 3 hour was ordered. An ultrasound last week noted an AFI of 24 cm. Normal is less than 20 cm. The fetus was noted to have extra fatty tissue around the body and has an estimated fetal weight of 4,300 g. The patient is very uncomfortable and can only sleep sitting up in a chair. Given the clinical situation an induction is started and 24 hours later she is in second stage of labor.

43. In anticipation of a possible postpartum hemorrhage due to the prolonged induction and macrosomia, which of the following options is best for the prevention of excess blood loss?

   (A) oxytocin 10 units IM if bleeding exceeds 500 cc
   (B) type and cross 2 units of packed red blood cells
   (C) epidural anesthesia to facilitate manual removal of the placenta if needed
   (D) two 18-guage IV lines
   (E) 600 $\mu$g of prostaglandin E1 (misoprostol) given per rectum after delivery of the placenta

44. What is the best option in preparation for a possible shoulder dystocia given the fetal macrosomia?

   (A) check the mother's glucose by finger stick every 2 hours
   (B) type and cross for 2 units packed red blood cells
   (C) request extra attendants in the room for delivery to help with McRoberts maneuver
   (D) delivery in the operating room to facilitate emergency cesarean delivery if needed
   (E) epidural anesthesia so the mother can let the fetus labor down without the urge to push

45. If the patient has a cesarean delivery, during early postpartum recovery, what is the best level for her $O_2$ saturation?

   (A) no minimum $O_2$ saturation as long as she has stable vital signs
   (B) 90%
   (C) 94%
   (D) 96%
   (E) the same as her predelivery $O_2$ saturations

# Answers and Explanations

1. **(D)** The change is one of relaxation of the ligaments, allowing more mobility at the sacroiliac and symphyseal joints and on occasion some instability. Whether or not these changes truly add to pelvic size has not been determined, but they seem to allow passage more easily, perhaps by accommodation.

2. **(C)** Clinical pelvimetry cannot directly measure the midplane of the pelvis, but its capacity can be estimated by the evaluation of the sacrosciatic notch, the ischial spines, and the concavity of the sacrum. Parallel pelvic sidewalls and a wide pubic arch are crucial to the outlet evaluation. The pelvic inlet cannot be assessed by clinical pelvimetry.

3. **(C)** The interspinous diameter is the lateral distance between the ischial spines. The ischial spines should not be too prominent on pelvic examination. The distance is generally considered to be the smallest pelvic diameter and the "obstetric limit" in preventing or allowing delivery. Thus one wants it to be at least 9 to 11 cm.

4. **(C)** A common misconception is that the fetal head follows a straight line through the pelvis. On the contrary, it describes nearly a 90° angle following the pelvic axis. The pelvic axis (curve of Carus) reflects a line in the center of the pelvic inlet (directing it posterior into the sacrum), then caudally toward the center of the outlet (extending the head). The classic mechanisms of labor can be better understood through a knowledge of the pelvic axis.

5. **(E)** In vertex presentations, the relation of the occiput to the maternal pelvis determines the position. The position of the occiput can be detected by finding the posterior fontanel. As it is on the left lateral side of the mother and the sagittal suture is transverse, the position is LOT.

6. **(E)** The pudendal block is often used for delivery or minor surgery on the vulva. The pudendal nerve can be blocked either transvaginally or percutaneously through the buttock. The latter route may be used in the presence of a Bartholin's abscess without causing pain during vaginal manipulation.

7. **(E)** The pudendal nerve is blocked near the ischial spines. This block will not interfere with uterine contractions and will provide anesthesia to the perineum. Because there is considerable overlap of innervation, midline infiltration anterior to the rectum is needed to provide the best block.

8. **(A)** Suture to prepare perineal lacerations is chosen on pain produced as well as dissolving in a reasonable time—weeks not many months. Studies show that Dexon and Vicryl (undyed should be used) cause the least inflammation and least discomfort. PDS and Monocryl are not used because they take too long to absorb.

9. **(B)** Fetal depression is the best reason to minimize the use of barbiturates in labor. For example, after a dose of thiopental is given, it will reach the fetal circulation in 2 to 3 minutes. A dose of 250 mg will have little effect on an

otherwise healthy infant, but it does have some effect. All the other distractors have been claimed. Remember, a barbiturate alone is a poor substitute for a true analgesic agent. It seldom is given in large enough doses to truly sedate or narcotize the mother, but when given with narcotics, it certainly can. Anesthetic and analgesic effects on the fetus are a never-ending source of controversy. There is no clear-cut "best" anesthetic or analgesic regimen for delivery. Judgment should be used, subject to local availability.

10. **(B)** This value is greater than that generally estimated by the obstetrician. In fact, the classic definition of postpartum hemorrhage is more than 500 mL at delivery and in the ensuing 24 hours—obviously a gross mistake. If the maternal reserves are good; however, there will be little change in the postpartum hematocrit unless the blood loss is substantially more than 500 mL. Blood loss is often difficult to measure without completely weighing sponges, drapes, and towels.

11. **(D)** A distinct boundary exists between the thin lower segment and the thicker upper uterine segment. It can easily be identified at the time of cesarean section if labor has progressed for some time. Retraction rings generally occur only when labor has been obstructed for quite some time. This ring can obstruct labor at times (pathologic retraction ring or Bandl's ring).

12. **(D)** The most common presentation is cephalic. Position is the relationship between the denominator of the fetus (occiput in cephalic presentations) and the planes of the birth canal.

13. **(C)** Generally, the fetus assumes an attitude with the arms and legs crossed in front of the body and the back curved in a convex manner. The head is generally flexed for best delivery. The cord usually occupies the space between the extremities.

14. **(E)** Fourteen-hour labors are average, but there is a great deal of variation. However, marked prolongation of any stage merits reevaluation to determine the reason. A systematic way to look at dysfunctional labor patterns is to see if there is a problem with the power (uterine contractions), passenger (fetal size and position of presenting part), and passageway (bony pelvic, full bladder, etc.). Warning signs must be observed to prevent catastrophe. Labor curves can give an excellent indication as to the diagnosis of abnormalities and prediction of when delivery will occur.

15. **(E)** By considering both frequency and intensity during a time period, an evaluation of contractile forces can be made. Quality of the contractions must also be known. Palpation or external monitoring cannot be used. Internal monitors must be used to accurately determine the pressure measurement. By convention >200 Montevideo units in 10 minutes is considered adequate.

16. **(D)** Pressures produced by the uterine fundus around the placenta have been measured at 300 mm Hg. Such pressure is enough to stop uterine bleeding and is a physiologic protective mechanism.

17. **(C)** A theory to explain the initiation of labor is that lysosomes containing phospholipase A become unstable at term due to decreased progesterone. The phospholipase A is released and causes release of arachidonic acid from phosphatidylglycerol found in the fetal membranes. The arachidonic acid then forms prostaglandins that initiate myometrial contractions. This is one of several theories regarding the initiation of labor. None have been shown to be completely satisfactory in explaining the phenomenon.

18. **(C)** When engagement has occurred, the inlet is adequate for that particular head. The midplane or outlet may not be. Also, the attainment of zero station by the head does not automatically imply engagement, although the head usually is engaged. If molding has changed the normal skull measurements, the presenting part may be at zero station before the greatest biparietal diameter of the head passes the pelvic inlet.

19. **(C)** This condition usually corrects itself as the head seeks the largest area in the pelvis.

Posterior asynclitism means the sagittal suture is closer to the sacrum. This may occur as the head seeks more room.

20. **(C)** *Bloody show* is a term used to describe the blood-tinged mucus that often precedes labor by a few hours to days. It is not pathologic and bleeding is not profuse. It occurs as a result of tearing of small veins in the cervix secondary to cervical effacement and dilatation in preparation for labor.

21. **(D)** Placental accretion markedly inhibits placental separation. If the uterus does not contract well postpartum, it may not exert sufficient force to shear the placenta from the decidua of the uterus. This will keep the uterus from contracting to close uterine sinusoids, resulting in heavy bleeding. The change in uterine configuration that occurs during and after delivery is the cause of placental separation. The lack of change from a discoid to globular shape should raise the concern for an undiagnosed twin.

22. **(E)** The lack of bleeding and shape of the uterus are clues that the placenta has not yet separated. The firm uterus makes retroplacental bleeding unlikely. Gentle massage to stimulate uterine contractions will probably result in placental separation, after which expulsion will occur rapidly. Pulling on the cord may avulse it from the placenta or even invert the uterus. The use of methergine may cause a strong tetanic contraction that can trap the placenta.

23. **(D)** Because of a rapid onset of action and a rapid metabolism, oxytocin should be closely monitored during its administration. Its IV use can cause transient hypotension that may be especially dangerous in patients with heart disease. The half-life of oxytocin is about 3 minutes. Why oxytocin does not always work to induce contractions is unknown.

24. **(E)** Although in some conditions a face presentation may deliver vaginally, cesarean section is the best option for this patient with thick meconium, a higher station with poor prenatal care, and a large infant.

25. **(D)** The Bishop score was originally developed to evaluate patients prior to induction of labor. It predicts the ease of inducibility based on cervical dilatation, effacement, consistency, position, and station of the vertex. Scores of 0 to 3 are assigned for each parameter, with higher total scores predicting a more favorable prognosis for induction. This patient's score is 6, indicating that the cervix is becoming ripe.

26. **(C)** This woman is in the latent phase of labor, which is the period between regular contractions and the onset of more rapid cervical dilatation (active phase). Latent phase is considered prolonged when it lasts longer than 20 hours in the nullipara and more than 14 hours in the parous woman. This primigravida has had 14 hours of latent-phase labor, which is not considered prolonged. Most authorities recommend therapeutic rest, if any action is to be taken.

27. **(B)** This gravida is in the active phase of labor, when there is an increased rate of cervical dilatation. This occurs by 4-cm dilation for most women. No cervical change after 2 hours is defined as an active-phase arrest. Arrest is a term used in situations where no change in a process has been noted over a period of time (commonly in 1–2 hours). Dilatation is used to describe the dilation of the cervix and descent refers to the movement of the presenting part through the pelvic axis.

28. **(B)** An appropriate step in the evaluation of abnormal labor patterns is the determination of the adequacy of uterine contractions, which can be done accurately with the use of an intrauterine pressure catheter. Since this patient's uterine activity is suboptimal, augmentation with oxytocin is indicated.

29. **(E)** Routine episiotomy is no longer performed. Episiotomy can be useful to expedite deliveries in the setting of fetal heart rate abnormalities or to enable appropriate maneuvers in relieving a shoulder dystocia. There is no evidence that episiotomy reduces the likelihood of pelvic relaxation later in life. Furthermore, recent studies have demonstrated an increased likelihood of

third- or fourth-degree lacerations after cutting an episiotomy.

30. **(D)** The ability of uterine muscle to retract allows a progressive diminution of the intrauterine cavity size, which gradually expels the fetus through the thinned-out lower segment and vagina. The upper segment contracts while the lower segment and cervix thins out and dilates to result in expulsion of the fetus. Uterine muscle is unique in function.

31. **(B)** Uterine bleeding is minimized postpartum by contraction of the myometrium and not by an increase in clotting factors. Women of high parity are at risk for uterine atony. Gravidas with severe pre-eclampsia are volume contracted and are less tolerant of excessive blood loss. Significant changes in pulse and blood pressure generally do not occur until large amounts of blood have been lost. Atony and retained placenta, followed closely by genital tract lacerations, are the most common causes of postpartum hemorrhage. Accreta is a very rare cause.

32. **(D)** Indications for induction of labor include prolonged pregnancy, diabetes mellitus, Rh isoimmunization, pre-eclampsia, premature or prolonged rupture of membranes, chronic hypertension, placental insufficiency, and suspected intrauterine growth retardation. Ideally, the fetus should be mature and the cervix should be favorable or "ripe": anterior, well effaced (50% or more), and dilated 1 to 2 cm. The head should also be well down in the pelvis. There are, unfortunately, no guarantees of delivery based on cervical assessment alone. Contraindications to induction include clear cephalopelvic disproportion, placenta previa, transverse lie, breech presentations, multiple gestation, and grand multiparity. Also any surgery on the uterus that has entered the uterine cavity through the upper active portion of the uterus. Such surgeries could include myomectomy, cornual resection from a cornual pregnancy, or a classical (vertical uterine) incision.

33. **(D)** Speculum examination revealing vaginal pooling, demonstrating an alkaline pH on nitrazine paper, is suggestive but may have other conditions in which there is no definite rupture of membranes; ferning on microscopic examination after drying on a slide confirms rupture of membranes. Pelvic examination may suggest this as well because, as the cervix dilates, palpation of amniotic membranes covering the presenting part (or an absence of the membranes) is usually possible. Coombs' test is a serologic test evaluating maternal sensitization to fetal red blood cells.

34. **(B)** This patient has premature rupture of membranes. Using the risk-based approach, she should receive GBS prophylaxis, since rupture of membranes is greater than 18 hours. Other criteria for administering antibiotics would be maternal fever greater than or equal to 100.4°F or a history of a previous birth of an infant with GBS disease. To minimize infectious complications for both the patient and her infant, she should be delivered promptly, but labor augmentation rather than cesarean section is indicated. If a rapid PCR testing for GBS is available, antibiotics should probably be started while waiting for the result of rapid testing.

35. **(E)** The uterus often changes in its profile when the fetal head drops. In primigravidas, lightening usually occurs prior to the onset of labor, whereas in multigravidas, it often occurs after the onset of labor. This engagement usually occurs after 37 weeks' gestation.

36. **(A)** This stage begins with the onset of true labor. Complete cervical dilation is one criterion that must be met for the application of forceps. No "pushing" should occur before full dilation.

37. **(C)** This stage ends with the delivery of the placenta. It includes placental separation and expulsion and should usually be accomplished within 20 minutes after the fetus is delivered. Otherwise, the cervix may partially close, entrapping the placenta.

38. **(B)** This stage covers that period of time during which the soft tissues of the perineum are distended by the fetus. It should not take longer than 2 hours or 20 normal uterine contractions,

with good maternal voluntary effort. Prolongation is an indicator of fetal–pelvic disproportion or poor maternal effort.

39. **(E)** The four classic maneuvers give much information regarding the presentation of the fetus. One palpates successively the fundus, the small parts, the suprapubic area, and the area of the anterior inlet. Leopold's maneuvers should be performed from 36 weeks onward.

40. **(C)** External cephalic version is performed in an attempt to avoid vaginal breech delivery or cesarean section for malpresentation. It involves rotation of the fetus through the maternal abdomen. Reported success ranges from 60% to 75%.

41. **(A)** The McRoberts maneuver promotes delivery of the anterior shoulder. It involves hyperflexion of the maternal legs onto the maternal abdomen, which results in ventral rotation of her pelvis to maximize the size of the outlet.

42. **(D)** Control of the fetal head to prevent its rapid expulsion with concomitant perineal and dural tearing is important. Pushing is stopped and a gentle lift applied through the perineum to slowly deliver the head in a controlled manner.

43. **(E)** To prevent postpartum hemorrhage, the best method would be to give misoprostol per rectum. Waiting to give oxytocin is ill advised. Oxytocin is best given at the time of delivery, and for this patient 10 units may be a small amount—an IV infusion would be a better option. Extra IV lines, and type and crossing blood, are important preparations but will not prevent a hemorrhage. Use of methergine if there have been no hypertensive issues works well and through a different mechanism than the rhythmic contractions by oxytocin or prostaglandin medications.

44. **(C)** This patient is at risk for shoulder dystocia. Being obese and having a fetus with extra adipose tissue and extra amniotic fluid are all warning signs. In addition her 1 hour was 138. Using a cutoff of 140 will only identify 80% of gestational diabetics. In very obese women, many clinicians will use 130 as a cutoff for the 50-g screen. In regards to management checking maternal blood sugars will not help with a shoulder dystocia, nor will having extra blood available. Delivery in the operating room may make matters worse, as it is often difficult to maneuver morbidly obese women on an operating room table. The extra attendants will be most valuable to help flex her thighs for the McRoberts.

45. **(C)** This woman is at risk for hypoxia from sleep apnea with her morbid obesity. $O_2$ saturation is an essential part of her immediate postoperative recovery, should she have a cesarean section. Most anesthesiologists will recommend using 94% as a cutoff for her $O_2$ saturations. If she has long-term sleep apnea giving to much oxygen is problematic, because she will be using low oxygen for her respiratory drive instead of high $CO_2$. Her predelivery level will not be as helpful as a guide because of her obstetric problems.

# CHAPTER 11

# Abnormal Labor and Delivery

## Questions

**DIRECTIONS (Questions 1 through 53): For each of the multiple choice questions in this section, select the lettered answer that is the one *best* response in each case.**

1. What is the maximum normal time for the second stage of labor in a primigravida without anesthesia?

    (A) 20 minutes
    (B) 60 minutes
    (C) 120 minutes
    (D) 240 minutes
    (E) no normal maximum

2. You are asked to consult on a 26-year-old woman (gravida 2, para 1) with a prior cesarean section because of breech positioning. She is at term. The nurse has plotted the labor curve (see Figure 11–1). What is the initial step in the evaluation and treatment of the most likely cause of this labor curve?

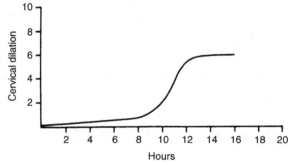

**Figure 11–1.**

    (A) administer oxytocin
    (B) assess pelvic adequacy
    (C) give sympathetic block
    (D) rupture membranes
    (E) perform cesarean section

3. Which of the following is the most common indication for primary cesarean section?

    (A) dystocia
    (B) prolapsed cord
    (C) diabetes
    (D) toxemia
    (E) malpresentation

4. Preterm rupture of the membranes is most strictly defined as spontaneous rupture at any time prior to which of the following?

    (A) a stage of fetal viability
    (B) the second stage of labor
    (C) the 32nd week of gestation
    (D) the onset of labor
    (E) the 37th week of gestation

5. You are examining a term patient in the labor and delivery (L&D) suite. Which of the following signs and symptoms is most likely to indicate ruptured membranes?

    (A) vaginal pool pH of 6.5
    (B) yellow-green color on nitrazine test
    (C) ferning on a specimen from the vaginal pool
    (D) superficial squamous cells in the vaginal pool
    (E) copious leakage on pants or underwear

6. Which of the following factors tends to increase the average duration of labor?

    (A) increasing parity
    (B) increasing age of the mother
    (C) decreasing size of the baby
    (D) occiput posterior (OP) position of the baby
    (E) ambulation

7. A fetus presents in breech position and is delivered without assistance as far as the umbilicus. The remainder of the body is manually assisted by the obstetrician. What is this called?

    (A) version and extraction
    (B) spontaneous breech delivery
    (C) partial breech extraction
    (D) total breech extraction
    (E) Pipers to the aftercoming head

8. A 28-year-old G3P2002 patient presents at 38 weeks' gestation. A fetus was felt to be in breech position as judged by information gained through Leopold's maneuvers. The fetus was well down in the pelvis, and the uterus was irritable. Pelvimetry was within normal limits, and the estimated fetal weight was 7$\frac{1}{2}$ lb and ultrasound confirms a frank breech with a well-flexed head and AFI of 14 cm. Assuming the provider has adequate experience in each of the following, what would not be offered to the patient as an approach to delivery management?

    (A) cesarean section
    (B) external cephalic version
    (C) internal podalic version
    (D) vaginal breech delivery
    (E) expectant management

9. Transverse lie in a multipara at term in labor is best treated by which of the following?

    (A) external version
    (B) internal version and extraction
    (C) oxytocin induction
    (D) cesarean delivery
    (E) abdominal support to effect position change

10. A 30-year-old methamphetamine user presents to L&D in active labor. She has had no prenatal care, but says she is 9$\frac{1}{2}$ months. You check fetal position and feel face and nose. You are concerned, because the most common associated condition with a face presentation is which of the following?

    (A) anencephaly
    (B) hydrocephaly
    (C) prematurity
    (D) placenta previa
    (E) oligohydramnios

11. A patient has entered spontaneous premature labor at 28 weeks' gestation. During the vertex delivery, one should do which of the following?

    (A) recommend epidural anesthesia to control delivery
    (B) perform an episiotomy
    (C) use prophylactic forceps
    (D) use vacuum extraction
    (E) allow spontaneous vaginal birth

12. A patient becomes suddenly unresponsive during active labor. The absolute diagnosis of amniotic fluid emboli is made by which of the following?

    (A) chest pain
    (B) chest X-ray
    (C) amniotic debris in the pulmonary circulation
    (D) the presence of consumptive coagulopathy
    (E) electrocardiogram (ECG) changes

13. Which of the following is a contraindication to the use of oxytocin for stimulating labor?

    (A) fetal demise
    (B) hypertonic uterine dysfunction
    (C) hypotonic uterine dysfunction
    (D) twin gestation
    (E) estimated fetal weight less than 5 lb

14. In which of the following cases might internal podalic version be indicated?

    (A) vertex delivery of the first twin and breech presentation of the second twin
    (B) term transverse lie with cervix completely dilated and membranes intact
    (C) double footling breech
    (D) impacted shoulder presentation
    (E) compound presentation

15. A 34-year-old woman (gravida 4, para 3) at $38\frac{1}{2}$ weeks whose pregnancy is complicated by gestational diabetes is in labor. The head delivers, but the shoulders do not follow. An efficacious method of delivery for a shoulder dystocia includes McRoberts maneuver. McRoberts maneuver is described as which of the following?

    (A) fundal pressure
    (B) extreme flexion of the maternal thighs
    (C) rotation to an oblique position after delivery of posterior arm
    (D) strong traction on the head
    (E) rotation of the posterior shoulder to the anterior

16. A 29-year-old G4P3003 with three prior C-sections is diagnosed with a placenta accreta at 28 weeks during follow-up ultrasound of a low anterior placental location. When is placenta accreta most likely to cause bleeding?

    (A) during the first stage of labor
    (B) prior to labor
    (C) because of consumption coagulopathy
    (D) after amniotic membrane rupture
    (E) during attempts to remove it

17. The risk of serious infection transmitted by blood transfusion is greatest for which of the following?

    (A) hepatitis C
    (B) Creutzfeldt–Jakob disease
    (C) human immunodeficiency virus (HIV)
    (D) syphilis
    (E) hepatitis B

18. If blood must be given without adequate cross-matching, what is the best type to use?

    (A) AB Rh-positive
    (B) AB Rh-negative
    (C) O Rh-positive
    (D) O Rh-negative
    (E) A Rh-positive

19. Which of the following factors is associated with small infants?

    (A) mothers with untreated gestational diabetes
    (B) multiparity
    (C) large parents
    (D) maternal smoking
    (E) postdate pregnancy

20. A 28-year-old G1P0 presents in active labor at term. Her history is remarkable only for a LEEP 4 years prior for HGSIL. The labor was complicated by complete effacement of the cervix and descent of the vertex at +1 station. However, the cervix did not dilate. A dimple may be noted at the external os. What is this condition called?

    (A) uterine dystocia
    (B) conglutinate cervix
    (C) cervix condupulare
    (D) sacculated uterus
    (E) vasa previa

21. A 26-year-old woman is first seen at 28 weeks' gestation. Her history and physical are normal except for the presence of a 2-cm posterior cervical leiomyoma. The patient is relatively asymptomatic. Which of the following is the best management for this patient?

    (A) myomectomy at 36 weeks
    (B) myomectomy now with steroids and tocolysis
    (C) progesterone therapy to decrease the myoma size
    (D) elective cesarean delivery at term
    (E) watchful waiting

22. After a low forceps delivery for fetal intolerance, a mother continues to have excessive vaginal bleeding despite a well-contracted uterus. Which of the following locations is most likely to be the site of a vaginal laceration after an instrumented delivery?

    (A) extending off the cervix
    (B) anterior upper third under the pubic symphysis
    (C) posterior upper third from an incompletely evacuated rectum
    (D) lateral middle third over the ischial spines
    (E) posterior middle third over the coccyx

23. A patient sustained a laceration of the perineum during delivery. It involved the muscles of the perineal body but not the anal sphincter. Such a laceration would be classified as which of the following?

    (A) first degree
    (B) second degree
    (C) third degree
    (D) fourth degree
    (E) fifth degree

24. A 19-year-old primiparous woman develops postpartum hemorrhage unresponsive to oxytocin and uterine massage. Her infant was 8.5 pounds. She has bled 750 cc. What is the most likely diagnosis?

    (A) laceration(s) of cervix or vagina
    (B) placenta accreta
    (C) uterine inversion
    (D) ruptured uterus
    (E) coagulopathy

25. A woman develops bleeding at 5-cm dilation with fetal distress. You perform a cesarean birth and find a couvelaire uterus. Which of the following causes a couvelaire uterus?

    (A) enlargement and invasion by placental tissue into the uterus
    (B) uterine, retroflexion, and adherence to the cul-de-sac peritoneum of the uterine serosa

    (C) a congenital anomalous development of the uterus
    (D) intramyometrial bleeding
    (E) Intrauterine infection

26. Which of the following situations has the greatest risk for the mother and infant?

    (A) rupture of an intact uterus
    (B) rupture of a previous uterine scar
    (C) pathologic contraction ring
    (D) dehiscence of a uterine scar
    (E) cervical laceration

## Questions 27 and 28 apply to the following patient

A 35-year-old woman (gravida 7, para 5, abortus 1) is in the active phase of labor with the vertex at −1 station. She complains of abdominal pain with the contractions. At the height of one contraction, the pain becomes very intense. Following this intense pain, uterine contractions cease. The maternal systolic BP drops 15 mm Hg.

27. What is the best course of action?

    (A) immediately perform a pelvic examination
    (B) place the patient on her side and reassure her
    (C) manage expectantly
    (D) begin oxytocin
    (E) perform an ultrasound

28. On abdominal examination, you discover a firm mass in the pelvis. It does not feel like the presenting fetal part. What is the most likely cause of the firm mass?

    (A) the placenta
    (B) a uterine fibroid
    (C) the contracted uterus
    (D) the fetal head
    (E) a pelvic kidney

29. A woman without prenatal care in labor at 38 weeks has a breech presentation. As the breech is expelled, a spina bifida is noted. The head does not deliver. With this history, what is the most likely problem?

    (A) hydrocephaly
    (B) cephalopelvic disproportion (CPD)
    (C) fetal goiter
    (D) missed labor
    (E) incompletely dilated cervix

30. Epidural anesthesia is preferable in which maternal condition?

    (A) to avoid maternal valsalva with bearing down in mother with previous cesarean section
    (B) multiple gestation
    (C) maternal cardiac disease
    (D) compound presentation
    (E) premature labor with a fetus <28 weeks

31. A patient in labor with a systolic BP of 125 mm Hg has just been given a saddle block. While lying on her back pushing on the delivery table, the level of the block stabilized at T10, fetal heart tones (FHTs) show a bradycardia to 105 bpm. However, her blood pressure drops to 90 mm Hg systolic. Which of the following is the most likely cause of these symptoms?

    (A) high spinal block
    (B) ruptured uterus
    (C) cardiac failure
    (D) amniotic fluid embolism
    (E) supine hypotensive syndrome

32. Which of the following indications most likely predict a classic cesarean section as opposed to a traditional transverse lower uterine segment cesarean section?

    (A) maternal Crohn's disease
    (B) vertical skin incision, unknown previous uterine incision
    (C) 26-week gestation with a breech presentation

    (D) fundal myoma
    (E) twins, with the first baby in a breech presentation

33. Which of the following situations would be likely to have the complication of a contracted pelvis?

    (A) Marfan's disease
    (B) long-standing maternal drug use
    (C) pendulous abdomen in a primigravida
    (D) morbidly obese multigravida
    (E) short maternal stature

34. The pathologic retraction ring of Bandl is most commonly associated with which of the following?

    (A) premature labor
    (B) uterine fibroids
    (C) obstructed labor
    (D) precipitate labor
    (E) multiple gestation

35. You are called to L&D to consult on a 23-year-old primiparous patient. The fetus has been at −2/−1 station for 4 hours with no dilation past 6 cm. Contractions are firm every 5 minutes. FHTs are reassuring with occasional early deceleration. EFW is 8 lb. You believe her pelvis is adequate. What is the next step?

    (A) forceps delivery
    (B) cesarean section
    (C) therapeutic rest
    (D) intrauterine pressure catheter to determine Montevideo units
    (E) parenteral analgesics

36. Term labors lasting less than 3 hours are associated with which of the following conditions?

    (A) decreased fetal morbidity
    (B) less maternal morbidity
    (C) increased fetal morbidity
    (D) primiparous labors
    (E) twins

**37.** You are delivering a 22-year-old woman's (gravida 2, para 0010) twin pregnancy at 38 weeks. The first baby is 6 $\frac{1}{2}$ lb estimated fetal weight and vertex. The second baby is estimated at 6 lb and breech. In discussing complications of internal podalic version, you discuss which of the following with the patient?

(A) fecal contamination

(B) postpartum hemorrhage

(C) perineal tear

(D) undiagnosed hydrocephaly

(E) fetal trauma

**38.** Your patient has been in labor for over 12 hours and has developed a temperature of 101.2°F. Pulse is 110 bpm. The fetal heart rate is 180 with good variability. The labor is progressing adequately. Which of the following is your next step in management?

(A) intravenous (IV) hydration

(B) antibiotics

(C) oxytocin

(D) fetal scalp sampling

(E) cesarean delivery

**Questions 39 and 40 apply to the following patient:**

A laboring patient receiving oxytocin for augmentation of labor suddenly clutches her chest in pain. Amniotic fluid embolus (AFE) is suspected.

**39.** The initial signs and symptoms occurring with AFE include which of the following?

(A) cyanosis and respiratory distress

(B) renal disease

(C) fever

(D) coagulopathy

(E) tumultuous labor and contractions

**40.** Treatment for AFE may include which of the following?

(A) hysterectomy

(B) oxygen and respiratory support

(C) antibiotics

(D) corticosteroids

(E) avoidance of prostaglandins

**41.** You are checking a 22-year-old primigravida in active labor. Labor has lasted 14 hours. She is 8-cm dilated and at 0 station. As the fetal head has descended, the shape has changed. Which of the following is the most likely etiology?

(A) cephalohematoma

(B) molding

(C) subdural hematomas

(D) hydrocephalus

(E) caput succedaneum

**42.** A 42-year-old G4P2012 has had a complicated prenatal course due to chronic hypertension and Type 2 diabetes. She also has adult onset asthma made worse with aspirin. Because of worsening hypertension an induction was initiated. She dilated to 5 cm and then did not progress further over the next 3 hours. Labor dystocia is likely due to which of the following issues?

(A) maternal hypertensive disorders

(B) ineffective uterine contractions

(C) maternal pulmonary disease

(D) hyperglycemia

(E) electrolyte imbalance

**43.** Certain patients are more likely than others to have uterine atony and hemorrhage after delivery. Circumstances that predict possible increased bleeding postpartum include which of the following situations?

(A) prolonged labor

(B) primigravidas

(C) hypertensive disorders

(D) pudendal anesthesia for delivery

(E) obesity

44. You have just delivered an 18-year-old woman (gravida 1, para 0). She is pre eclamptic. Her uterus is soft with moderate-to-heavy bleeding. Examination reveals no laceration. You diagnose uterine atony. Which of the following is the best management option?

    (A) 0.2-mg intramuscular (IM) ergonovine (Methergine)
    (B) 0.2-mg oral ergonovine
    (C) 10 units of oral oxytocin
    (D) 250 $\mu$g prostaglandin F2-alpha orally
    (E) 20 units of IV oxytocin

45. A 31-year-old healthy woman (gravida 3, para 2) is in labor at 40 weeks' gestation. Her first delivery was a low transverse cesarean for breech; the second was an uncomplicated VBAC. Her vital signs have been stable. Her epidural is functioning and she is lying on her side. When the cervix was approximately 7-cm dilated and the fetus was at −1 station, she developed tachycardia to 120 and a drop in blood pressure from 115/60 to 70/30. She has become dizzy upon sitting up. FHTs are 130. No bleeding is evident. The hematocrit is reported at 35%. What is your primary diagnosis?

    (A) vasa previa
    (B) pulmonary embolus
    (C) chorioamnionitis
    (D) supine hypotensive syndrome
    (E) ruptured uterus

**Questions 46 through 48 apply to the following patient:**

A 27-year-old G3P3 has delivered a 9.5lb female after a 21-hour labor in which contractions were augmented with oxytocin. The placenta delivered intact. Her perineum has a second-degree laceration.

46. As you begin to repair the perineum, you also have the nurse administer which of the following?

    (A) misoprostol per vagina
    (B) misoprostol per rectum
    (C) oxytocin orally

    (D) prostaglandin F2-alpha IM
    (E) oxytocin IV

47. After repair of the laceration, the patient continues to bleed heavily. She has lost 350 cc of blood. At this step you should assess uterine tone and do which of the following?

    (A) inspect the cervix and upper vagina for lacerations
    (B) do a manual exploration of the uterus for retained products of conception
    (C) do a bedside ultrasound to evaluate for retained products
    (D) place a second large bore IV line
    (E) place a foley catheter

48. After 45 minutes, the patient has lost 1,400 cc. The uterus is very "boggy" and does not contract well. Pulse is 105 bpm, blood pressure is 95/58, and oxygenation is 98%. Studies show a hemoglobin of 7.2 with a hematocrit of 22%, a platelet count of 95,000. What should be your next step?

    (A) recheck of the hematocrit
    (B) evaluate for HELLP syndrome
    (C) prepare for laproscopy
    (D) transfer 2 units packed cells and 2 units fresh frozen plasma
    (E) evaluate for von Willebrand's disease

**Questions 49 and 50 apply to the following patient:**

A 17-year-old G2P0AB woman with no prenatal care at 29 weeks' gestation presents with painful contractions and pressure. Her cervix is 3 cm, 60% effaced, and breech at −2 station. There is no evidence of ruptured membranes. Her contractions are every 3 minutes. FHT are 150 with accelerations. Maternal vital signs are temperature 36.8 degrees, pulse 96, BP 110/72.

49. What should you do?

    (A) perform amniocentesis to rule out chorioamnionitis
    (B) begin tocolytic agents
    (C) do a fetal fibronectin
    (D) observe to look for cervical change
    (E) give IV hydration

**50.** The patient continues to contract, and a repeat pelvic examination is notable for a cervix of 3 cm, 90%. What should you do?

(A) give antenatal steroids
(B) start antibiotics
(C) give IV sedation
(D) give IV hydration
(E) prepare for a cesarean delivery

**51.** Match the following fetal heart rate tracing (Figure 11–2) with the descriptive term that best fits the situation.

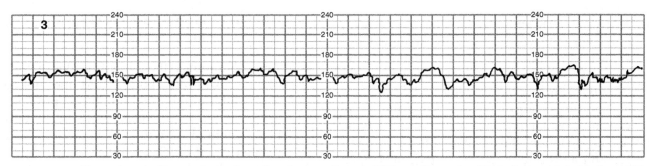

**Figure 11–2.** (Reproduced with permission from Cunningham F, et al. *Williams Obstetrics*, 23rd ed. New York: McGraw-Hill, 2010, p. 418.)

(A) early decelerations
(B) late decelerations
(C) normal tracing
(D) poor variability
(E) sinusoidal pattern

**Questions 52 and 53 apply to the following patient:**

A GP woman at 38 weeks' gestation presents with contractions of minimal strength but occurring every 2 to 3 minutes lasting 45 to 50 seconds. The FHTs are reactive and reassuring. Her cervix is soft, 1cm dilated, 25% effaced, and the vertex is at −1 station. Her cervix is unchanged since yesterday when she was seen in clinic.

**52.** With what is this labor pattern is consistent?

(A) prodromal labor
(B) normal uterine wake sleep cycles
(C) primary arrest of labor
(D) secondary arrest of labor
(E) tachysystole

**53.** The patient states that she is exhausted and has not slept or eaten in 2 days. Her mother demands that you do something. What is your best plan of management?

(A) admit her to L&D and begin oxytocin
(B) admit her to L&D and begin misoprostol for cervical ripening
(C) send her home with reassurance
(D) have her walk for 1–2 hours and recheck
(E) admit and give her medication to rest and for pain

**DIRECTIONS (Questions 54 and 55):** The following group of questions is preceded by a list of lettered options. For each question, select the one lettered option that is *most* closely associated with it. Each lettered option may be used once, multiple times, or not at all.

(A) rupture of a classic uterine scar
(B) dehiscence of a uterine scar
(C) spontaneous rupture of an intact uterus
(D) cervical tear
(E) traumatic rupture of the intact uterus

**54.** A G5P5 patient develops marked bleeding after delivery of the infant that continues as severe hemorrhage after the spontaneous delivery of the placenta that appears intact on inspection. The bladder is empty. The uterine fundus is firm at the umbilicus. She has an epidural.

**55.** A 25-year-old G3P2 with prior low transverse cesarean delivery is found to have a paper thin lower uterine segment covered with only peritoneum at the time of a repeat cesarean section. She has no bleeding.

56. A 28-year-old G4P2 presents in labor at 37 weeks. You examine her and feel the nose and mouth of the fetus, with the chin closest to the maternal symphysis. She is 5 cm, 100% effaced, 0 station, external heart tones are reassuring, and EFW is 6 ½ lb. What should you do?

    (A) perform a cesarean delivery
    (B) allow labor to progress
    (C) give an epidural and very gently manually rotate the baby to vertex
    (D) give low-dose oxytocin until the head rotates to vertex
    (E) prepare and administer amnioinfusion

57. What position is this baby in (Figure 11–3)?

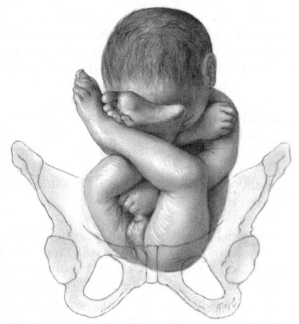

**Figure 11–3.** (Reproduced with permission from Cunningham F, et al. *Williams Obstetrics*, 23rd ed. New York: McGraw-Hill, 2010, p. 528.)

    (A) double breech lie
    (B) Frank breech presentation
    (C) double footling breech presentation
    (D) complete breech presentation
    (E) compound presentation

58. During the induction of labor of a 41.5-week multigravida woman, with misoprostol, the mother begins to feel increasing pelvic pressure and low back pain. FHTs are reassuring and maternal vital signs are p-92, BP 110/68, R-18; T-37 contractions are every 2 to 3 minutes and moderate. Her cervix is 2 cm 50%, −2 station with blood tinged mucus. What does this situation represent?

    (A) impending rupture of the uterus
    (B) normal early labor
    (C) tachysystole
    (D) misoprostol syndrome
    (E) primary arrest of labor

59. What is the most favorable clinical scenario for a successful trial of labor after cesarean birth?

    (A) only one previous cesarean delivery
    (B) anesthesia immediately available
    (C) a previous vaginal delivery
    (D) clear amniotic fluid
    (E) carefully induced labor between 39 and 40.5 weeks' gestation

# Answers and Explanations

1. **(C)** An exact time for optimum labor cannot be established, but prolonged labor leading to maternal exhaustion, often secondary to a disproportion, can lead to increased fetal morbidity. The accepted time for the second stage is usually 2 hours. This makes observation of labor curves and fetal monitoring essential parts of the management. If the patient has been effectively pushing for more than 2 hours without significant progress, one should review the 3 Ps: Power, Pelvis/Passageway, and Passenger—to be sure that there are no contraindications to a vaginal delivery such as a macrosomic infant or abnormal presentation. If none are found continuing to let the second stage continue longer is reasonable.

2. **(B)** The pattern is one of secondary arrest of labor. CPD is the most likely cause. Therefore, the first step is the evaluation of the pelvis/passageway in relationship to the estimated fetal weight. Be sure that bladder is empty. Persisting to attempt a delivery through an inadequate pelvis is always contraindicated.

3. **(A)** The most common indications for primary cesarean section are CPD and uterine inertia, which are the reasons for dystocia. The most common reason for all cesarean sections is the history of a prior cesarean section.

4. **(E)** Preterm rupture of membranes refers to rupture before 37 weeks' gestation. Arguments exist as to the most appropriate therapy for preterm rupture of membranes. If it occurs early in gestation, one must balance the risk of infection against the risk of prematurity if labor is induced. The greatest risk is intrauterine or fetal infection. Premature rupture is prior to the onset of labor and has nothing to do with gestational age.

5. **(C)** The pH of amniotic fluid is alkaline, 7.0 to 7.5, and the nitrazine paper should turn blue or blue-green. However, blood will cause this reaction also. Superficial squamous cells are found in the normal vagina. Drainage on the patient's underwear could be vaginal secretion or urine. Ferning is the fern-like crystal pattern created by the drying of vaginal pool fluid. It is present when there is a high saline concentration and supports the diagnosis of rupture of membranes.

6. **(D)** The length of labor generally lessens with increasing parity. The age of the mother alone does not affect labor. Smaller babies generally have a shorter second stage of labor. The OP position generally increases the total length of labor by 60 to 120 minutes.

7. **(C)** Partial breech extraction is a safe and effective means of delivering a breech. Piper forceps (specifically designed for the aftercoming head) may also be applied to the aftercoming head for control. Spontaneous delivery is also possible. Total breech extraction typically is done for the second twin. In this case, the feet of the second fetus are grabbed and pulled through the cervix with the rest of the body being delivered with manual traction.

8. **(C)** Current data suggest that a woman with breech presentation at term should be offered cesarean delivery. The Multisite Term Breech

Delivery Study found higher morbidity to the fetus in this situation. However, subsequent studies and review of the data interpretation of the Term Breech Delivery Study that revealed significant flaws have challenged the concept that a C-section is clearly best. It is now accepted that waiting for delivery (conservative management) since there can be a small possibility of a spontaneous version is acceptable. Also if the clinical expertise is available the use of external version and even a planned vaginal breech delivery are options. An internal breech version and extraction is done only for second twins.

9. **(D)** Often, a classic or vertical uterine incision is the wisest choice, as extracting the infant through a low transverse incision may be extremely difficult. The purpose of abdominal delivery is to avoid fetal trauma. An inadequate uterine incision would defeat this intention.

10. **(A)** Anencephalics often have face presentation because of the lack of a cranium. Breeches are common with prematurity and hydrocephalus. Placenta previa does not allow a presenting part in the pelvis.

11. **(E)** Vertex premature births may proceed spontaneously. In fact, use of a vacuum extraction may injure a premature infant presenting by vertex. The use of forceps or episiotomy does not protect the fetus from injury during a vaginal delivery.

12. **(C)** Ready access to the pulmonary vessels is available while placing a Swan–Ganz catheter to monitor the patient. Another way of diagnosing amniotic fluid emboli is finding debris in blood from the right heart. However, presumptive diagnosis is made from suggestive signs and symptoms that include abrupt onset of hypotension, hypoxia, and consumptive coagulopathy, and treatment is then begun which is primarily supportive.

13. **(B)** An absolute contraindication to the use of oxytocin is hypertonic uterine dysfunction. Oxytocin tends to increase hypertonic uterine dysfunction in the hypertonic uterus. Hypo-

tonic uterine dysfunction is the principal indication for oxytocin. A dead fetus will obviously not be adversely affected. If the uterus can tolerate labor, oxytocin can be used judiciously with close fetal monitoring in twin gestation, preterm infant or intrauterine growth restriction.

14. **(A)** The only indication for internal podalic version that is at all likely to occur is the second twin. A transverse lie with a completely dilated cervix and intact membranes is extremely rare. Also at term risk of developing into a head entrapment is real. A prolapsed cord with fully dilated cervix, unengaged vertex, and recently ruptured membranes is another possible indication, but this situation would be extremely rare also. Generally, cesarean section is a safer and more expeditious procedure.

15. **(B)** Shoulder dystocia creates an obstetric emergency. One must know what to do because no time will be available to read about it if it occurs. Many maneuvers have been described—all with fair success. You should know McRoberts maneuver, which is extreme flexion of the thighs. Others include suprapubic pressure and rotation of the posterior shoulders and delivery of posterior arm.

16. **(E)** A dictum in obstetrics is that a partially separated placenta bleeds. One that is not separated generally does not bleed. The bleeding occurs when attempts are made to deliver the placenta. Placenta accreta may require hysterectomy. Accretas are commonly associated with prior C-section or uterine surgery that violates nitabuch layer thereby allowing trophoblasts to invade the myometrium.

17. **(A)** Fortunately, the most feared infection (HIV) is the most rare, estimated at 1:300,000. Hepatitis is still the greatest risk for infection, although currently all blood for transfusion is checked for hepatitis B antigen, syphilis, and HIV among others.

18. **(D)** O-negative blood should not have A or B antigens, nor should it sensitize or cause a reaction with the D antigen of the Rh system.

**19. (D)** Smoking tends to cause a decrease in fetal size. Although people with mild, uncontrolled diabetes such as gestational diabetes have large children, severe diabetics tend to have "small-for-dates" infants. In multiparous patients, there is a tendency for subsequent children to be slightly larger. In postdate pregnancies, infants often continue to grow.

**20. (B)** One may start the cervical dilation by gently tearing the center of the cervix, after which dilation usually proceeds rapidly. This is a rare situation, and manual dilation is rarely indicated. There is no uterine dystocia since there has been complete effacement and descent to +1. Vasa previa is the umbilical cord over the cervix and this would not prevent cervical dilation. A sacculated uterus is caused by the persistent entrapment of the pregnant uterus in the pelvis causing marked thinning of the lower uterine segment to accommodate the fetus.

**21. (E)** In the absence of factors necessitating immediate action, the patient should be followed closely until the dangers of prematurity are past. Decision as to the mode of delivery will depend on the position and size of the tumor. Myomectomy during pregnancy may precipitate labor and is almost always a contraindication. Myomas may also undergo red (hemorrhagic) infarction during pregnancy, causing pain and bleeding.

**22. (D)** Excluding perineal tears in the lower third, the most likely position for vaginal tears is over the ischial spines. This site should be specifically examined. Suburethral and high lateral fornix areas should also be routinely examined, as well as the cervix.

**23. (B)** The usual classifications do not include fifth-degree tears. Some use fourth degree as being through the rectal mucosa, while others use third degree with extension to the rectum to designate the most severe laceration. An anatomic repair in layers without devitalizing of tissue should ensure good healing. First degree involves only the skin or vaginal mucosa. Second degree involves extends into the fascia and muscles that surround the vagina.

**24. (A)** Massage and oxytocin are a good regimen for uterine atony and may make even a ruptured uterus stop bleeding for a short time. After uterine atony, the next most common cause of bleeding postpartum is a laceration. Therefore, all postpartum bleeders should be reexamined to rule out such tears.

**25. (D)** The uterus can be enlarged because of extravasation of blood between the myometrial fibers. This is most commonly caused by placental abruption. If severe, this bleeding may inhibit uterine contractions, though such severity is quite rare. If stable and not expanding, the intramyometrial hematoma is best left alone! Coagulopathy and lack of specific bleeding sites dictate conservative therapy.

**26. (A)** Maternal mortality from rupture of an intact uterus may be as much as 10%. The infant's prognosis is much worse. Obstruction or hyperstimulation is the most common etiology. The dehiscence of a prior C-section scar often is an incidental finding at C-section from a failed treat of labor after C-section (TOLAC). Rupture of a prior uterine scar depending on where it can be as dangerous to mother and infant as the rupture of an intact uterus. A cervical laceration can result in significant maternal blood loss but tends not to injure the infant.

**27. (A)** This is a classic example of uterine rupture. If rupture has occurred, fetal mortality is very likely and one should anticipate the possibility of rapid onset of severe maternal shock. Emergent C-section delivery and mechanical methods will stop the maternal bleeding. Massive vascular support is often necessary to save the mother's life due to blood loss and DIC. A stat C-section may save the infant although fetal death is common in this setting.

**28. (C)** With the history of severe pain and cessation of contractions, the fetal head is probably no longer in the pelvis and the diagnosis of uterine rupture is more certain. Evaluation and treatment must be rapid.

**29. (A)** Spina bifida is noted in approximately one-third of fetuses with hydrocephaly. Its presence in the situation described should immediately warn of the defect. This can become a very difficult problem if no further assessment of the degree of hydrocephalus has been made.

30. **(C)** Epidural analgesia is often employed in women to prevent any bearing-down urges when the fetus descends onto the pelvic floor. Of these choices, maternal cardiac disease is the only option where that might be necessary. With the continuous epidural, the force of the uterine contractions is adequate to bring the presenting part to the perineum, where a vacuum or forceps may be used to assist delivery.

31. **(E)** The supine hypotension can be relieved by putting the patient on her side or pushing the uterus off of the great vessels to allow adequate cardiac return and aortic flow. Increased fluid administration and medication can both be used to elevate blood pressure.

32. **(C)** Physical factors making lower segment dissection difficult or time consuming certainly favor vertical incisions. Premature breech fetuses may present with a poorly developed lower uterine segment and a fetal head size that is typically larger than the breech, thus necessitating a vertical uterine incision. Maternal Crohn's and twins would not affect site of uterine incision.

33. **(E)** Short maternal stature of the choices given is a potential sign of a contracted pelvis. Other choices include face presentation, bone and mineral disease, and previous history of pelvic orthopedic trauma. Prior knowledge of borderline or absolute pelvic contraction can avert disaster. A good clue is an abnormal labor curve.

34. **(C)** If a prolonged obstructed labor is neglected, a thin and overdistended uterine segment may rupture. Cesarean section should be performed before a pathologic retraction ring has time to develop. In attended labor, Bandl's ring has become a rarity.

35. **(D)** This patient fills the picture of secondary arrest of labor. With contractions every 5 minutes oxytocin is likely indicated, given that she has not progressed in 4 hours. An intrauterine pressure catheter placement to verify adequate power is being achieved. Once adequate or no progress has been made then the diagnosis may be CPD and then a C-section may be needed. At this time there is no indication for cesarean section. The cervix is not dilated so forceps are not appropriate. Analgesics are reasonable but would not help labor.

36. **(B)** Precipitate labors have an increased rate of fetal brain damage and hypoxia and an increased maternal morbidity of postpartum hemorrhage and lacerations. Primiparous and twin delivery typically take much longer than 3 hours.

37. **(E)** Fetal trauma can occur, but if the procedure is done only for indicated reasons, such as delivery of the second twin, it should not be a major factor. Rupture of the lower uterine segment is a potential danger, especially if the segment is thinned out.

38. **(B)** IV antibiotics are indicated for infection. Cesarean delivery and oxytocin are not necessary if labor is progressing well. Although by giving the antibiotics by IV will result in IV hydration, which is not the primary intervention.

39. **(A)** The sudden onset of dyspnea, cyanosis, and shock during labor should make one immediately consider AFE, aspiration of gastric content, or heart failure. Immediate cardiorespiratory support should be given. The coagulopathy is almost pathognomonic for AFE but will not occur immediately. Primary concerns are respiratory support and prompt delivery of the infant to potentially save the infant and improve maternal respiratory status.

40. **(B)** Hysterectomy is only for uterine hemorrhage from DIC despite intervention of no use and will only add operative insult. Immediate use of corticosteroids is also of minimal benefit. Positive end expiratory pressure assisted respiration may be lifesaving in pulmonary edema from either cause. Steroids or antibiotics do not have significant value in this scenario. Prostaglandins may be used as appropriate for hemorrhage.

41. **(B)** Subdural hematomas, although they may occur, generally do not contribute to any marked change in shape. Cephalohematoma is a possibility, although it is unlikely to occur at this station. Molding is the most likely cause. Caput succedaneum is the part of the fetal head over the cervical os that becomes edematous. It usually attains a thickness of only a few millimeters but in case of prolonged labors it may become thicker. By looking at the location of the caput, one can determine the position of the vertex.

42. **(B)** One can think of dystocia as occurring because of some abnormality of the powers, the passenger, or the passage. Electrolyte imbalance, or other maternal issues such as maternal hypertensive disease play no known direct role.

43. **(A)** Other predictors of increased postpartum bleeding include past history of atony and high parity. Atony, injuries, and retained placental fragments are by far the most common. Obesity or hypertension alone is not a significant cause.

44. **(E)** Ergot derivatives should not be given in patients with hypertension, and oxytocin is not effective orally, though it has, in the past, been given by the buccal route. Prostaglandin F2-alpha is given IM.

45. **(E)** Although it is unusual for labor to persist with a ruptured uterus, it must be included in the differential. Vasa previa would cause immediate fetal distress. Pulmonary complication and anesthetic complication are also possibilities but do not account for all the signs. The mother has no apparent respiratory problems. Supine hypotension should not occur on her side.

46. **(E)** After delivery of the baby, it is appropriate to administer oxytocin. Since she has an IV line is receiving pitocin, and this is the best route. Misoprostol is a second-line alternative given orally as well as rectally but not per vagina as she would expel it with the postpartum bleeding. At this point IM F2-alpha is not needed. Oxytocin is not given orally.

47. **(A)** The patient's continued bleeding signals a problem. It is not yet a true hemorrhage (>500 cc); however, the next step is to make sure the fundus is firm and check for other sources of bleeding including cervix and vagina. The large infant and long labor will predispose to uterine atony as well.

48. **(D)** At this point the patient has developed a significant postpartum hemorrhage. Her vital signs are changing and her hemoglobin is low. A Foley catheter should be placed as well as a second IV line (16 guage preferably). She should be transfused at least 2 units of PRC. Current recommendations are 2:1 or 1:1 ratio of packed red blood cells (PRBC) to fresh frozen plasma. Laparoscopy is contraindicated. The low platelets are most likely from wash out not severe preeclampsia. And a recheck of the hemocult at this time is an unnecessary delay.

49. **(B)** The patient presents in preterm labor with a very premature infant. At 3-cm dilation, further observation is inappropriate. At 3-cm dilated the accuracy of the fibroection assay is less helpful. In addition if she just had a digital examination the test may be invalid. Amniocentesis is reasonable if there are signs of infection. However these are not obvious signs of infection. IV hydration is good for uterine irritability but with advanced dilation at this gestational age tocolytics are more important. Tococystic agents are indicated while assessment is begun.

50. **(A)** As her cervix changes antenatal steroids should be given, if they have not been given previously. If her labor stops cesarean delivery is unnecessary.

51. **(C)** This is a normal tracing or Category I with the new classification. There is no deceleration and variability is good. A sinusoidal pattern would contain regular–repetitive oscillations. They are not present here.

52. **(A)** This pattern is typical of prodromal or "false labor." Prior to cervical change there is not any arrest either primary or secondary. The contractions are less than 5/10 minutes, thus no tachysystole.

53. **(E)** Because she is exhausted and not in labor, the best option is pain relief and rest. Inducing labor

in a 38-week primiparous woman with an unfavorable cervix is an invitation for a poor outcome and is contraindicated. More walking will not help and given her second visit to us (seen earlier in clinic) she should be given something for relief.

54. **(D)** A deep cervical tear or vaginal laceration is the most likely cause of the bleeding in the situation described. Laceration probably occurred with dilation by the fetal head that provided some compression until delivery. The observation of marked bleeding that started prior to placental separation is concerning for lacerations as a source. Good visualization and assistance are often necessary to recognize and correct the problem. Lower segment rupture can also cause bleeding during the third stage but is extremely uncommon. In addition, the likelihood further decreases if the fundus contracts firmly.

55. **(B)** Dehiscence is not uncommon in low transverse scars. The fetal membranes remain intact, and labor can proceed normally if there is no obstruction. The risk of rupture is increased, however. Unless transvaginal examination is performed after normal delivery, these scar defects may never be found. Current recommendations are not to perform a transvaginal uterine exploration unless there is bleeding.

56. **(B)** The baby is mentum anterior. The pelvis is adequate and the baby is of reasonable size (not too large). Since FHTs are good it is reasonable to allow labor to continue as some of these fetuses will convert to vertex and some deliver spontaneously. If mentum posterior there is no way these infants can negotiate the pelvic curve and rarely deliver vaginally.

57. **(B)** This is a frank breech. A compound presentation usually refers to a hand and vertex simultaneously. In complete breech, both hips and one or both knees are flexed. An incomplete breech has one or both hips not flexed and the knee and foot is below the breech. A footling breech is a subtype of the incomplete breech.

58. **(B)** This is not tachysystole or ruptured uterus. These are all signs of normal early labor not an arrest of labor. Tachysystole is more than five contractions in 10 minutes.

59. **(C)** Rupture of the uterus after previous C-section occurs in approximately 0.5% of women. Successful trial of labor is defined as a vaginal birth after labor. The factor most strongly associated with successful trials is a previous vaginal birth. Spontaneous labor (vs. induced) and a C-section for breech versus CPD are also factors that indicate an increased likelihood of success.

# Operative Obstetrics

## Questions

1. A 23-year-old woman (gravida 1, para 0), approximately 6 weeks pregnant, comes to your clinic for treatment. A home pregnancy test was positive 1½ weeks ago. She has developed bleeding over the past 2 days. What is the most likely cause of the bleeding?

   (A) hydatidiform mole
   (B) abruptio placentae
   (C) ectopic pregnancy
   (D) abortion
   (E) uterine rupture

**Questions 2 through 4 apply to the following patient:**

A 19-year-old woman presents with 3 days of dark spotting and mild cramping at 9 weeks' gestation. An ultrasound notes a viable 9-week gestation with no obvious problems in the uterus or ovaries. You explain that she has a threatened abortion. She and her partner are concerned about what will happen if the pregnancy does not miscarry.

2. She asks about the risk of the fetus being abnormal. Which of the following can be said about the risk?

   (A) the same as in patients without bleeding
   (B) slightly increased
   (C) moderately increased
   (D) markedly increased
   (E) 99–100%

3. What should therapy for threatened abortion include?

   (A) progesterone intramuscular (IM)
   (B) dilation and curettage (D&C)
   (C) prolonged bed rest
   (D) restricted activity
   (E) prostaglandin suppositories

4. What may be the result of high doses of progesterone for threatened abortion?

   (A) save the fetus
   (B) keep the placenta alive
   (C) keep the corpus luteum functioning
   (D) cause habitual abortion
   (E) cause retention of a dead fetus

5. A 19-year-old has been bleeding intermittently for 26 weeks. She presents with a change to dark bleeding and minimal cramping for 4 days. Your clinic ultrasound notes an intrauterine fetal demise. She is distraught. She would prefer to let "nature take its course." She asks if there is any risk to her. What do you explain as the only significant risk?

   (A) a positive human chorionic gonadotropin (hCG) titer
   (B) systemic allergies
   (C) bone marrow depression
   (D) coagulopathy
   (E) toxemia

6. A 19-year-old G1P0 patient complains of spotting and right-side pain. She had a positive urine pregnancy test 3 weeks ago. Ultrasound does not identify an intrauterine pregnancy. On laparoscopy 125 cc of blood is seen in the pelvis. There is minimal blood from the tube and a small bit of tissue is recovered floating free in the peritoneal cavity. This pregnancy is likely which of the following?

   (A) spontaneous abortion
   (B) delivery
   (C) tubal abortion
   (D) decidual cast
   (E) Arias-Stella phenomenon

**Questions 7 through 9 apply to the following patient:**

A 26-year-old woman whose last menstrual period (LMP) was 2½ months ago develops bleeding, uterine cramps, and passes tissue per vagina. Two hours later, she is still bleeding heavily.

7. What is the most likely diagnosis?

   (A) twin pregnancy
   (B) threatened abortion
   (C) inevitable abortion
   (D) premature labor
   (E) incomplete abortion

8. The bleeding is most likely due to which of the following?

   (A) retained products of conception
   (B) ruptured uterus
   (C) systemic coagulopathy
   (D) vaginal lacerations
   (E) bleeding hemorrhoids

9. What is the indicated procedure?

   (A) hysterectomy
   (B) vaginal packing
   (C) compression of the hemorrhoids
   (D) intravenous (IV) fibrinogen
   (E) uterine curettage

**Questions 10 through 12 apply to the following patient:**

A 24-year-old woman (gravida 2, para 0, abortus 1) is seen in the emergency department because of vaginal bleeding and abdominal cramps. Her LMP was 10 weeks ago. History is unrevealing except for an induced abortion 2 years ago without complications. She presently denies instrumentation for abortion. Physical examination reveals a BP of 110/70 mm Hg, pulse 120, and temperature 101.8°F. The abdomen is tender with slight rebound in the lower quadrants. The pelvic examination reveals blood in the vault and a foul-smelling discharge from the cervix, which is dilated to 2 cm. The uterus is 8- to 10-week size and tender, and no adnexal masses are palpated.

10. What is the most likely diagnosis?

   (A) choriocarcinoma
   (B) hydatidiform mole
   (C) pelvic inflammatory disease (PID)
   (D) septic abortion
   (E) twisted ovarian cyst

11. Ring forceps through the cervix removed necrotic-appearing tissue. Which of the following laboratory studies would you consider most important to obtain prior to instituting antibiotic therapy?

   (A) white blood cell (WBC) count and hematocrit (Hct)
   (B) type and Rh
   (C) coagulation screen
   (D) Gram stain and culture
   (E) abdominal X-ray

12. Which of the following is definitive initial therapy in this case?

   (A) curettage after antibiotics
   (B) hysterectomy
   (C) bed rest and antibiotics
   (D) hysterotomy
   (E) outpatient antibiotics

13. Which of the following patients would be at greatest risk for ectopic pregnancy?

   (A) a healthy woman on birth control pills for longer than 18 months' duration

   (B) a woman with past history of three incidents of PID

   (C) a woman with history of endometriosis

   (D) a healthy woman with irregular menses

   (E) a woman with past history of several urinary tract infections (UTIs)

14. A 28-year-old G3P0AB2 has a quantitative hCG of 2,850. She has spotting and abdominal pain. An ultrasound shows fluid in the cal de sac and no intrauterine pregnancy. What is the most likely site of an ectopic pregnancy?

   (A) external fallopian tube

   (B) ovarian surface

   (C) mesosalpinx

   (D) ampulla of the fallopian tube

   (E) interstitial portion of the fallopian tube

15. During laparoscopy to rule out ectopic pregnancy, a tubal pregnancy is found. If untreated, where will the tube most commonly rupture?

   (A) urachus

   (B) bladder

   (C) space of Retzius

   (D) large bowel

   (E) peritoneal cavity

16. An intrastitial (cornual) pregnancy is discovered on ultrasound, and it is verified by laparoscopy. Which of the following best describes the condition?

   (A) It rarely exceeds 4 weeks' gestation.

   (B) It is generally more dangerous than an ampullary ectopic pregnancy.

   (C) It requires hysterectomy.

   (D) It is quite common.

   (E) It is extrauterine.

17. Four months after a loop electrosurgical excision procedure (LEEP) with an endocervical curettage, a 21-year-old presents with abdominal pain. Her uterus is slightly enlarged, pregnancy test is positive. She has no adnexal masses and is slightly tender over the bladder. An ultrasound detects a small cervical pregnancy without heart tones, but with an oblong yolk sac. After explaining to your patient the issue, which of the following do you recommend?

   (A) immediate delivery per vagina

   (B) transfuse as needed until viability of fetus is assured

   (C) cesarean section

   (D) chemotherapy with methotrexate

   (E) estrogen injections and bed rest

18. You are called to the operating room. The general surgeons have operated on a woman to rule out appendicitis and they find signs of an abdominal pregnancy with a 14-week fetus and placenta attached to the omentum. What is the best course of action in this case?

   (A) removal of both fetus and placenta

   (B) laparoscopic ligation of umbilical cord

   (C) removal of the fetus only

   (D) closely follow until viability and then deliver by laparotomy

   (E) IV methotrexate and removal of the fetus

19. What is the best diagnostic sign indicating an abdominal pregnancy?

   (A) positive pregnancy test

   (B) ultrasound view not demonstrating uterine wall between fetus and bladder

   (C) abnormal position of the fetus

   (D) lateral X-rays showing fetal parts overlying the maternal spine

   (E) uterine contractions with oxytocin administration

20. During a laparotomy for a suspected ectopic pregnancy in a 24-year-old woman who wishes to bear children, you find a ruptured left tubal ectopic with about 400 mL of blood in the peritoneal cavity. The other tube appears normal and the ovaries are uninvolved. What is the accepted treatment?

    (A) bilateral salpingectomy
    (B) left salpingectomy or salpingostomy
    (C) bilateral salpingo-oophorectomy (BSO)
    (D) hysterectomy and left salpingectomy
    (E) right salpingectomy

21. Application of forceps is appropriate in which of the following situations?

    (A) breech at +3 station, cervix completely dilated, membranes ruptured
    (B) vertex at +1 station, cervix completely dilated, membranes intact
    (C) mentum anterior, +3 station, cervix completely dilated, membranes ruptured
    (D) transverse lie, +3 station, cervix completely dilated, membranes ruptured
    (E) vertex at +3 station, cervix +9 cm dilated, membranes ruptured

22. Anticipating success, an obstetricion has made a concerted attempt to deliver a patient using forceps. The attempt fails. How is the procedure termed?

    (A) an incomplete delivery
    (B) a trial of forceps
    (C) malapplication of forceps
    (D) failed forceps
    (E) high forceps

23. You are delivering a woman (gravida 3, para 2) with two previous successful vaginal births. The woman has been in labor for 12 hours with a 10-hour first stage. The second stage of labor has lasted approximately 1 hour 14 minutes. The baby is doing well without any evidence of distress and of an appropriate size (approximately 8 lb). The mother has had an epidural and is tired from pushing, and you decide to apply forceps. After pelvic examination, forceps are applied to the presenting part of a term pregnancy, but the lock does not properly articulate even with gentle maneuvering. What should you do?

    (A) rotate the forceps
    (B) apply enough pressure to lock the forceps
    (C) exert traction
    (D) reapply the forceps
    (E) remove the forceps and perform cesarean delivery

24. There are many relative contraindications to the use of vacuum extraction for delivery if all else is appropriate. What would be an acceptable scenario for application of a vacuum extractor?

    (A) nonvertex presentation
    (B) fetal coagulopathies
    (C) cervix is 9 cm dilation with fetal intolerance of labor
    (D) fetal prematurity <35 weeks
    (E) fetal scalp electrode

**Questions 25 through 27 refer to the following patient:**

A 19-year-old primigravida at term has been in active labor for 4 hours. The membranes have just ruptured; the station is −3, fetal heart tones (FHTs) are 140 and regular, and the cervix is dilated 4 cm. Contractions are every 5 minutes and last approximately 40 seconds.

25. What is the next step in management?

    (A) patient ambulation
    (B) oxytocin augmentation
    (C) cesarean section
    (D) clinical pelvimetry and estimation of fetal size
    (E) turn the patient on her side

26. The patient continues to have infrequent contractions. Your clinical pelvimetry is within normal limits. Estimated fetal size is 7½ lb. Pelvic findings are unchanged. What is the next step in management?

(A) determine the maternal hydration status

(B) patient ambulation

(C) oxytocin infusion

(D) cesarean section

(E) await vaginal delivery

27. Three hours later, the cervix is 5-cm dilated and the contraction pattern is irregular despite significant oxytocin infusion. The station is –2 and the head is molded. The FHTs are normal. What is the next step in management?

(A) Duhrssen's incisions

(B) forceps delivery

(C) increased oxytocin

(D) heavy sedation

(E) cesarean section

28. You are counseling a couple in your clinic who desire VBAC (vaginal birth after cesarean section). Her baby is in a vertex presentation, appropriate size for 37 weeks, and her previous low transverse procedure was for breech presentation. In providing informed consent, in which of the following ways do you explain the risk of uterine rupture?

(A) less than 1%

(B) between 2% and 5%

(C) 15–20%

(D) dependent on the length of her labor

(E) dependent on the location and proximity of the scar site to the placental implantation

29. A pregnant woman at 32 weeks is brought to the emergency department after a motor vehicle accident with abdominal trauma. The fetus is dead and the mother is in shock. You diagnose an abruption and go to the operating room with trauma surgeons for a possible C-section delivery. You find bleeding into the myometrium beneath the uterine serosa. In severe cases, what is the cause of abruptio placentae?

(A) uteroplacental apoplexy

(B) uterine rupture

(C) minimal effect on fetal heart rate

(D) adnexal torsion

(E) disseminated intravascular coagulopathy (DIC)

30. Vaginal examination is contraindicated in which situation during pregnancy?

(A) carcinoma of the cervix

(B) gonorrhea

(C) prolapsed cord

(D) placenta previa

(E) active labor with ruptured membranes >6 hours

31. A 30-year-old woman (gravida 4, para 2, abortus 1) has been seen in the emergency department at 29 weeks' gestation because of the sudden onset of painless vaginal bleeding that soaked four perineal pads and has now ceased. The mother's vital signs and Hct are normal, and the FHTs are regular at 140 bpm. At this time, what should you do?

(A) perform a double setup examination

(B) order an ultrasound examination

(C) perform a cesarean section

(D) send the patient home on bed rest

(E) hospital observation with tocolysis as necessary

**Questions 32 and 33 apply to the following patient:**

32. A 35-year-old married woman (gravida 4, para 3, abortus 0), who now is at approximately 36 weeks' gestation, developed copious, painless, vaginal bleeding 2 hours prior to admission. On examination, the uterus appears soft and nontender. FHTs are 140 and regular, the vertex is floating, and there is no evident bleeding or signs of ruptured membranes. Maternal vital signs are stable. What is the most likely diagnosis?

(A) carcinoma of the cervix

(B) placenta previa

(C) abruptio placentae

(D) vasa previa

(E) hematuria

33. What is your next step in management?

    (A) amniocentesis for lung maturity studies
    (B) ultrasound for placental localization
    (C) continued hospital monitoring
    (D) very gentle vaginal examination of the fornices with care not to go through the os
    (E) speculum examination to visualize the cervix

34. Which woman is most likely to have placenta previa at 32 weeks with vaginal bleeding?

    (A) 19-year-old, gravida 1, para 0, vertex presentation
    (B) 24-year-old, gravida 2, para 1, breech presentation
    (C) 34-year-old, gravida 5, para 3, abortus 1, vertex presentation
    (D) 36-year-old, gravida 7, para 6, abortus 0, transverse lie
    (E) 28-year-old, gravida 3, para 1, abortus 1, breech presentation

35. The safest, most precise, and simplest method of placental localization is which of the following?

    (A) auscultation
    (B) ultrasonography
    (C) radioisotope study
    (D) abnormal palpation
    (E) soft tissue X-ray

36. A G7P6 patient presents in advance labor with a Frank breech presenting on the perineum. The vaginal breech delivers without difficulty until the head that becomes entrapped by the cervix. To release the head you need to perform Duhrssen's incisions, which are classically made at which position(s) on the cervix?

    (A) 8 o'clock
    (B) 9 and 3 o'clock
    (C) 10, 2, and 6 o'clock
    (D) 12 and 6 o'clock
    (E) anterior to the fetal chin and posterior to the occiput

**Questions 37 and 38 apply to the following patient:**

A walk-in patient has presented in labor with a double footling breech. As the buttocks are delivered, a meningomyelocele is seen. There is sudden arrest of progression, and the head cannot be delivered. Examination reveals a large mass above the pubis abdominally. Vaginal palpation confirms the impression of a grossly enlarged head.

37. What is the most probable diagnosis?

    (A) anencephaly
    (B) diabetic infant
    (C) hydrocephaly
    (D) huge goiter
    (E) polycystic kidneys

38. Internal version and extraction at term is indicated in which of the following?

    (A) face presentation mentum posterior
    (B) shoulder presentation in early labor
    (C) persistent brow
    (D) the second twin
    (E) transverse lie

**Questions 39 and 40 apply to the following patient:**

A pregnant patient at 37 weeks' gestation complains of nausea, anorexia, and upper midabdominal pain for 10 hours. Her physical examination is negative except for diffuse abdominal tenderness. Her temperature is 101°F, pulse 90, BP 110/60, FHTs 140, Hct 38, and WBC 11,900. Urinalysis is negative for protein and red blood cells (RBCs) are present.

39. What is the most likely diagnosis?

    (A) appendicitis
    (B) ureteral stone
    (C) degeneration of a myoma
    (D) eclampsia
    (E) pyelonephritis

40. On further evaluation, probable appendicitis is diagnosed. What is the treatment?

    (A) antibiotics and observation
    (B) cesarean section at the time of appendectomy
    (C) 24–48 hours of observation
    (D) immediate laparotomy and appendectomy if appendicitis is found
    (E) amniocentesis and if negative for infection—antibiotics without surgery

41. A 25-year-old patient at 27 weeks' gestation has complained of nausea, dull right flank pain persistent for 2 days, and mild diarrhea. She presently complains of pain in the mid right abdomen and flank. On examination, the pulse is 90, temperature is 100°F, and BP is 120/70 mm Hg. Her chest is clear, uterus is midway between the xiphoid and umbilicus and nontender, with FHTs at 140. Pelvic examination is within normal limits, as is the rest of the physical. Urinalysis reveals 50 to 100 WBCs/high power field (HPF). HCT is 37, WBC is 11,800. Which diagnosis is most likely?

    (A) duodenal ulcer
    (B) volvulus
    (C) degenerating leiomyoma
    (D) placental abruption
    (E) pyelonephritis

42. A 36-year-old woman (gravida 5, para 3, abortus 1) is first seen for her present pregnancy at 21 weeks' gestation. History and examination are within normal limits. A routine Pap smear is taken, which returns as high-grade squamous intraepithelial lesion (SIL) [cervical intraepithelial neoplasia (CIN) III]. What should you do?

    (A) repeat the Pap smear
    (B) advise abortion with cone biopsy or hysterectomy in 4–6 weeks
    (C) wait until after delivery and obtain another smear
    (D) perform a cesarean hysterectomy with wide vaginal cuff
    (E) perform colposcopy and biopsy

43. In a similar patient, a cone biopsy is performed. The cone specimen is obtained with a diagnosis of carcinoma in situ and free surgical margins. What is your advice?

    (A) follow the patient to term and allow vaginal delivery
    (B) perform a radical hysterectomy
    (C) perform a cesarean hysterectomy with wide vaginal cuff
    (D) give 6,000 rads whole-pelvic irradiation after delivery by cesarean section
    (E) perform a cesarean section at term

44. A 32-year-old woman is seen at 10 weeks' gestation. History and physical are normal except for the presence of a 9- to 10-cm simple asymptomatic cystic adnexal mass. What should be your management?

    (A) immediate laparotomy and further indicated surgery
    (B) repeat ultrasound in 4–6 weeks and then determine management plan
    (C) immediate total abdominal hysterectomy (TAH) and BSO
    (D) suppression of the cyst by estrogens
    (E) transcutaneous needle aspiration under ultrasound guidance

45. A pregnant patient at 18 weeks is found by biopsy to have carcinoma of the breast. What is the most appropriate management?

    (A) abortion and immediate irradiation
    (B) abortion and immediate breast surgery with node evaluation
    (C) immediate abortion, breast surgery with node evaluation, and irradiation
    (D) surgery on the breast, node, evaluation, and irradiation as indicated following delivery
    (E) conservative observation until after delivery at term

**46.** Treatment for severe abruptio placentae includes which of the following?

(A) heparin

(B) blood replacement and expectant management

(C) steroid therapy for pulmonary maturity

(D) monitoring of plasma fibrinogen and tocolysis with a calcium channel blocker (not a beta-mimetic)

(E) delivery

# Answers and Explanations

1. **(D)** The bleeding from any of these options may be profuse or minimal. Abortion is the most common. Up to one-third of all pregnancies are thought to end in early spontaneous abortion. Uterine rupture is very unlikely to cause bleeding in the first trimester.

2. **(B)** There is a small but definite risk of fetal abnormality in any pregnancy. An early threatened abortion, as defined by bleeding only, does not appear to significantly increase the long-term risk of abnormality if an abortion does not occur. There is an increased risk of preterm delivery, low birth weight, and perinatal mortality. Bleeding after 16 weeks may be of greater significance.

3. **(D)** Reassurance and pelvic rest are the best modes of therapy. These modalities are not proven but are accepted care. Prolonged bed rest is not warranted. The patient should be followed to document continued uterine growth and viable products of conception. Ultrasound is of great help for this.

4. **(E)** Because pregnanediol drops when the fetoplacental unit dies, it was thought that progesterone was therapeutic. However, the true etiology was the death of the fetus. Giving more progesterone did not result in viability. It did inhibit myometrial activity, resulting in retained products of conception. If the fetus is alive, high doses of 19 norprogestins may be virilizing. Progestins are occasionally used to support a failing corpus luteum cyst.

5. **(D)** The ability of the blood to clot should be checked prior to performing a treatment for a fetal demise. DIC triggered by the release of tissue thromboplastins is usually a problem 3 to 4 weeks after fetal death.

6. **(C)** Rare, if the fetus and placenta are viable, the placenta may implant on some other peritoneal structure, and, rarely, an abdominal pregnancy may result. Many more ectopic gestations than is generally realized may terminate as tubal abortions or simply be reabsorbed. Decidual cast is the sloughing of the endometrial decidual reaction of a pregnancy no matter where the pregnancy is located. This is pasted per cervical os. The Arias-Stella phenomenon are pathological changes noted that verify presence of a pregnancy often not in the uterus.

7. **(E)** An incomplete abortion is diagnosed if some, but not all, of the products of conception are passed. Often, bleeding can be severe. Evacuation should stop the bleeding and pain. Although a twin pregnancy is possible, once the individual pregnancy has passed the bleeding should stop. Threatened abortion is when there is spotting or cramping but no cervical dilation. This becomes an inevitable abortion when there is certain dilation. Premature labor is diagnosed once the pregnancy has reached 24 weeks' gestational age.

8. **(A)** A partially separated placenta will bleed profusely. If completely separated, the uterine contractions tend to occlude blood vessels and

pass the tissue. Therapy is therefore directed at placental removal.

9.  **(E)** The indicated therapy is to completely empty the uterus to allow the myometrium to contract. Vaginal packing will often not stop uterine bleeding and does not address the primary cause. Hysterectomy would be used as a last resort. Suction is safer and more effective than sharp curettage, good anesthesia and appropriate setting are essential. Broad-spectrum antibiotics are also indicated. Since hemostasis is from uterine contraction provision of fibrinogen does not impact the bleeding. If the bleeding is not excessive and patient is stable, a medical completion might be considered.

10. **(D)** In the presence of missed menstrual periods, bleeding, cramping, enlarged, tender uterus; discharge; and fever; septic abortion is the first diagnostic possibility. Aggressive evacuation of the uterus and IV administration of antibiotics are indicated in this potentially life-threatening problem.

11. **(D)** Cultures should always be obtained prior to antibiotic therapy in the setting of a septic abortion. Blood cultures from septic abortions often reveal anaerobes. The other tests should be ordered also, but their results will not be changed by antibiotics. Therapy, however, is begun on an empiric basis prior to the return of culture results. Abdominal ultrasound is used to rule out a gas forming infection such as clostridia.

12. **(A)** Early curettage after adequate antibiotics is the standard. Waiting for the patient to become afebrile to perform the curettage allows the infected material to remain in the uterus, and the patient may get worse instead of better. The infection must be evacuated promptly.

13. **(B)** Endosalpingitis, creating blind pockets in the tubal mucosa, is recognized as the leading predisposing factor for the development of ectopic pregnancies. Women on birth control pills or with irregular menses or endometriosis are not necessarily predisposed. The prompt and

aggressive treatment of pelvic infection is designed to prevent tubal damage and maintain fertility.

14. **(D)** The ampulla is the most common site. Often, the ectopic embryo can be removed without removing the tube, but tubal function is occasionally compromised. After one ectopic pregnancy, the probability of having another is about 10%. Future fertility also declines.

15. **(E)** Rupture into the peritoneal space may cause a hemoperitoneum. Less commonly, rupture into the broad ligament can also occur, resulting in a broad ligament hematoma without free blood in the peritoneal cavity. Tubal rupture generally will occur at about 8 to 10 weeks' gestation, producing rapidly progressive symptoms.

16. **(B)** Interstitial pregnancies are rare—generally less than 2% of all ectopic pregnancies. However, because of their placement and large blood supply, they can grow quite a bit prior to rupture and then bleed massively. Because of the large uterine defect caused by rupture, hysterectomy may be (but is not always) necessary.

17. **(D)** The lower uterine segment and cervix do not constrict blood vessels well because they do not contract down, as does the fundus. Therefore, bleeding from the attempted surgical removal of a cervical gestation can be immense. Hysterectomy is a safe method of management but results in sterility. If the pregnancy is diagnosed early, other forms of management, including uterine artery embolization and medical treatment (chemotherapy), have been employed with success.

18. **(C)** The maternal mortality from abdominal gestation is quite high. Usually, an abdominal fetus should be removed as soon as diagnosed. Removing the placenta adds to the risk of hemorrhage. Despite the complications, the placenta is best left in situ unless its entire blood supply can be visualized and occluded without harming the mother. This may be done with the use of methotrexate or embolization.

19. **(B)** Positive pregnancy tests and abnormal fetal positions are not specific. Uterine contractions should not be felt after oxytocin if the pregnancy is abdominal. X-rays may or may not help. One must be aware of oblique views, which may project the fetal skeleton over the maternal spine. Hysterograms may be definitive but may be damaging if the fetus is in utero. Ultrasound is safer but subject to error also.

20. **(B)** Left salpingo-oophorectomy would also be acceptable, especially if the ovary is involved in the mass, or if there is a strong likelihood of compromising its blood supply by removing the tube and ectopic pregnancy. Every effort is now made to save the ovary and, many times, the tube. In many instances, the ectopic pregnancy can be "shelled out" and the tube repaired to preserve fertility.

21. **(C)** For forceps to be applied, several criteria must be met, among them being that the head must be engaged (i.e., fetus must present by the vertex or by face with chin anterior; the cervix must be completely dilated and the membranes ruptured). In a breech delivery, forceps can be used once the body is delivered to assist on delivery of the after-coming head. Application of forceps in other situations is dangerous to both the mother and the fetus.

22. **(D)** Usually, such an event is traumatic for mother, child, and surgeon. A trial of forceps, which implies good application and moderate traction, is an acceptable procedure. If no progress is made, the trial is discontinued and a cesarean section performed. To persist with forceps constitutes poor judgment. If forceps do not work a vacuum should not be attempted, as that leads to significantly increased morbidity when done as a subsequent procedure.

23. **(D)** If the forceps do not apply easily and lock securely without undue pressure, the probability exists that they are not properly applied. Position of the head should be rechecked and the forceps should be reapplied before any traction or maneuvers are attempted. To do a C-section

for maternal fatigue is not indicated at this time.

24. **(E)** The indications for vacuum extraction are the same as those for forceps delivery, namely the head must be engaged, it must be a vertex presentation, the position of the fetal head must be precisely known, the cervix must be completely dilated, the membranes must be ruptured, and there should be no cephalopelvic disproportion (CPD). Although forceps can be applied to a mentum anterior face presentation, the vacuum should not be used on the face for obvious reasons. If the fetus is very small, the vacuum does not fit well and there is increased risk of vascular rupture and bleeding, which is also a problem with fetal coagulopathies or after scalp sampling. It is reasonable to attempt a vacuum extraction (VE) after routine monitor with a scalp electrode.

25. **(D)** With the head at a high station, one should be alert to the possibility of CPD and must also check for a prolapsed cord after membrane rupture. A primigravida in labor with an unengaged head is a high-risk patient. The pelvis should be evaluated. Clinical pelvimetry and evaluation of fetal size is indicated as well as fetal position/presentation to rule out an occiput posterior (OP) or face presentation.

26. **(C)** Incoordinate uterine action may give rise to poor labor progression. Some authorities feel that oxytocin is contraindicated if the contractions do not have fundal dominance. Moving the patient about with a high head and ruptured membranes may lead to prolapse of the cord. Many, however, would attempt a trial of judicious oxytocin stimulation, especially as the contraction pattern is suboptimal.

27. **(E)** Forceps are contraindicated with an incompletely dilated cervix. Despite all efforts, the labor is not progressive. Abdominal delivery is indicated after these attempts have been made and progress is less than 1.2 cm/h with no real descent. Duhrssen's incisions are cuts in the cervix at 6, 10, and 2 o'clock position for an entrapped

after-coming fetal head in a vaginal breech delivery.

28. **(A)** VBAC has an upward of 70% success rate. The risk of rupture is <1%. Catastrophic rupture when the fetus is extruded into the mother's abdomen is also less than 1%.

29. **(A)** *Uteroplacental apoplexy* and *Couvelaire uterus* are terms used to describe the same process. The hematoma may spread via the broad ligament and tubes and, if extensive, may lead to decreased uterine muscle efficiency. The uterus may need to be removed. If hematomas are stable, they need not be evacuated. Such a degree of abruption would almost always result in fetal distress.

30. **(D)** No one believes how much a placenta previa can bleed until it happens. Ultrasound has helped immensely in the management of this difficult problem. Double setup examination (a pelvic examination in the operating suite with the preparations for an emergent C-section as needed) may be used to diagnose the condition acutely in viable pregnancies. In other situations, such as premature pregnancies, ultrasound is the best way to diagnose a previa rather than risk precipitating a major bleed may allow time to temporize. Cervical examination in the presence of cervical cancer or cervical infection is rarely going to cause a significant bleed or complication. In the setting of a possible prolapsed cord, an examination to verify the diagnosis and then to elevate the presenting part off the cord is indicated. Although a patient with premature rupture of membranes not in labor should not have a cervical examination due to the increase risk of infection. However, once the patient is in active labor there is no contraindication of labor.

31. **(B)** Placenta previa must be ruled out, but this should not be done by pelvic examination at this time. If a previa is present, a pelvic examination may precipitate massive bleeding, making cesarean section mandatory. At 29 weeks' gestation, the fetus has a good chance of survival if further insults do not occur. The placenta should be localized by ultrasound and expectant treatment instituted if placenta previa is found and no further severe bleeding occurs. The limits of what constitutes acceptable blood loss are often hard to define and should be determined prospectively. Blood should be ordered and an IV started.

32. **(B)** The history is classic for placenta previa. An older, multiparous woman in late gestation with painless copious vaginal bleeding and a floating presenting part must be evaluated for placenta previa. Carcinoma of the cervix would be rare. Abruption often will have pain, and bleeding from vasa previa is statistically uncommon, especially with intact membranes and a normal fetal heart rate.

33. **(B)** At this point a definitive diagnosis should be made. Amniocentesis may be warranted later, but ultrasound to denote placental position should be performed. A digital examination is contraindicated, and a speculum examination will not give the necessary information.

34. **(D)** Both multiparity and increasing age tend to predispose to placenta previa, although age appears to be more important. Malpresentation, especially if no part of the fetus occupies the true pelvis, should also alert one to the possibility of previa. Ultrasound is the easiest way to make the diagnosis.

35. **(B)** Ultrasound has no radiation hazard, nor does it require intravascular injections. Ultrasound can also be used to determine fetal size and locate intraperitoneal masses. Most centers have ultrasound available in their labor and delivery areas.

36. **(C)** Classically, three incisions are made—one each at 2, 10, and 6 o'clock. These positions avoid the major blood supply that are located at 3 and 9 o'clock position and allow a vaginal repair. However, the use of Duhrssen's incisions should be extremely rare.

37. **(C)** The combination of breech presentation, meningomyelocele, and enlarged head make hydrocephaly the most likely diagnosis.

38. **(D)** Persistent face and brow, as well as transverse lie with shoulder presentations, can best

be delivered by cesarean section. Internal version has few indications and is a difficult procedure, even for those with a great deal of experience. One of the few indications is for the delivery of a second twin. In this situation with entrapment of the head after delivery of the buttocks is no longer a candidate for an internal version. Although cutting through the cartilage at the pubic symphysis may be an action of desperation for delivery of the head by opening the pelvic curvature, this is a dismal situation to have occur.

39. **(A)** Eclampsia requires convulsions or coma, and even preeclampsia would most probably be ruled out by negative proteinuria and normal BP. The patient's fever points more to appendicitis. Increased WBC is not necessary to make the diagnosis of appendicitis. In fact the common symptoms of appendicitis in the nonpregnant patient are commonly not seen in the pregnant patient. Pyelonephritis is possible but not as likely with no costovertebral angle (CVA) pain or pyuria. Pyelonephritis can cause gastrointestinal symptoms and is relatively common in pregnancy.

40. **(D)** The presence of pregnancy makes the diagnosis of appendicitis more difficult because many signs are changed. Pain, for example, may not be in the right lower quadrant. Nausea and vomiting, fever and chills may not be evident. The treatment is immediate laparotomy and appendectomy if there is significant suspicion for appendicitis is important for the maternal and fetal well-being. Delivery of the infant if no evidence of sepsis is not indicated.

41. **(E)** Early pyelonephritis can cause just such symptoms. There is no good evidence for abruptio placentae or degenerating myoma. Gastrointestinal disease such as ulcer or volvulus will not cause a markedly abnormal urinalysis.

42. **(E)** Obtaining a histologic specimen is best done by colposcopically directed biopsy. A Pap smear is only a screening tool and a definitive diagnosis is needed prior to contemplating treatment. Agreement exists as to the need for histologic examination in the immediate future. Directed

biopsy is usually best when performed with colposcopic guidance. Small cervical biopsies pose no threat to the pregnancy.

43. **(A)** If invasive disease is ruled out, vaginal delivery can be safely accomplished. Conization may predispose to cervical abnormalities of either premature dilation or lack of dilation, but such late complications are rare. Bleeding or premature labor may be a significant complication. A primary C-section does not improve outcome even if hysterectomy is indicated eventually. A peripartum hysterectomy is a risk for significant operative hemorrhage and inability to get an adequate vaginal cuff for optimal treatment.

44. **(B)** There is a very slight risk that the cyst is a carcinoma or will obstruct labor. There is a greater risk that it will undergo torsion. Surgery early in pregnancy (first trimester) markedly increases the chance of abortion. If there is no immediate need to operate (i.e., the mass is unlikely to be cancer) the surgery may be done after 16 weeks. However, the mass may also be followed.

45. **(D)** Pregnancy does not seem to influence the long-term prognosis of breast carcinoma. Both surgery and chemotherapy can be done prior to delivery, but radiation therapy is not recommended because of scatter, which may exceed the allowable fetal dose. The only reason for an abortion is due to maternal decision after complete counseling regarding treatment options and prognosis.

46. **(E)** Blood replacement should keep the patient out of shock and the urine output adequate, but it should not be given until the clinical condition warrants. Blood replacement should be directed at the necessary components, for example, packed cells, platelets, and fresh frozen plasma. Delivery should occur as soon as is safe. Coagulopathy is common, and replacement of blood products is often necessary. Fresh or freshly frozen serum contains coagulation factors. Cryoprecipitate is the major source of fibrinogen. Platelets may also be needed. Heparin is contraindicated, as is delay of delivery to give steroids.

# Puerperium

## Questions

1. A previously energetic woman complains of crying, loss of appetite, difficulty in sleeping, and feeling of low self-worth, beginning approximately 3 days after a normal vaginal delivery. These feelings persisted for approximately 1 week and then progressively diminished. Which of the following is the best term to describe her symptoms postpartum?

   (A) blues
   (B) manic depression
   (C) neurosis
   (D) psychosis
   (E) schizoid affective disorder

2. A patient has just delivered her first child after an uncomplicated pregnancy and term vaginal delivery. She is anxious to breast-feed. As part of her postpartum discharge counseling, she should be told that few things interfere with lactation, but she should avoid which of the following?

   (A) Depo-Provera
   (B) frequent suckling
   (C) high dose ($\geq 50$ $\mu$g estradiol) oral contraceptive pills
   (D) Levonorgestrel intrauterine device (IUD)
   (E) progestin-only oral contraceptive pill (minipill)

3. At delivery, a perineal laceration tore through the skin of the fourchette, vaginal mucous membrane, and the fascia and perineal muscles of the perineal body but not the anal sphincter or mucosa. This should be recorded in the medical record as what type of laceration?

   (A) first-degree
   (B) second-degree
   (C) third-degree
   (D) fourth-degree
   (E) complete

4. A patient is being discharged from the hospital following an uncomplicated vaginal delivery. Discharge counseling and plans would include which of the following?

   (A) discontinue prenatal vitamins
   (B) no driving for 4 weeks
   (C) no coitus for 6 weeks
   (D) return to work only after 6 weeks of maternity leave
   (E) rubella immunization for nonimmune patients

**Questions 5 through 7 apply to the following patient:**

A 24-year-old patient (gravida 2, para 2) has just delivered vaginally an infant weighing 4,300 g after a spontaneous uncomplicated labor. Her prior obstetric history was a low uterine segment transverse cesarean section for breech. She has had no problems during the pregnancy and labor. The placenta delivers spontaneously. There is immediate brisk vaginal bleeding of greater than 500 cc.

5. Although all of the following can be the cause for postpartum hemorrhage, which is the *most* frequent cause of immediate hemorrhage as seen in this patient?

    (A) coagulopathies
    (B) retained placental fragments
    (C) uterine atony
    (D) uterine rupture
    (E) vaginal and/or cervical lacerations

6. In this patient with a significant postpartum bleed, when should transfusions be started?

    (A) after the loss of 750 cc of blood
    (B) before giving other volume expanders
    (C) before using prostaglandin $E_2$ ($PGE_2$)-alpha
    (D) if the patient becomes hypotensive despite other volume expanders
    (E) when packed cell volume (PCV) is <30%

7. After a significant period of hypovolemic shock, the bleeding was controlled and the vascular volume replaced. Estimates of blood loss were over 2,500 cc. The patient apparently recovered well. However, she was unable to breast-feed and gradually noted breast atrophy and no resumption of menses. Later, she developed constipation, slurred speech, and moderate nonpitting edema. Which of the following is the most likely diagnosis?

    (A) acute tubular necrosis (ATN)
    (B) amenorrhea–galactorrhea syndrome
    (C) Asherman's syndrome (uterine synechiae)
    (D) pituitary tumor
    (E) Sheehan's syndrome (pituitary necrosis)

**Questions 8 and 9 apply to the following patient:**

8. A patient calls your clinic complaining of continued heavy vaginal bleeding. She had an "uncomplicated" vaginal birth 2 weeks ago of her second child. What is the most likely diagnosis from the following differentials?

    (A) coagulopathies
    (B) retained placental fragments
    (C) uterine atony
    (D) uterine rupture
    (E) vaginal lacerations

9. The most efficacious treatment of persistent uterine hemorrhage in the second to fourth week of the puerperium, as observed in this patient is which of the following?

    (A) dilation and curettage (D&C)
    (B) Ergotrate
    (C) high doses of estrogen
    (D) high doses of progesterone
    (E) uterine packing

10. The postpartum nurse calls about a patient who had an uncomplicated vaginal delivery 12 hours ago. She is concerned that the patient has the following findings. Which of them should be of most concern to you?

    (A) abdominal rigidity
    (B) leukocytosis of 16,000
    (C) proteinuria
    (D) a pulse rate of 60
    (E) a single temperature of 100.4°F

11. A patient had a prolonged labor requiring a C-section in the setting of chorioamnionitis. She has continued with spiking temperatures despite antibiotics and a diagnosis of postpartum pelvic thrombophlebitis is being made. She suddenly complains of chest pain and dyspnea. Which of the following tests will be most helpful to diagnose a pulmonary embolism?

    (A) arterial blood gas
    (B) auscultation of the chest
    (C) chest x-ray

(D)  electrocardiogram (ECG)

(E)  spiral computed tomography (CT) scan

**Questions 12 through 15 apply to the following patient:**

An 18-year-old patient finally delivered a 4,000-g infant vaginally. Her prenatal course was complicated by anemia, poor weight gain, and maternal obesity. Her labor was protracted, including a 3-hour second stage, a mid-forceps delivery with a sulcus laceration, and a third-degree episiotomy.

12.  Which of the following is the greatest predisposing cause of puerperal infection in this patient?

(A)  coitus during late pregnancy

(B)  iron deficiency

(C)  maternal exhaustion

(D)  poor nutrition

(E)  tissue trauma

13.  She develops a persistent fever of 101°F on the third day postpartum. What is the most likely etiology?

(A)  cholecystitis

(B)  endometritis

(C)  mastitis

(D)  pneumonia

(E)  thrombophlebitis

14.  If this infection spreads to include the supporting connective tissues of the uterus, what is it called?

(A)  parametritis

(B)  peritonitis

(C)  phlebothrombosis

(D)  pyemia

(E)  thrombophlebitis

15.  Puerperal infection may be spread by several routes. Which of the following is the most common route that results in serious complication of a septic thrombophlebitis?

(A)  arterial

(B)  direct extension

(C)  fomites

(D)  lymphatic

(E)  venous

16.  A patient who is 12 hours postpartum develops a temperature of 104°F, a tender uterus, and increased lochia without an odor. Her pregnancy course had been complicated only by limited and inconsistent prenatal care. Your antibiotic choice needs to be sure to cover which of the following organisms?

(A)  *Bacteroides*

(B)  *Beta-streptococcus*

(C)  *Escherichia coli*

(D)  *Gonococcus*

(E)  *Staphylococcus*

17.  Bacteria can be cultured from most endometrial cavities 2 to 3 days postpartum in patients who are asymptomatic. The anaerobic organism most commonly found is which of the following?

(A)  *Beta-streptococcus*

(B)  *Clostridium*

(C)  *E. coli*

(D)  *Peptococcus*

(E)  *Peptostreptococcus*

18.  During childbirth classes, a patient should be told which of the following regarding breast-feeding?

(A)  Breast milk is a major source of immunoglobulin G (IgG).

(B)  Most ingested drugs that are soluble in maternal blood do not cross into breast milk.

(C)  Mother's milk contains a large amount of iron.

(D)  The postpartum period of lactation is a time of above-normal fertility.

(E)  Prolactin stimulates milk production and breast development.

19. A 16-year-old patient delivered a term infant yesterday. She is placing the child for adoption and is not going to breast-feed. She asks for something to suppress lactation. What is simplest and safest method of lactation suppression?

    (A) breast binding, ice packs, and analgesics
    (B) bromocriptine
    (C) deladumone
    (D) Depo-Provera
    (E) oral contraceptive pills

20. A patient presents 1-week postpartum with complaints of her right breast being engorged, hot, red, and painful. She reports a fever of 101°F. If her breasts were cultured, which of the following is the most likely organism to be found?

    (A) aerobic *Streptococcus*
    (B) anaerobic *Streptococcus*
    (C) *E. coli*
    (D) *Neisseria*
    (E) *Staphylococcus aureus*

21. A class C diabetic patient delivers at term. It is important to check her blood sugar levels immediately postpartum, since there may be a decrease in the insulin requirements of diabetic patients. This can be partly explained by which of the following?

    (A) decreased activity
    (B) decrease in plasma chorionic somatomammotropin [hCS or human placental lactogen (hPL)]
    (C) decrease in plasma estrogen
    (D) decrease in plasma progesterone
    (E) increased food intake

22. Immediately after the completion of a normal labor and delivery, the uterus should be which of the following?

    (A) at the level of the symphysis pubis
    (B) boggy
    (C) discoid
    (D) firm and rounded
    (E) immobile

23. A patient had a vaginal delivery of a 4,500-g infant after a prolonged second stage. She is now unable to void. Each of the following could be a reason and can be initially treated with Foley placement. Which of the following can represent a most serious etiology of inability to void in the immediate postpartum period?

    (A) anesthesia
    (B) edema
    (C) emotions
    (D) hematoma
    (E) overdistention of the bladder

24. Average blood loss from an uncomplicated vaginal delivery, when carefully measured, has been found to be which of the following?

    (A) g<200 mL
    (B) approximately 350 mL
    (C) approximately 550 mL
    (D) approximately 750 mL
    (E) approximately 1,000 mL

25. The decidual layer is divided into several parts, pregnancy. The remaining layer can be damaged with a curettage for retained placenta. Which of the following is the part that should remain?

    (A) decidua capsularis
    (B) decidua vera
    (C) zona basalis
    (D) zona functionalis
    (E) zona spongiosa

**Questions 26 and 27 apply to the following patient:**

A 20-year-old woman (gravida 1) has just delivered. After expression of the placenta, a red, raw surface is seen at the vaginal introitus. Simultaneously, the nurse states that the patient is pale and her BP is 70/40 mm Hg. External bleeding has been of normal amount.

26. Which of the following would be the most likely diagnosis?

    (A) ovarian cyst
    (B) ruptured uterus

(C) second twin

(D) uterine inversion

(E) vaginal rupture

27. Emergency treatment would initially consist of which of the following?

(A) delivery of the infant

(B) exploratory laparotomy

(C) immediate hysterectomy

(D) immediate replacement of the fundus

(E) massive blood transfusion

28. A 21-year-old G1 now P1 has had a vaginal delivery of a 2,700-g infant. Her labor was complicated by severe pre-eclampsia. Bimanual massage of the uterus and intravenous oxytocin do not control her postpartum hemorrhage. What is the next best intervention?

(A) B-Lynch suture

(B) D&C

(C) Ergotrate

(D) packing the uterus

(E) prostaglandin $F_2$ ($PFG_2$)-alpha

# Answers and Explanations

1. **(A)** Short-term feelings of depression, commonly called postpartum blues, occur in 85% of women for a short time in the immediate postpartum period. This is a mild disorder that is usually self-limited, but if it persists, it may represent postpartum depression. Then medical intervention, including antidepressant therapy, is beneficial. If it is associated with severe symptoms of psychoses, suicidal thoughts, or delusions, consultation with a psychiatrist should be obtained immediately. In the situation of postpartum psychosis, both the woman and the infant are in danger of harm. If a woman has experienced postpartum depression or psychosis in a prior pregnancy or if she has depression or psychosis when not pregnant, she is at increased risk for a postpartum reoccurrence.

2. **(C)** Birth control pills containing high pharmacologic amounts of estrogens have been shown to decrease milk production, as has chronic smoking. Low doses of progestins alone do not appear to have this effect. Even higher doses of progestin as found in Depo-Provera given postpartum do not seem to increase problems with breast-feeding. Estrogen is needed for milk production, but high levels are inhibiting. Suckling is a stimulus to milk production. However, the use of lower dose combination oral contraceptive pills ($\leq 30$ $\mu$g estrogen) is an option once breast-feeding is well established.

3. **(B)** A second-degree tear does not involve the anal sphincter. Third-degree lacerations involve the anal sphincter, and fourth-degree lacerations include the sphincter and the rectal mucosa. Any laceration should be carefully repaired and examined after repair for the integrity of the anal sphincter and the rectal mucosa. Currently if a laceration is not actively bleeding and is not a third or fourth degree, more providers are opting not to repair a laceration if it is well approximated since the actual sutures can cause more discomfort than the laceration.

4. **(E)** The woman's comfort and desire should serve as the basis for resumption of coitus, although it is probably best to wait until the vaginal bleeding has stopped to decrease the risk of infection. After a vaginal delivery, a patient should be able to resume normal activities within days. The recommendation for 4 to 6 weeks of maternity leave is more due to decreased energy levels and time to adjust to parenting role rather than true medical indications. Prenatal vitamins, especially ones with iron supplementation, are helpful and should be continued for 2 to 3 months postpartum. Postpartum is an excellent time to immunize for rubella.

5. **(C)** Uterine atony accounts for by far the greatest number of bleeding incidents accounting for up to 70% of postpartum hemorrhages. Potential trauma is obvious in the process of a delivery but usually does not cause this much bleeding. Also, in the case of significant lacerations, the bleeding is often evident prior to the delivery of the placenta. Coagulopathy is possible in cases of abruption or severe hypertension but typically does not cause immediate hemorrhage unless there are significant lacerations. Uterine rupture, given this patient's history, is a definite possibility but still is less common than atony. Uterine inversion is an uncommon event and is

more likely to follow a delay in placenta separation with traction on the cord. With the macrosomic infant she likely had an overdistended uterus, which increases her risk of atony.

6. **(D)** A great danger exists in letting a patient become hypovolemic in the face of continued bleeding. Most deaths from maternal hemorrhage can be traced to inadequate blood replacement (too little, too late). Do not allow blood loss to get out of hand. By the same token, transfusion involves many risks. It should be performed judiciously. Uterine massage and bimanual compression, Ergotrate, dilute oxytocin IV, and PGF2-alpha should all be tried for uterine atony. Surgical removal of placental fragments or repair of laceration should be done as needed.

7. **(E)** Anterior pituitary necrosis from postpartum hemorrhage with significant shock will cause the loss of gonadotropins, thyroid-stimulating hormone (TSH), and adrenocorticotropic hormone (ACTH), generally in that order. Lack of breast milk is usually the first clue. Amenorrhea may be the second sign. Sheehan syndrome is a rare occurrence when good postpartum management prevents or adequately treats blood loss and prevents shock. ATN would have presented early postpartum with extremely dilute urine and evidence of hypovolemia. Asherman's syndrome is the scarring of the endometrial cavity after a D&C, especially in the situation of a postpartum hemorrhage. The symptoms are confined to postpartum amenorrhea with or without cramping, depending on whether it is only an outlet obstruction. Forbes–Albright syndrome (amenorrhea–galactorrhea syndrome) is usually associated with a pituitary tumor and not with pregnancy. Galactorrhea is also associated with this syndrome.

8. **(B)** Early bleeding is most often due to atony or lacerations. Late continued profuse bleeding, even several weeks following delivery, may be due to retained placenta. Other causes may be subinvolution of the uterus, infection, and/or choriocarcinoma. Ultrasound is indicated for diagnosis and a D&C for therapy if needed.

9. **(A)** Retained placenta and subinvolution of the placental sites are common causes of late puerperal bleeding. Ergotrate causes cramping, but does not often resolve the problem. Severe hemorrhage can occur during a D&C and should be anticipated in high-parity women possibly because the placenta is implanted lower in the uterus with each subsequent pregnancy. The possibility of removing all of the endometrium and creating Asherman's syndrome must be kept in mind, especially if there is an infection. Placental polyps and gestational trophoblastic disease are rare causes that should be remembered. Uterine packing will not remove the retained placental fragments. Unless there is severe atony, estrogen will not help.

10. **(A)** A leukocytosis of up to 25,000 may occur immediately postpartum with no other signs of infection and is likely due to the stress and exertion of labor and delivery. A low pulse rate is commonly seen. Proteinuria can be expected, especially following a difficult labor. This is likely due to bladder trauma from the descending vertex causing bruising or lochia mixing with the urine when collected. Two temperatures of >100.4°F are required prior to diagnosing a postpartum endomyometritis. True abdominal rigidity is not normal during the puerperium. This is concerning for abdominal bleeding which could represent a uterine rupture.

11. **(E)** Of the tests listed, spiral CT is the best. Pulmonary emboli usually cause decreased $PO_2$ and may cause cardiac right-axis shift, pulmonary avascular areas, and pleural effusion. Blood gases and auscultation are not very specific or sensitive for PE. Pulmonary angiography, which will usually reveal filling defects from embolic phenomena, is more specific but is costly and takes longer. Spiral CT is rapidly becoming the diagnostic test of choice since it is accurate, low risk for the patient, and relatively quick to obtain. Anticoagulation is the mainstay of therapy. About one-half of the pulmonary emboli during pregnancy originates in the pelvic veins.

**12. (E)** Devitalized tissue forms an excellent culture medium for bacteria, especially anaerobic forms. Meticulous surgical technique will help to decrease the incidence of infection, as will careful selection of surgical materials. However, the act of repair with the foreign body reaction of the suture and constriction of blood flow by too tight a repair may also contribute to an infectious complication. For that reason many superficial lacerations that have adequate hemostasis are not being repaired.

**13. (B)** One must look at the wound if a fever arises following surgery. After a delivery, the wound or raw surface always includes the uterus, and infection must be actively ruled out. Mastitis may occur but is usually later. Although pneumonia, cholecystitis, and thrombophlebitis may cause a fever, these are relatively uncommon. Urinary tract infection (UTI) is another very likely source of the fever.

**14. (A)** Parametritis, or pelvic cellulitis, may be secondary to genital tract lacerations, thrombophlebitis, or direct invasion by pathogenic bacteria. It is treated in a similar fashion to nonpuerperal pelvic infection.

**15. (E)** Thrombophlebitis is associated with about 40% of fatal cases of puerperal sepsis. Fomites are objects that are not in themselves infected, but they can carry an infecting organism from one place to another. Direct extension is always a possibility but not the most likely one.

**16. (B)** Although puerperal infectious morbidity definition states to "ignore" the first 24 hours, high temperatures such as 104°F must be addressed. This may be associated with a very aggressive infectious source. The lack of foul odor would imply aerobic bacteria. Coverage for group A and group B streptococcus is critical. Also, pediatrics should be notified of this development since it may alter their management of the newborn.

**17. (E)** Most endometrial bacteria appear to be contaminants rather than causing a clinical infection, as patients tend to remain asymptomatic and have a normal postpartum course. However, if a fever occurs, the most likely cause is metritis. Anaerobic bacteria require meticulous culture technique to be recovered. *E. coli* and *Streptococci* are facultative bacteria. Since techniques for acquiring a noncontaminated endometrial sampling for culture are difficult, cultures are not routinely done. Instead a broad-spectrum antibiotic that covers the common pathogens is initiated empirically.

**18. (E)** Prolactin stimulates milk production. Breast milk is very low in iron, and supplementation is needed for breast-fed babies. Anemia can also be present in babies fed only cow's milk. Although the time of lactation is one of subnormal fertility, breast-feeding cannot be claimed as a highly effective method of birth control. Most drugs will enter breast milk; therefore, one must consider this when counseling and prescribing for breast-feeding mothers. IgA is the primary antibody contained in breast milk and appears to prevent many gastrointestinal infectious complications for newborns.

**19. (A)** Multiple hormonal interventions have been tried. These predispose to thromboembolic phenomena and have a significant occurrence of rebound engorgement as the hormonal influence decreases. Bromocriptine, via a decrease in prolactin levels, was tried, but there was an association with hypertension, stroke, and seizure with its use. The safest treatment is a binder of the breast, ice packs, and analgesics for the first week postpartum.

**20. (E)** *S. aureus* is the most common etiologic agent in postpartum mastitis. Mastitis is rare in the nonnursing mother. It is usually transmitted by the nursing infant who is already colonized. Treatment of mastitis includes antibiotics, continuance of nursing, and drainage of any abscess. Argument exists as to the method of skin incision for drainage of breast abscesses. Circumareolar skin incisions following Langer's skin lines are advocated by some for cosmetic reasons. A deep abscess can be opened radially after the skin incision is made. Identification of possible nosocomial infection is important since infants may be colonized by nursery staff in the hospital who are carriers of resistant strains of

*Staphylococcus* and other organisms. Fewer authorities now recommend the discontinuance of nursing, although the need to empty the breast is still emphasized.

21. **(B)** Both human chorionic somatomammotropin (hCS), often called placental lactogen, and pituitary somatomammotropin levels remain low immediately postpartum. As they have marked anti-insulin effects, the rapid loss may account for part of the decrease in the insulin requirement often seen in postpartum diabetic patients. Also, placental insulinase is no longer present. One should be careful not to give too large an insulin dose, which might precipitate insulin shock in the postpartum patient.

22. **(D)** The uterus may be discoid prior to the separation of the placenta, but after the third stage of labor, it should be rounded and firm at the level of the umbilicus. A soft or boggy uterus usually signifies lack of tonus and the diagnosis of atony.

23. **(D)** Trauma causing hematoma large enough to cause inability to void is potentially a serious complication postpartum. A pelvic examination should be done whenever there is urinary retention postpartum. Delivery usually causes some trauma to the base of the bladder and trigone, and edema and ecchymosis are common. Anesthesia and/or overdistention may result in poor bladder function for varying periods of time, but all of these will usually resolve with a short time of catheterization. Prolonged bladder distention can cause pain, detrusor injury, and uterine atony with delayed hemorrhage.

24. **(C)** Estimates of blood loss are often 250 mL. However, measurements have shown that a blood loss of 500 to 600 mL is quite common. This amount will not result in a hematocrit drop in most women. This is because the expanded blood volume during pregnancy is like having two autologous units for transfusion. Immediate postpartum hemodynamic changes provide rapid compensation.

25. **(C)** The zona basalis remains to give rise to new endometrium. Some of the basal endometrium is located between myometrial fibers and will usually remain, even after a D&C. This layer rapidly regenerates. If it is removed in a vigorous D&C, one will have Asherman's syndrome.

26. **(D)** Uterine inversion is a rare occurrence, and shock is often out of proportion to blood loss. Immediate recognition is important in the treatment. Ruptured uterus and ovarian cyst would not be seen at the introitus. Vaginal rupture would not be a mass but heavy bleeding. A second twin would not be red and raw.

27. **(D)** Immediate replacement is the quickest and most effective therapy. If recognized early before administering postpartum oxytocin or contraction of the lower uterine segment, replacement is easy. If it is allowed to persist, surgical repair may be required. Bleeding and hypotension out of proportion to blood loss are the greatest dangers. If there is a delay in replacement, aggressive volume expansion is necessary.

28. **(E)** Uterine packing has little place in modern obstetrics as a first-line treatment for early postpartum hemorrhage. It causes uterine distention when the desired effect is contraction of the muscle fibers to occlude bleeding vessels. A B-Lynch suture involves an exploratory laparotomy and would be done just prior to proceeding with a hysterectomy if the bleeding is not controlled. A D&C is useful if one feels that retained placental fragments are causing the bleeding. Although Ergotrate is very effective for treating uterine atony, they can cause a dangerous increase in blood pressure in women who are already hypertensive.

# CHAPTER 14

# Newborn Assessment and Care

## Questions

**DIRECTIONS (Questions 1 through 43): For each of the multiple choice questions in this section, select the lettered answer that is the one *best* response in each case.**

1. An infant is born and at 5 minutes it has a vigorous cry, a heart rate of 105, movement of all four extremities, grimacing with stimulation, and has bluish hands and feet. What is the Apgar score of this infant?

    (A) 10
    (B) 9
    (C) 8
    (D) 7
    (E) 6

2. Newborns who are allowed to remain at room temperature immediately after delivery rather than warmed by skin-to-skin contact with mom or placement in a warmer are at risk for the development of which of the following?

    (A) metabolic acidosis
    (B) metabolic alkalosis
    (C) respiratory acidosis
    (D) respiratory alkalosis
    (E) pneumonia

3. Which of the following is the most common cause of failure to establish effective respiratory effort in the newborn?

    (A) fetal acidosis
    (B) fetal immaturity
    (C) upper airway obstruction
    (D) congenital laryngeal stenosis
    (E) infection

4. A patient with no prenatal care presents in labor claiming to be at 43 weeks of gestation. Which of the following neonatal findings would support the diagnosis of a postmature infant?

    (A) anemia
    (B) increased subcutaneous fat
    (C) long fingernails
    (D) vernix
    (E) fusion of the fetal eyelids

5. Five infants are admitted to the newborn nursery after uncomplicated vaginal deliveries. Which of the following newborns would be classified as high-risk and merits closer monitoring?

    (A) 3,500 g, 39 weeks' gestation, Apgar score 8/9
    (B) 2,650 g, 41 weeks' gestation, Apgar score 7/8
    (C) 3,800 g, 41 weeks' gestation, Apgar score 7/8
    (D) 3,100 g, 38 weeks' gestation, Apgar score 7/9
    (E) 2,650 g, 37 weeks' gestation, Apgar score 7/9

6. A 2-day-old newborn has a mild degree of hyperbilirubinemia. What is the most appropriate next step in management?

   (A) observation only
   (B) exposing the infant to light
   (C) O-negative packed red blood cells (RBCs) given as an exchange transfusion
   (D) spinal tap
   (E) soy-based formula feeding

7. On the 5th day of life, how would the weight of a term infant that weighed 7 lb, 8 oz at birth be expected to change?

   (A) increased 6–8 oz
   (B) increased 2 oz
   (C) remained the same
   (D) decreased 2 oz
   (E) decreased 5–7 oz

8. The first-time mother of a newborn would like to know about the care of the umbilical cord stump. When does the umbilical cord stump of a newborn most frequently slough off?

   (A) 2nd day after delivery
   (B) 5th day after delivery
   (C) 10th day after delivery
   (D) 15th day after delivery
   (E) 21st day after delivery

9. A term infant is delivered via cesarean delivery as a double-footling breech. It is noted to have an Apgar score of 3 at 1 minute and later to be irritable and restless. The infant's muscles are rigid, and the anterior fontanel bulges. The infant develops progressive bradycardia. What is the most likely cause of these findings?

   (A) brain stem injury
   (B) infection
   (C) congenital abnormality
   (D) neonatal sepsis
   (E) intracranial hemorrhage

10. A heroin-abusing woman presents to labor and delivery and has a precipitous vaginal delivery of a term infant who has poor respiratory effort and Apgar scores 2/4/6. Rather than simply sedation from narcotic abuse, what is the most likely finding in a neonate with intrapartum asphyxia?

    (A) alkalemia
    (B) hypoxia
    (C) hypocapnia
    (D) tachycardia
    (E) increased anal sphincter tone

11. Continued apnea in the newborn most often results from which of the following?

    (A) maternal infection
    (B) epidural anesthesia
    (C) central nervous system (CNS) depression
    (D) maternal hyperventilation
    (E) naloxone administration

12. After a delivery complicated by a shoulder dystocia, a newborn is found to have paralysis of one arm with the forearm extended and rotated inward next to the trunk. These findings are most consistent with which of the following?

    (A) damage to the C8–T1 nerve roots
    (B) neonatal asphyxia
    (C) damage to the brachial plexus
    (D) fracture of the clavicle
    (E) comminuted fracture of the humerus

13. Within the first minute after delivery, the baby does not breathe spontaneously. The heart rate is 80 to 90 bpm. There is some movement, with pale and limited irritability. What is the most appropriate next step in management?

    (A) dry and warm the newborn
    (B) slap the baby's back gently at first, then vigorously if necessary
    (C) ventilate the infant by mask
    (D) do external cardiac massage
    (E) administer intravenous bicarbonate ($NaHCO_3$) via umbilical vein

14. When faced with the delivery of a premature newborn, the normal resuscitation should be altered to routinely include which of the following?

    (A) assisted ventilation
    (B) minimal handling
    (C) systemic antibiotic prophylaxis
    (D) nikethamide
    (E) intravenous bicarbonate (NaHCO₃)

15. At a new obstetrics visit, a nulliparous patient shares her fears of having a neonatal death because her mother had a child with a neonatal death. In counseling the patient, you explain that, in the United States, which of the following is the most common factor associated with neonatal death?

    (A) birth injury
    (B) prematurity
    (C) congenital malformations
    (D) metabolic diseases
    (E) intrauterine growth restriction

16. A premature newborn exhibits rapid grunting respiration, chest retraction, and a diffuse infiltrate in the lung fields demonstrated on chest X-ray. What is the most likely cause for these findings?

    (A) pneumococcal pneumonia
    (B) neonatal sepsis
    (C) respiratory distress syndrome (RDS)
    (D) congestive heart failure (CHF)
    (E) hypoglycemia

17. After a normal labor and delivery of monozygotic twins at 35 weeks of gestation, one is found to be polycythemic, and the other small and markedly anemic. What is the most likely etiology of this phenomenon?

    (A) acute fetal bleeding
    (B) fetal cardiac failure
    (C) inadequate maternal iron intake
    (D) placental anastomosis
    (E) Rh incompatibility

18. Approximately 2 days after delivery, an apparently healthy newborn male infant develops an intracranial hemorrhage. Vital signs are normal. His hematocrit and white blood cell (WBC) counts are normal, but platelets are slightly decreased. The bleeding time is normal for age, but the prothrombin time is greatly prolonged. Blood type is A, Rh-negative. What is the most likely explanation for these findings?

    (A) unrecognized birth trauma
    (B) sepsis
    (C) erythroblastosis fetalis
    (D) hemophilia
    (E) hemorrhagic disease of the newborn

19. A premature newborn is found to have abdominal distention, ileus, and bloody stools. An abdominal x-ray shows excessive gas in the bowel and free air under the diaphragm. What is the most likely diagnosis?

    (A) appendicitis
    (B) toxic megacolon
    (C) peptic ulcer disease
    (D) necrotizing enterocolitis
    (E) diabetic enteropathy

20. A male infant is delivered with very little amniotic fluid. He is noted to have low-set ears, contractures of the extremities, and prominent epicanthal folds. He does not void and dies during the first day of life. What is the most likely diagnosis?

    (A) glycogen storage disease
    (B) renal agenesis
    (C) talipes equinovarus
    (D) anencephalus
    (E) trisomy 18

21. Fetal anencephaly is commonly associated with which of the following?

    (A) pituitary hyperplasia
    (B) oligohydramnios
    (C) bradycardia
    (D) adrenal hypertrophy
    (E) postterm labor

22. What is the most common manifestation of fetal anoxic brain injury?

   (A) choroid plexus hemorrhage
   (B) rupture of the cerebral vein at the junction of the falx and tentorium
   (C) mental retardation
   (D) cerebral palsy
   (E) hemiplegia

23. Neurologic abnormalities are found in greatest proportion in infants with which of the following?

   (A) high Apgar scores and normal birth weight
   (B) low Apgar scores and normal birth weight
   (C) low Apgar scores and low birth weight
   (D) high Apgar scores and high birth weight
   (E) low Apgar scores and high birth weight

24. An infant was born 10 hours previously to a mother whose membranes ruptured 27 hours prior to delivery. The mother was febrile in labor. The infant develops respiratory distress, apnea, and an unstable blood pressure. What is the most likely explanation of this infant's symptoms?

   (A) group A streptococcus
   (B) group B streptococcus
   (C) listeriosis
   (D) herpetic encephalopathy
   (E) infant rubella

25. A patient who is a practicing veterinarian is concerned about contracting toxoplasmosis from her feline patients. In counseling the patient, what do you note as the most common sequela of a fetal toxoplasmosis infection?

   (A) phocomelia
   (B) anencephaly
   (C) mental retardation
   (D) ambiguous genitalia
   (E) respiratory distress in the first 24 hours of life

26. While counseling a mother on the risks of a child having a trisomy 21 after second-trimester screening, you note that the general background incidence of significant fetal malformations (birth defects) is approximately which of the following?

   (A) <1%
   (B) 3–5%
   (C) 7–9%
   (D) 10–13%
   (E) 14–18%

27. Widespread use of thalidomide in Europe in the mid-1980s was clearly associated with birth defects. As thalidomide has been reapproved by the FDA for certain indications, it is important that all women in the reproductive age who are prescribed this medication or whose partner is taking thalidomide use very effective contraception. This is because when used in the first trimester, thalidomide is associated with phocomelia, which is defined as a defect in the development of which of the following?

   (A) color vision
   (B) the digits
   (C) the long bones
   (D) the great vessels
   (E) the cytochrome P450 system

28. A child is born with genital ambiguity. The genital folds (scrotum and labia minora) are adherent in the midline, and there is severe hypospadias. The parents ask you about the gender of their child. Your best response, based on the information given, should be which of the following?

   (A) The child has female pseudohermaphroditism and should be raised as female.
   (B) The diagnosis is most likely testicular feminization and the child should be raised as a male.
   (C) This is called an incomplete scrotal raphe and the child should be raised as a male.

(D) It is likely the child has vaginal atresia but should be raised as a female

(E) While the sex of rearing will most likely be female, assignment must await further investigation.

29. A patient who reports episodes of binge drinking in the first trimester wants evaluation of the fetus for fetal alcohol syndrome so she might terminate the pregnancy if it is affected. You inform her that antenatal testing is unable to detect the physical manifestations of fetal alcohol syndrome and it is associated with which of the following?

(A) fetal hypospadias

(B) postmaturity

(C) midfacial hypoplasia

(D) macrosomia

(E) congenital cataracts

30. The perinatal death rate is defined as which of the following?

(A) deaths in utero of fetuses weighing 500 g or more per 1,000 population

(B) the sum of the fetal death rate and neonatal death rate per 1,000 live births

(C) infant deaths (younger than 1 year) per 1,000 live births

(D) deaths in utero of fetuses weighing 1,000 g or more per 1,000 births

(E) fetal and neonatal deaths occurring after 36 weeks' gestation and until 3 months of life, expressed per 1,000 population

31. A patient with no prenatal care delivers shortly after arriving in the labor and delivery suite. Fetal prematurity would be suggested by finding which of the following?

(A) labia majora that are in contact with one another

(B) one or both testes in the scrotum

(C) fingernails that extend to or beyond the fingertips

(D) breast tissue palpable

(E) lanugo hair

32. Which of the following is the most common cause of a "large-for-gestational age" (LGA) infant?

(A) maternal diabetes

(B) congenital abnormalities

(C) in utero infections

(D) erroneous last menstrual period (LMP)

(E) maternal hypertension

**Questions 33 and 34 refer to the following patient:**

You deliver an infant who has a moderate shoulder dystocia and at 1 minute it does not cry, as well as has flexed extremities, irregular respiration, a bluish color, and a heart rate of 90 bpm.

33. What is the most appropriate Apgar score for this infant?

(A) 1

(B) 3

(C) 5

(D) 7

(E) 9

34. At 5 minutes after resuscitation efforts, the infant has a pink body, blue fingers, vigorous cry and active motion, good respiration, and heart rate of 120 bpm. What is the most appropriate Apgar score for this infant?

(A) 1

(B) 3

(C) 5

(D) 7

(E) 9

35. A Simian line or crease is most closely associated with which of the following?

(A) Turner syndrome

(B) Down syndrome

(C) cri du chat syndrome

(D) Klinefelter syndrome

(E) trisomy 13

36. A mother presents with no prenatal care and proceeds to deliver an apparently term infant with a normal trunk, shortened arms, short bowlegs, a globular skull, and blue sclerae. This collection of neonatal findings is most suggestive of which of the following?

    (A) Wilson's copper storage disease
    (B) Down syndrome
    (C) fetal drug exposure
    (D) congenital rickets
    (E) osteogenesis imperfecta

37. You deliver a preterm appropriately grown infant at approximately 36 weeks' gestation. Active resuscitation is begun and it becomes apparent that endotracheal intubation is needed. Based on the infant's gestational age of 36 weeks and estimated weight of 2,500 g, what is the most appropriate endotracheal tube size (inside diameter, mm)?

    (A) 2.0
    (B) 2.5
    (C) 3.0
    (D) 3.5
    (E) 4.0

38. Antimicrobial therapy is routinely applied to the eyes of newborns to prevent blindness caused by which of the following?

    (A) *Neisseria gonorrhoeae*
    (B) *Chlamydial* conjunctivitis
    (C) *Herpes simplex*
    (D) Group B streptococcus
    (E) *Hemophilus Ducreyi*

39. While counseling a patient who is in preterm labor at 28 weeks, you review a number of strategies to minimize adverse outcomes. In this discussion, you note that which of the following interventions has been shown to reduce the rate of intraventricular hemorrhage in preterm neonates?

    (A) antibiotics
    (B) corticosteroids
    (C) magnesium sulfate

    (D) artificial surfactant
    (E) calcium channel blockers

40. A 16-year-old G1P0 patient who is a recent immigrant from Mexico presents at 24 weeks' estimated gestational age (EGA) with a recent onset of a rash. It is determined to be rubella. You reassure her that an in utero infection with rubella virus is unlikely to result in congenital rubella syndrome when it occurs after how many weeks of pregnancy?

    (A) 9 weeks
    (B) 11 weeks
    (C) 13 weeks
    (D) 15 weeks
    (E) 17 weeks

41. Which of the following neonatal findings would suggest congenital rubella syndrome rather than a congenital cytomegalovirus infection?

    (A) thrombocytopenia
    (B) hepatosplenomegaly
    (C) fetal growth restriction
    (D) cataracts
    (E) hemolytic anemia

42. What is the most common cause of clonic seizures in the initial 24-hour newborn period?

    (A) hypoxic–ischemic encephalopathy
    (B) intracranial hemorrhage
    (C) infection
    (D) hypoglycemia
    (E) drug withdrawal

43. What is the approximate caloric need of a normal full-term infant through the first year of life?

    (A) 25 kcal/kg/d
    (B) 50 kcal/kg/d
    (C) 75 kcal/kg/d
    (D) 100 kcal/kg/d
    (E) 125 kcal/kg/d

# Answers and Explanations

1. **(B)** The Apgar scoring system, described by anesthesiologist Virginia Apgar in 1952, is a technique to assess the well-being of a newborn. An Apgar score is awarded to the infant at 1 and 5 minutes of life. In some cases, the Apgar score may be assessed again at 10 minutes of life or beyond. The infant gets a score of 0, 1, or 2 points in each of five categories: heart rate, respiratory effort, reflex irritability, muscle tone, and color. An Apgar score of 3 or less at 5 minutes in infants is associated with an increased risk of anomalies or developmental problems (goes from 0.3% to 1%). The change from 1 to 5 minutes is a good indicator of the successful neonatal resuscitation. See Table 14–1.

TABLE 14–1. Apgar Scoring

| Signs | Points Scored | | |
|---|---|---|---|
| | 0 | 1 | 2 |
| Heartbeats per minute | Absent | Slow (<100) | Over 100 |
| Respiratory effort | Absent | Slow, irregular | Good, crying |
| Muscle tone | Limp | Some flexion of extremities | Active motion |
| Reflex irritability | No response | Grimace | Cry or cough |
| Color | Blue or pale | Body pink, extremities blue | Completely pink |

2. **(A)** The normal infant who is cool will resist metabolic acidosis and maintain pH by compensatory respiratory alkalosis. If the infant is in trouble from asphyxia, it may be unable to compensate, and the acidosis is accentuated. Ventilation will usually restore normal function. A common error in the resuscitation of infants is to do the resuscitation on a cold table rather than in an infant warmer.

3. **(C)** In the majority of infants, respiratory effort will be initiated between 30 and 60 seconds after birth. Fetal acidosis, drugs given to the mother, upper airway obstruction, a premature infant, pneumothorax, congenital anomalies, infection, and trauma can all be severe enough to inhibit an infant's respiratory effort. The cause must be sought and corrected. Most often, the cause is upper airway obstruction by fluids and mucus, which may be easily cleared by bulb suction.

4. **(C)** Other identifying features are decreased subcutaneous fat, wrinkled skin, decreased vernix, polycythemia, dehydration, and meconium staining. Such infants are classically described as having the features of "a little old man." If good nutrition is maintained throughout pregnancy, an infant of a long gestation can be macrosomic. Fusion of the eyelids is characteristic of a very immature fetus.

5. **(B)** This infant is undergrown or small for dates (SGA). He has grown too slowly in utero and may have been nutritionally compromised for some time. Postmaturity and growth retardation are risks often found together, often with poor infant outcomes.

6. **(B)** As bilirubin pigment appears to break down in ultraviolet light, such treatment may keep it from reaching a dangerous level that could necessitate an exchange transfusion. Putting the bassinet in daylight is treatment enough for some; others will need a special treatment system exposing them to higher levels of ultraviolet light.

7. **(E)** The normal newborn will lose 5 to 7 oz of his birth weight soon after delivery and gain it back by 10 days postpartum. He should then continue to gain weight rapidly. Feeding generally does not go well at first, accounting for the weight loss.

8. **(C)** Mothers often ask how long the umbilical stump will remain and what to do to care for it. Leaving it open and washing the area with soap and water seems to be adequate care. The umbilical stump should be cultured in cases of neonatal sepsis. It will normally slough spontaneously in about 10 days.

9. **(E)** The breech delivery, bulging fontanel, and progressive worsening of the condition all point to CNS bleeding. A subdural hematoma should be treated by immediate aspiration. The breech places the newborn at greater risk for head entrapment and resultant trauma even with an abdominal delivery. Also, it has been noted that infants that are breech at term have a higher risk of congenital anomalies.

10. **(B)** Asphyxia is a condition in which the arterial blood is hypoxic, acidotic, and hypercapnic. The heart rate is decreased and the anal sphincter may relax, causing loss of meconium. It is often associated with cooling of the infant, narcosis, brain hemorrhage, or metabolic acidosis.

11. **(C)** Drugs, fetal immaturity, fetal trauma, fetal anomalies, fetal infection, and fetal hypoxia are the major causes of newborn apnea. Most of these result in depression of the fetal CNS. Naloxone, stimulation, and assisted ventilation are all used to overcome apnea.

12. **(C)** In the newborn, both Erb's and Klumpke's paralysis usually result from trauma to the brachial plexus during a difficult delivery. The brachial plexus is made of C5, T6, C7, C8, and T1, C2. Klumpke's paralysis affects only the hand and involves C7, C8, and T1. Ptosis and miosis can also occur if sympathetic fibers of these nerves are involved in the injury. The injury most often occurs when pressure on the fetal head and neck (and therefore the brachial plexus) is too great. Lateral pressure on the head during vertex delivery (especially with shoulder dystocia) or hyperextension of the arms over the head during breech birth may cause this injury. This is also called Duchenne's paralysis.

13. **(C)** This is a moderately to severely depressed infant (estimated Apgar score 2–4). Respiration must be established. Gentle or rough handling is unlikely to help. If the baby is hypoxic, respiration by assisted ventilation is the key to helping the neonate. Establishing effective ventilation will speed the heart, and acidosis will correct with ventilation.

14. **(B)** Minimal handling, a warm environment, and supplemental oxygen are indicated for any premature newborn, with more vigorous resuscitation and treatment utilized only as indicated by the fetal condition. Drugs to stimulate respiration have not proven to be effective and may be dangerous.

15. **(B)** Prematurity from whatever etiology is the most common factor associated with neonatal death. Respiratory difficulty is often the major problem with these infants. However, many organs can fail in these small infants. Although intrauterine growth restriction is often associated with premature delivery or pregnancies with poor outcomes, growth restriction by itself does not appear to be an independent factor in neonatal death. The second most common cause of neonatal death is congenital malformations.

16. **(C)** RDS is most common in premature infants and is due to a decreased amount of phospholipid surfactants in the alveoli. It is treated with assisted ventilation and artificial surfactant.

17. **(D)** One twin can get a progressively larger amount of blood than the other because of placenta anastomoses. This is called twin–twin transfusion and classically results in one small, anemic twin and one large, plethoric twin who is subject to CHF. Acute fetal bleeding could cause anemia but should not result in significant size discrepancy. Poor maternal iron stores or an Rh incompatibility would affect both infants.

18. **(E)** The time to onset of the bleeding associated with a normal bleeding time and with a prolonged prothrombin time points to hemorrhagic disease of the newborn. The infant has hypoprothrombinemia as a result of low placental transport of vitamin K. Infants of mothers with epilepsy are at an increased risk for this disease. Infants of those mothers should be given supplemental vitamin K at birth. Routine administration of vitamin K is recommended for all neonates. Vitamin K in small doses given to the mother in labor or the infant at the time of delivery is prophylactic for hemorrhagic disease of the newborn. One milligram of vitamin K given to the infant is also used in therapy of hemolytic disease of the newborn.

19. **(D)** Necrotizing enterocolitis is a disease seen in both low-birth-weight and premature infants. The cause is unknown, but it is believed that the cause is related to immaturity of the gastrointestinal system rather than ischemia, as previously thought. It can be prevented by administration of immunoglobulin. In mild forms, the disease can be treated by dietary restriction; in severe forms, the bowel may need to be resected.

20. **(B)** Defects in the urinary system are associated with defects in the genital tract, low-set ears, and other anomalies. Low-set ears and cardiac defects are also seen in trisomy 18. Ultrasound studies performed during pregnancy will reveal oligohydramnios.

21. **(E)** In fetuses with anencephaly, the pituitary is either absent or markedly hypoplastic. Whether the lack of adrenocorticotropic hormone (ACTH) causes the associated adrenal atrophy is disputed. Lack of an intact CNS delays the onset of labor. There is no effect on fetal heart rate. Face presentations are common with anencephaly; because of the lack of a cranium, the head will not stay flexed. Fetal CNS malformations tend to occur with pregnancies in very young or very old mothers. Diabetics also are at increased risk, unless the hydramnios caused by the fetal inability to swallow prompts labor earlier.

22. **(A)** Ventricular hemorrhages from the choroid plexus are the result of hypoxia. Rupture of the great cerebral vein at the junction of the falx and tentorium is more likely to occur from mechanical trauma and to result in subdural hematomas and/or dural tears. Studies suggest that the majority of cases of cerebral palsy occur before birth or are acquired after birth as a result of factors such as sepsis or fever. Cerebral palsy due to birth anoxia is much less common than choroid plexus hemorrhage.

23. **(C)** This concept is both important and logical. The premature or undergrown infant who is depressed at birth has a higher incidence of neurologic abnormalities than term normal-weight, high-Apgar infants. In some cases, both the newborn's low birth weight and poor Apgar scores are the result of an underlying process that results in neurologic abnormalities as well; that is, the low Apgar and birth weight are the result, not the cause, of the infant's developmental problems. Long-term follow-up is needed.

24. **(B)** Mothers are often asymptomatic carriers (urine, rectum, or vagina) of group B beta-hemolytic streptococci. Half of the newborns are colonized at the time of delivery. Early overwhelming sepsis occurs in about 1 in every 100 of the infants of colonized mothers. This is the reason why authorities recommend antibiotic prophylaxis in culture-positive or high-risk mothers during labor. Listeriosis and *Salmonella* can cause infant sepsis but are very rare. Rubella is not associated with sepsis at birth but of serious indolent infectious sequelae both before and after birth.

25. **(C)** Cerebral calcification, chorioretinitis, and head size abnormalities are also found in infants following a toxoplasmosis infection. Fortunately, not all infants of infected mothers are affected. Some also show only mild effects.

26. **(B)** About 3% to 5% have clinically significant malformations, and about 1% die. Congenital malformations account for a significant proportion of perinatal deaths.

27. **(C)** The defects in the extremities may be of varying severity. Most of the infants are of normal intelligence and survive. Thalidomide (the most potent human teratogen known) made the public aware of this drug-induced anomaly.

28. **(E)** Sex assignment can be very difficult in the case of the infant with ambiguous genitalia. Generally, three categories of children fit this problem: female pseudohermaphrodites, male pseudohermaphrodites, and those with genetic or metabolic gonadal abnormalities. When the abnormality is severe, the female sex is usually assigned because the female pseudohermaphrodite can often have normal fertility and sexual function; the male pseudohermaphrodites in most cases can have neither. While there is great pressure to assign a gender in the delivery room, further investigation of the genital structures present, as well as the infant's chromosomal makeup, must be established before the optimal sex of rearing is assigned.

29. **(C)** When one drug is abused, it is likely two or more are used. In illicit drug users, the incidence of polydrug abuse has been estimated as up to 75% of all users. From the aspect of neonatal malformation, alcohol abuse is most commonly associated with midfacial hypoplasia and behavioral/social problems. It has also been associated with brain, spine, and cardiac defects. Prematurity and growth restriction are also common. Congenital cataracts are more typical of infants exposed to viral infections early in gestation.

30. **(B)** Perinatal deaths refer to both fetal and neonatal deaths, and the rate is calculated per 1,000 live births. It has been often proposed as an indirect measure of the quality of perinatal care. Although neonatal death is more clearly defined as death within 28 days of birth and fetal death is death prior to birth, individual states will vary on whether the pregnancy must have reached 20, 24, or 28 weeks EGA or fetal size must be >500 g to be considered an intrauterine fetal devise (IUFD) and if any signs of life irrespective of gestational age, makes a birth a neonatal death. It is these inconsistencies that

make it hard to compare state-to-state statistics and nation-to-nation performance.

31. **(E)** Preterm infants have lanugo hair, rudimentary nails, no palpable breast tissue, gaping labia, and undescended testes. Dubowitz scale utilizing these and other characteristics is accurate to about ± 2 weeks.

32. **(A)** LGA implies that the infant who has been in utero for whatever length of time has grown more than normal during that period. Diabetes in the mother will result in episodes of excessive increased glucose available for fetal growth, but the mother does not have much, if any, small vessel disease that may adversely affect placental transport and fetal growth. Thus, the overall effect is likely an LGA infant. Congenital anomalies, intrauterine infection, and maternal hypertension will cause SGA infants.

33. **(B)** This infant is in a high-risk category and needs close attention and respiratory assistance. The Apgar score is 3, suggesting severe CNS depression that may be temporary with adequate resuscitative support.

34. **(E)** Given the high hematocrit of most newborns, it is very difficult for them to saturate it all with oxygen to make their fingers pink. There is no prognostic difference between an Apgar score of 9 and an Apgar score of 10.

35. **(B)** Trisomy 21 is more common with older mothers. The children also have hypotonia, epicanthal folds, Brushfield spots, a furrowed tongue, and a distal axial triradius. The developmental retardation may be mild to severe.

36. **(E)** Osteogenesis imperfecta is characterized clinically by short limb dwarfism, a large head with wide fontanels, poorly ossified or unossified calvarium, hypotonia, hyperlaxity of ligaments, prominent eyeballs and blue sclerae and a small nose with a depressed bridge. On radiographic imaging, osteoporosis and multiple fractures are common. Wilson's disease and Down syndrome are not associated with limb defects. Congenital rickets is rare in developed

countries and is not associated with craniofacial abnormalities of this type. While drugs such as thalidomide are associated with phocomelia (limb shortening), they generally do not cause the cranial abnormalities found here.

37. **(D)** The most appropriate endotracheal tube size for this infant would be 3.5 mm. Tubes 3.5 to 4.0 mm are appropriate for infants greater than 38 weeks, while a 3.0-mm tube would be most appropriate for infants between 28 and 34 weeks (1,000–2,000 g). When the newborn is less than 1,000 g or 28 weeks' gestation, a 2.5-mm tube should be used.

38. **(A)** While chlamydial infections can result in conjunctivitis, neonatal blindness is most often the result of gonococcal ophthalmia neonatorum. Infections by the herpes virus or Group B streptococcus are associated with encephalitis. *Hemophilus ducreyi* is rare and is the causative organism in chancroid.

39. **(B)** Antenatal corticosteroid therapy is associated with a reduction in the rate of neonatal respiratory distress and a reduction in the incidence of intraventricular hemorrhage. Antenatal antibiotic and calcium channel blockers are associated with an increased latency in cases of preterm rupture of the membranes or preterm labor, respectively. Recent studies indicate that magnesium sulfate may have a protective role in reducing the rate of neonatal encephalopathy, but it does not appear to independently reduce the rate of hemorrhage. Surfactant therapy reduces the risk of RDS, but it can be used only after delivery.

40. **(E)** While fetal infection after rubella exposure actually rises with gestation age after 20 to 22 weeks, congenital rubella syndrome does not occur after 17 weeks. The highest rate of congenital rubella syndrome is associated with infections occurring before 11 weeks and the rate declines thereafter. Infants born with a congenital rubella infection can continue to shed virus for many months after delivery, posing a threat to other infants, children, and susceptible adults who come in contact with them.

41. **(D)** Thrombocytopenia, hepatosplenomegaly, fetal growth restriction, and anemia are common to congenital infections by both rubella and cytomegalovirus. Cataracts, however, are more typical of rubella exposure.

42. **(A)** While all of the listed options can cause clonic seizures in the newborn, the most common cause (60%) of seizures in the first 24 hours of life is hypoxic–ischemic encephalopathy.

43. **(D)** The average caloric need of a normal fullterm infant through the first year of life is approximately 100 to 110 kcal/kg/d. Standard infant formulas and breast milk provide approximately 20 kcal/oz. Therefore, feedings of 150 to 180 mL/kg/d will provide the needed caloric intake for the average term infant.

# CHAPTER 15

# Infertility

## Questions

**DIRECTIONS (Questions 1 through 22): For each of the multiple choice questions in this section, select the lettered answer that is the one *best* response in each case.**

1. A 28-year-old woman and her partner present to their physician as they have not been able to achieve pregnancy during the past 1 year. Her partner, age 35, and she are both healthy and take no prescription medications. They are sexually active two to three times per week and do not use any contraception. Prior to initiating a potentially expensive infertility evaluation, they ask what percentage of reproductive-age couples are unable to conceive after 1 year of coitus without contraception?

   (A) 5
   (B) 15
   (C) 40
   (D) 60
   (E) 90

2. A 31-year-old infertility patient with regular ovulatory menstrual cycles has begun therapy with clomiphene citrate. Before she starts therapy, what information should you provide her regarding the medication?

   (A) Typically, the timing of ovulation is increased by a week.
   (B) Approximately 40% of patients will respond to clomiphene citrate with increased endometrial thickness.
   (C) The risk of multiple gestation is 25%.

   (D) Clomiphene citrate improves the fecundity rate principally through its effect on the endometrial lining.
   (E) Risk and side effects of clomiphene citrate include nausea, hot flushes, weight gain, and mood swings.

3. You are counseling a 30-year-old woman who wants to become pregnant. Which of the following is the most accurate method for her to time intercourse?

   (A) thermogenic shift in basal body temperature (BBT)
   (B) urinary luteinizing hormone (LH) kit testing
   (C) serum progesterone level
   (D) profuse, thin, acellular cervical mucus
   (E) mittelschmerz

4. In a young, obese, chronically anovulatory woman with an elevated LH:FSH (luteinizing hormone:follicle-stimulating hormone) ratio and polycystic-appearing ovaries, which of the following is the preferred initial method of ovulation induction?

   (A) metformin
   (B) human menopausal gonadotropins (hMGs)
   (C) pulsatile gonadotropin-releasing hormone (GnRH)
   (D) clomiphene citrate
   (E) bromocriptine mesylate

5. A patient with hypogonadotropic hypogonadism desires ovulation. What is the initial treatment of choice?

   (A) low-dose estrogen therapy
   (B) hMG therapy
   (C) bromocriptine mesylate
   (D) cyclic progesterone
   (E) clomiphene citrate

6. A woman who suffered from a severe postpartum hemorrhage and hypotensive shock that was associated with a placental abruption in a motor vehicle accident now has anterior pituitary failure (Sheehan syndrome). She wishes to have another child. Ovulation can be induced using which of the following hormonal therapies?

   (A) low-dose estrogen therapy
   (B) hMG injections
   (C) pulsatile GnRH
   (D) clomiphene citrate
   (E) bromocriptine mesylate

7. Different sex hormones have different effects on the cervical mucus. Which of the following statements accurately describes the effect of estrogen?

   (A) It decreases the water content of cervical mucus.
   (B) It decreases the palm-leaf crystallization pattern of mucus upon drying (ferning).
   (C) It decreases formation of glycoprotein channels, which favor sperm penetration.
   (D) It increases cervical mucus stretchability (spinnbarkeit).
   (E) It increases the amount of potassium chloride in the cervical mucus.

8. A patient who is now ovulating on clomiphene citrate has not conceived. You wish to do a postcoital test to see if there has been a negative cervical response to the anti-estrogen effects of the clomiphene citrate. She asks for information about the postcoital test (PCT). Which of the following best describes this test?

   (A) It predicts whether pregnancy can occur.
   (B) It correlates the number of sperm in the cervical mucus with the pregnancy rate.
   (C) It examines the ability of sperm to reach and survive in the mucus.
   (D) It is performed within 1 hour of coitus.
   (E) It is performed in the secretory phase of the cycle.

9. A 31-year-old patient is preparing to start in vitro fertilization (IVF) because of obstructed fallopian tubes. On hysterosalpingogram (HSG), it is noted that she has large dilated hydrosalpinges present bilaterally. What should be your next step?

   (A) The patient should begin her IVF treatment cycle.
   (B) The patient should repeat the HSG to confirm the result.
   (C) The patient should not be offered the opportunity to have IVF.
   (D) Bilateral salpingectomies should be done prior to starting IVF.
   (E) Her hydrosalpinges should be drained via transvaginal aspiration prior to starting IVF.

10. A 31-year-old G3P0Ab 3 woman is counseled to have an HSG for further evaluation of recurrent pregnancy loss and infertility? She has had three prior miscarriages requiring dilation and curettage. Otherwise, she is healthy. She has been attempting pregnancy for 13 months. Which of the following is the HSG likely to reveal given her history?

   (A) unicornuate uterus
   (B) distal tubal obstruction
   (C) proximal tubal obstruction
   (D) hydrosalpinx
   (E) intrauterine synechiae

11. A 33-year-old Asian woman complains of pelvic pain and amenorrhea associated with low-grade fever and weight loss. Physical examination demonstrates a tender pelvic mass. Surgical findings include dense pelvic adhesions, segmental dilatation of the fallopian tubes, and everted fimbria. Microscopic examination of the right fallopian tube shows proliferation of tubal folds with giant cells within the tube. Which diagnosis do these findings suggest?

   (A) endometriosis
   (B) adenocarcinoma
   (C) tuberculosis
   (D) gonorrheal salpingitis
   (E) salpingitis isthmica nodosa

12. A 27-year-old azoospermic male undergoes a testicular biopsy revealing normal seminiferous tubules. He is diagnosed with hypogonadotropic hypogonadism and receives FSH and human chorionic gonadotropin (hCG) injections. What is the minimal time required before repeating the semen analysis for spermatogenesis response?

   (A) 15 days
   (B) 30 days
   (C) 60 days
   (D) 90 days
   (E) 120 days

13. A patient's husband has had a previous vasectomy reversal. They have been attempting to achieve a pregnancy for a year without success. Which of the following tests should be considered primarily in this man?

   (A) Sims–Huhner test
   (B) hamster egg sperm penetration assay
   (C) sperm antibody testing
   (D) semen analysis
   (E) split ejaculate analysis

14. A couple with male infertility characterized by a semen analysis with a sperm count of 14 million/mL (low), 25% motility (low), and 23% normal forms (low) presents to your clinic. The husband's physical examination and hormone studies are normal. What is the most appropriate initial therapy?

   (A) clomiphene citrate
   (B) varicocelectomy
   (C) IVF
   (D) intrauterine insemination with washed husband's sperm
   (E) insemination with donor sperm

15. A 32-year-old male with oligospermia (low sperm count) has a history of fever accompanying painful swelling of the parotid gland and right testicle during high school. What is the most likely etiology of this condition?

   (A) cytomegalovirus
   (B) herpes simplex
   (C) varicella-zoster
   (D) mumps
   (E) influenza

16. A 43-year-old woman accompanied by her husband reports to you a history of pelvic adhesions and bilateral distal occlusion of both fallopian tubes with large hydrosalpinges. Both ovaries are buried in thick vascular adhesions. Adoption is not a consideration for the couple. What is the most appropriate recommended therapy for this couple?

   (A) gamete intrafallopian transfer (GIFT)
   (B) IVF using her own eggs
   (C) lysis of adhesions and surgical mobilization of the ovaries
   (D) ovulation induction using gonadotropins with intrauterine inseminations
   (E) IVF using donor eggs

17. During an ultrasound examination to harvest oocytes, the reproductive endocrinologist must be able to identify the position of the patient's ovaries. Which landmark is most helpful in locating the ovaries?

   (A) bladder
   (B) cul-de-sac
   (C) iliac vessels
   (D) uterus
   (E) rectum

18. A 33-year-old patient has incapacitating midline dysmenorrhea. Cyclic oral contraceptive pills previously had been unsuccessful and she gets only mild relief from analgesics. She wishes to retain her uterus in hope of becoming pregnant in the future. Which of the following current treatment options may be helpful for dysmenorrhea but should be avoided because of reducing her chances of successful future pregnancy?

(A) diagnostic laparoscopy
(B) continuous oral contraceptive pills (OCPs)
(C) levonorgestrel-releasing intrauterine system (Mirena)
(D) endometrial ablation
(E) depo-lupron

19. A woman has had three successive spontaneous abortions. She presents with a web printout of multiple therapies she wants to try. In your counseling you first let her know that without any treatment she is at risk of a fourth spontaneous abortion. Which of the following is the approximate percentage of risk?

(A) 0–5%
(B) 10–20%
(C) 30–50%
(D) 55–70%
(E) 75–90%

20. A patient with two previable pregnancy losses has been told that she likely has an incompetent cervix. She asks you to tell her about this entity. Which of the following can you correctly tell her?

(A) It is associated with first-trimester spontaneous abortions.
(B) It is easily diagnosed by precise measurement of cervical resistance to dilatation.
(C) It is characterized by painless dilatation of the cervix after the first trimester of pregnancy.
(D) It is inherited as an autosomal recessive disease.
(E) It is primarily treated by medical therapy.

21. You are counseling a couple about factors that can affect fertility. Which of the following factors adversely affect spermatogenesis?

(A) swimming
(B) exposure to cold
(C) febrile illness
(D) boxer shorts
(E) weekly intercourse

22. A 44-year-old woman is oligo-ovulatory and wants to conceive using her own eggs. Which of the following is the most predictive of diminished ovarian reserve as a result of age-related changes?

(A) serum early follicular phase FSH and estradiol levels
(B) serum early follicular phase FSH and LH levels
(C) serum progesterone during the late luteal phase
(D) serum inhibin B levels during the late luteal phase
(E) GnRH

DIRECTIONS (Questions 23 through 29): The following groups of questions are preceded by a list of lettered options. For each question, select the one lettered option that is most closely associated with it. Each lettered option may be used once, multiple times, or not at all.

Questions 23 through 25

Match the drug with its descriptor.

(A) clomiphene citrate
(B) bromocriptine mesylate
(C) hMGs
(D) GnRH
(E) dexamethasone
(F) GnRH analog

**23.** Dopamine agonist

**24.** Antiestrogen

**25.** Urinary metabolites of postmenopausal women

**Questions 26 through 29**

Match the procedure with its practical use.

    (A)  colposcopy
    (B)  laparoscopy
    (C)  hysteroscopy
    (D)  HSG
    (E)  ultrasound

**26.** A procedure that assesses both uterine cavity and tubal lumen

**27.** A procedure that visualizes pelvic endometriosis

**28.** A procedure that visualizes the uterine cavity

**29.** A procedure that detects ovum release from the follicle

# Answers and Explanations

1. **(B)** About 15% of reproductive-age couples are unable to conceive after 1 year of coitus without contraception. Eighty percent of couples achieve conception within 1 year, with 25% conceiving during the first month of unprotected coitus.

2. **(E)** The risks and side effects of clomiphene citrate include nausea, hot flushes, weight gain, and emotional liability. These side effects occur with relative frequency in 10% to 25% of patients. The risk of multiple gestation with clomiphene citrate is 7%. Clomiphene citrate acts on the hypothalamus as an antiestrogen to blunt the negative feedback of estrogen. It may also have negative effects on endometrial proliferation, thus causing a decrease in endometrial thickness. Typically, ovulation takes place at the expected time for an ovulatory woman.

3. **(B)** When used by a motivated individual, the urinary LH surge predicts ovulation within 24 hours in 87% of menstrual cycles. BBTs and endometrial decidualization rely on progesterone action to retrospectively identify ovulation. Profuse, thin, acellular cervical mucus results from high circulating estrogen levels unopposed by progesterone. It cannot distinguish between the presence of a dominant follicle or chronic anovulation. Mittelschmerz, the transient abdominal pain accompanying bleeding from the ovulatory follicle, does not occur in all women.

4. **(D)** Clomiphene citrate (CC) is the initial treatment for most anovulatory or oligo-ovulatory infertility. Approximately 80% of women will ovulate with CC. Metformin is an insulin-sensitizing agent that induces spontaneous ovulatory cycles in approximately 33% of women with insulin-resistant polycystic ovary syndrome (PCOS). In the largest trial comparing CC to metformin, live birth rates were higher with clomiphene than metformin therapy. A consensus group has recommended against the routine use of metformin except in women with glucose intolerance. Intramuscular administration of hMGs and intravenous pulsatile GnRH therapy are expensive and inconvenient. They are not the initial drugs of choice in a woman with an intact pituitary and functioning ovaries. Bromocriptine is useful in the setting of elevated prolactin which is not the case in PCOS.

5. **(B)** Absence of ovarian function due to hypothalamic dysfunction is characterized by low-normal circulating gonadotropin levels and is referred to as hypogonadotropic hypogonadism. Anovulation accompanying hypogonadotropic hypogonadism is associated with low circulating estrogen levels and is therefore unresponsive to CC. Ovulation can be established with pulsatile GnRH therapy or hMG administration. Bromocriptine is for suppression of prolactin when it is the cause for anovulation. Cyclic progesterone is used in cases of high estrogen due to chronically elevated FSH or LH by providing negative feedback to hypothalamic–pituitary axis.

6. **(B)** Sheehan syndrome is a condition in which the cells of the anterior pituitary responsible for FSH and LH production are no longer viable. Thus, the remnant pituitary will be unresponsive to increases in endogenous (CC) or exogenous (pulsatile) GnRH. These women

undergo successful ovulation with daily injections of hMG (a combination of 75 IU FSH and 75 IU LH) for an average length of time of 10 to 12 days, which directly stimulates folliculogenesis to create mature follicles and oocytes.

7. **(D)** Cervical mucus consists of multiple cross-linked glycoproteins. Although amounts vary with the menstrual cycle, 90% of cervical mucus consists of water and sodium chloride (NaCl). In the early follicular phase, a scant amount of cervical mucus is present. During the late follicular phase, a rise in circulating estrogen levels alters vascular epithelial permeability and increases the water content of cervical secretions. The mucus becomes profuse, thin, acellular, and clear, resulting in a high degree of stretchability (8–10 cm), referred to as spinnbarkeit, when pulled from the cervix, or stretched between a slide and a cover slip. The NaCl content of the mucus allows it to form a palm-leaf crystallization pattern upon drying, a phenomenon referred to as *ferning*. These properties of estrogen-stimulated mucus promote formation of glycoprotein channels favoring sperm penetration.

8. **(C)** The PCT, or Simms–Huhner test, examines sperm survival in cervical mucus and determines whether sperm are migrating into the female reproductive system. It does not predict whether pregnancy can occur. The test is performed after 2 days of sexual abstinence and 1 to 2 days before ovulation, when estrogen-stimulated cervical mucus is abundant. BBTs or the midcycle LH surge may be used to determine the timing of the PCT. Mucus is withdrawn from the endocervical canal within 8 hours of coitus and examined. The presence of any forwardly motile sperm in alkaline mucus suggests adequate coital technique and a normal cervical mucus–sperm interaction.

9. **(D)** The bulk of the evidence in the current literature suggests that the presence of large hydrosalpinges decreased the pregnancy success rate of IVF by approximately 50%. Thus, it is now standard practice to recommend bilateral resection of hydrosalpinges prior to initiating IVF to increase the couple's chances of success. Aspi-

rating the hydrosalpinges will simply result in refilling of the fallopian tubes with fluid.

10. **(E)** Hysterosalpingography entails injection of radiopaque dye through the uterus with fluoroscopic visualization of the uterine cavity and tubal lumen. The resulting HSG is useful in detecting uterine anomalies and fallopian tube occlusion in women with histories of repetitive spontaneous abortion and infertility. This woman has been able to conceive in the past but has had three spontaneous miscarriages and resultant D&Cs. She is at risk for intrauterine adhesions from those procedures. Although she could have the other conditions, she has been able to conceive, making anomalous uterus, tubal obstruction, and hydrosalpinx less likely.

11. **(C)** *Mycobacterium tuberculosis* is prevalent in several parts of the world, including the southeastern United States, Asia, Mexico, and Scotland. Intestinal tuberculosis used to be the source of most pelvic organ involvement, but now in the United States, it usually represents a secondary invasion, occurring by lymphohematogenous spread from a primary lung infection. Pelvic tuberculosis occurs in about 5% of patients with pulmonary disease. The tube may be studded with miliary implants, which should not be mistaken for Walthard's rests or metastatic cancer. Distinguishing features of this disease are extremely dense pelvic adhesions, segmental dilatation of the fallopian tubes, and everted fimbria, giving the tube the appearance of a "tobacco pouch." Peritoneal disease may cause ascites, while endometrial involvement may lead to amenorrhea.

12. **(D)** Spermatogenesis occurs over 72 days. Therefore, the earliest time period that sperm can be detected is 90 days but frequently requires longer observation periods.

13. **(D)** The most important part of the male infertility evaluation is a semen analysis. In this situation it is important to verify patency of vas deferens before expending additional funds on the more subtle aspects of sperm function. A semen specimen is obtained by masturbation

after 3 to 7 days of abstinence, or through intercourse using nonspermicidal silicon condoms. The sample must be kept warm and received by the laboratory within 1 hour. Occasionally, it is important to examine subtle aspects of sperm function by other methods. The sperm penetration assay evaluates the ability of human sperm to penetrate golden hamster eggs prepared to accept foreign sperm. A split ejaculate may be useful for some types of inseminations and collects the semen in two portions: the first portion containing the sperm-rich fraction and prostatic fluid, and the second portion containing seminal vesicle fluid with less sperm numbers. Detection of antibodies directed against sperm is helpful for rare cases of immunologic infertility. The Sims–Huhner test or sperm penetration assay of cervical mucus in vitro was developed to study sperm–mucus interactions but is rarely performed today.

14. **(D)** Appropriate initial therapy is intrauterine inseminations with husband's sperm. With mild-to-moderate male factor infertility, the success of inseminations is lower (5–15% per cycle). However, this method should be attempted before proceeding to donor sperm or IVF. If the couple requires IVF to successfully conceive, then the recommended procedure for IVF is intracytoplasmic sperm injection (ICSI). This is a procedure that involves the injection of single sperm into an oocyte to achieve fertilization. Varicocelectomy is helpful only after documentation of a varicocele.

15. **(D)** The RNA virus, paramyxovirus, is responsible for mumps. It causes parotid gland inflammation, which is occasionally accompanied by pancreatitis, orchitis, and encephalitis. Mumps orchitis can produce abnormalities in sperm quality and quantity, particularly if it occurs postpuberty. This is the most common complication of mumps in men, occurring in up to 38% of postpubertal males. Impaired fertility occurs in approximately 13% of men with orchitis but sterility is uncommon.

16. **(E)** Maternal aging and decreased ovarian reserve at age 43 precludes the use of GIFT or IVF as a reasonable therapeutic approach for this couple. Ovulation induction is not indicated because of the presence of severe tubal factor with bilateral hydrosalpinges. There is no need for lysis of adhesions due to the poor prognosis with this couple using the patient's own tubes and ovaries. Donor egg IVF would offer a one in two chance for pregnancy success in this couple.

17. **(C)** Reproductive endocrinologists generally use a needle to aspirate the ovarian follicles to obtain oocytes. This is most commonly done as an office procedure under ultrasound guidance. The technique of aspiration is generally unaffected by previous pelvic disease. In fact, the ovary that is immobilized by pelvic adhesions may be an easier target to hit than the one that is freely mobile. Since the ovaries are anatomically below the uterine corpus and just above the cul-de-sac, transvaginal aspiration is the method of choice for most clinicians. On routine scanning for ovarian position, the ovaries almost always are found to overlie the great vessels of the pelvis. These vessels are therefore used as a landmark during pelvic scanning.

18. **(D)** Dysmenorrhea is either primary—no organic or structural cause or secondary to some other condition such as uterine myomas, Pelvic Inflammatory Disease (PID), adenomyosis, or endometriosis. Strategies that have been shown to be successful in the treatment of dysmenorrhea include nonsteroidal anti-inflammatory drugs, combine oral contraceptives—both cyclic and continuous, progestins, including oral, Intramuscular (IM), and intrauterine device (IUD), laparoscopic treatment of endometriosis, depo-lupron treatment of endometriosis, and endometrial ablation. Endometrial ablation may increase the risk of infertility, miscarriage, preterm labor, antepartum hemorrhage, and abnormal placental attachment. It is therefore contraindicated in women who wish to maintain the possibility of fertility.

19. **(C)** The risk of first-trimester spontaneous abortion after three successive abortions, with a prior live birth is about 32% and with no prior live birth, it is 47% (30–55%). Inaccurate theoretical calculations performed over 50 years ago stated

that a woman with a history of three successive abortions had a 73% to 84% chance of aborting a subsequent pregnancy. The use of these inaccurate, pessimistic projections led to several empirical therapies for the treatment of recurrent abortion.

20. **(C)** The term incompetent cervix refers to the painless dilatation of the cervix during the second trimester or early third trimester of pregnancy. Prolapse of fetal membranes through the cervix is usually followed by expulsion of a living fetus that is too immature to survive. A careful history to determine whether these events occurred previously is required since precise methods to diagnose an incompetent cervix do not exist. Although a shortened cervical length or funneling during the second trimester increases the risk of incompetence its sensitivity and specificity is poor. The most common cause of incompetent cervix is trauma (e.g., dilatation and curettage, conization, and cervical amputation), although exposure to stilbestrol in utero has also been associated with this disorder. An incompetent cervix is usually treated by surgical cerclage (e.g., McDonald and Shirodkar), a procedure designed to restore the competency of the cervix.

21. **(C)** Several environmental factors, including occupations with prolonged sitting (truck drivers), febrile illness, use of jockey shorts, and hot baths or saunas may adversely affect spermatogenesis by increasing intratesticular temperature. The testes are located outside the abdomen because the optimal temperature for spermatozoa production is 1°F less than body temperature. Forty percent of infertile men have a varicocele, defined as dilation of the pampiniform plexus above the testis. Retrograde blood flow increases scrotal temperature and disturbs spermatogenesis. A varicocele also occurs in approximately 10% to 15% of the general population. Attempts to reduce scrotal temperature (e.g., use of boxer shorts) are commonly advised as part of the treatment of male infertility. Swimming should not harm spermatogenesis. Once the offending behavior is ceased, one must wait 90+ days to see if the behavior change has improved the sperm count.

22. **(A)** The most predictive test of diminishing ovarian reserve in a woman is the early follicular phase FSH and estradiol levels. Serum LH is not helpful. There is no evidence that luteal progesterone is predictive of ovarian reserve. Serum inhibin B levels have been implicated but remain less predictive than FSH and estradiol.

23. **(B)** Bromocriptine, a lysergic acid derivative, acts as a dopamine agonist, to inhibit prolactin release. In most women with elevated serum prolactin levels and amenorrhea–galactorrhea, bromocriptine restores normal menstruation within 6 weeks and causes cessation of galactorrhea by 13 weeks. Bromocriptine therapy also may diminish the size and symptoms of prolactin-secreting pituitary adenomas. Approximately 5% of patients terminate bromocriptine therapy due to nausea, headache, and faintness. These side effects may be minimized by taking the medication with food and by gradually increasing the bromocriptine dose to the appropriate level for the patient.

24. **(A)** CC is an oral antiestrogen that binds to estrogen receptors in the reproductive tract and hypothalamus. By inhibiting estrogen-negative feedback on FSH, clomiphene induces an elevation in circulating FSH levels, which stimulates folliculogenesis. Clomiphene therapy may be combined with midcycle hCG administration and luteal-phase progesterone supplementation. Its use may cause a reduction in cervical mucus and an abnormal endometrial biopsy due to antiestrogenic actions on the cervix and endometrium. The multiple birth rate associated with clomiphene therapy is about 5%, and most of these pregnancies are twin gestations.

25. **(C)** hMGs are derived from the urine of postmenopausal women. Commercially available ampules contain about equal amounts of LH and FSH. Intramuscular administration of hMGs is expensive and associated with a multiple birth rate of about 10%. Purified FSH, separated from urinary LH by immunochromatography, has become available.

26. **(D)** Hysterosalpingography detects intrauterine pathology and confirms tubal patency by

spill of dye from the tube into the peritoneal cavity. Radiopaque dye is used for the HSG and may be either oil or water soluble. Oil-soluble media produce a sharp image and transiently increase fertility in some women, perhaps by decreasing local macrophage activation or enhancing tubal ciliary action. Their use may be associated with granuloma formation and a 1% risk of pulmonary embolism that is usually asymptomatic. Water-soluble media are used when there is a history suggestive of tubal disease. Hysterosalpingography is performed shortly after menstruation to avoid radiation exposure to an early pregnancy. It should be postponed in women with suspected pelvic infection due to a 1% to 3% risk of exacerbating the disease.

27.  **(B)** Laparoscopy refers to the endoscopic visualization of the pelvic viscera. It can directly visualize pelvic disease and assess tubal patency by confirming spill of methylene blue dye from the tubal fimbria after its intrauterine injection (chromotubation). Laparoscopy identifies unsuspected pathology such as pelvic endometriosis in up to 50% of asymptomatic women with no other cause for infertility. It may also detect uterine anomalies of fusion such as a bicornuate uterus.

28.  **(C)** The uterine cavity can be assessed directly by hysteroscopy. During hysteroscopy, the uterine cavity is distended with a variety of media such as sterile saline or glycine. A scope is inserted and direct inspection of the cavity is performed. Surgical instruments may be used during hysteroscopy to treat abnormalities of the uterine cavity such as submucosal fibroids, uterine septum, or synechiae.

29.  **(E)** Ultrasound can detect ovum release from the follicle. Unfortunately, no procedure currently exists to detect ovum transfer into the fallopian tube.

# Clinical Endocrinology

## Questions

1. A 21-year-old athletic woman with diabetes on a low-dose oral contraceptive comes to your clinic with irregular menses and bilateral breast discharge. On examination, the discharge is expressed and galactorrhea is confirmed with fat globules seen microscopically. She currently takes metoclopramide (Reglan) for delayed gastric emptying. A random serum prolactin level is 65 ng/mL. Which of the following is most likely responsible for her hyperprolactinemia?

   (A) metoclopramide
   (B) pregnancy
   (C) oral contraceptive
   (D) pituitary adenoma
   (E) exercise

2. During pregnancy, the placenta and fetus actively contribute to the maternal hormone levels and impact the maternal–fetal unit physiology. Which of the following hormones decreases after the first trimester of pregnancy?

   (A) progesterone
   (B) prolactin
   (C) human chorionic gonadotropin (hCG)
   (D) human placental lactogen (hPL)
   (E) estriol

3. A 25-year-old woman who underwent menarche at 11 years of age presents with a history of irregular menstrual cycles over the last 12 months, increased weight gain, and bilateral pelvic pain. Transvaginal ultrasound shows large cystic adnexa, with cysts measuring 7 to 9 cm in size. A urine pregnancy test is negative. Her thyroid-stimulating hormone (TSH) level is 17 mIU/mL, and prolactin level is 10 ng/mL. Which of the following is the treatment of choice for this patient to regain normal menstrual cycles?

   (A) monophasic birth control pills
   (B) triphasic birth control pills
   (C) levothyroxine treatment
   (D) bromocriptine treatment
   (E) gonadotropin-releasing hormone (GnRH) agonist treatment

4. A 22-year-old woman with amenorrhea of 6 weeks' duration undergoes surgery for acute appendicitis. At the time of surgery, a 3-cm semisolid left ovarian cyst is discovered. It is vascular and appears to contain a blood-filled central cavity. A serum pregnancy test is positive. Which of the following is the most appropriate next step in this patient's management?

   (A) ovarian cystectomy
   (B) ovarian wedge resection
   (C) oophorectomy
   (D) salpingo-oophorectomy
   (E) no additional therapy indicated

5. A 25-year-old woman is having a severe intrapartum hemorrhage with hypovolumic shock. Which of the following symptoms is evidence of pituitary infarction?

   (A) infrequent urination
   (B) diarrhea
   (C) easy bruisability
   (D) lactation failure
   (E) perspiration

6. A 16-year-old girl has not experienced menarche. Examination shows absence of breast development and small but otherwise normal female pelvic organs. Which of the following diagnostic tests is most useful in determining the etiology of the amenorrhea?

   (A) serum follicle-stimulating hormone (FSH)
   (B) serum estradiol
   (C) serum testosterone
   (D) magnetic resonance imaging (MRI) of the head
   (E) ovarian biopsy

**Questions 7 and 8 apply to the following patient:**

An 18-year-old patient has not experienced menarche. Examination shows normal breast development and absence of a uterus.

7. Which of the following diagnostic tests is most useful in determining the etiology of the amenorrhea?

   (A) serum FSH
   (B) serum estradiol
   (C) serum testosterone
   (D) MRI of the head
   (E) ovarian biopsy

8. If congenital androgen insensitivity syndrome (testicular feminization) is diagnosed, it is caused by a defect in what aspect of androgen function?

   (A) synthesis
   (B) metabolism
   (C) receptor action

   (D) excretion
   (E) aromatization

9. An adult genetic male with 17-alpha-hydroxylase deficiency would have which of the following findings?

   (A) no breast development, uterus present, hypertension
   (B) no breast development, uterus present, hypotension
   (C) breast development, uterus absent, hypotension
   (D) no breast development, uterus absent, hypertension
   (E) breast development, uterus present, hypertension

10. A 28-year-old patient complains of amenorrhea after dilation and curettage (D&C) for postpartum bleeding. She denies any other complaints and did not require a blood transfusion at the time of her postpartum bleed. Which of the following is the most likely diagnosis?

   (A) gonadal dysgenesis
   (B) Sheehan syndrome
   (C) Kallmann syndrome
   (D) Mayer–Rokitansky–Küster–Hauser syndrome
   (E) Asherman syndrome

11. A 25-year-old woman experiences galactorrhea and amenorrhea of 8 weeks' duration with irregular vaginal bleeding. Which of the following serum assays should initially be performed?

   (A) hCG
   (B) progesterone
   (C) prolactin
   (D) FSH
   (E) luteinizing hormone (LH)

12. A 14-year-old girl complains of irregular vaginal bleeding. Her general examination and pelvic organs are normal. Which of the following is the most likely cause of anovulatory bleeding (dysfunctional uterine bleeding [DUB]) in this patient?

(A) hypothyroidism

(B) pituitary adenoma

(C) polycystic ovary syndrome (PCOS)

(D) congenital adrenal hyperplasia (CAH)

(E) hypothalamic immaturity

13. A 15-year-old girl is seen in the emergency department. She has a sudden onset of heavy vaginal bleeding. She has noted irregular, painless vaginal bleeding of 6 months' duration. Her medical history is unremarkable, and she is not sexually active. Physical and pelvic examinations are normal, but blood is coming through the cervical os. A serum pregnancy test is negative, and complete blood cell count has hematocrit of 37% (normal 35% to 45%) and normal white blood cell and platelet counts. Which of the following is the best course of immediate action?

(A) observation

(B) estrogen therapy

(C) progesterone therapy

(D) nonsteroidal anti-inflammatory therapy

(E) D&C

14. An 18-year-old woman comes to your clinic with irregular cycles since menarche and mild hirsutism. She is not interested in pregnancy or contraception. Her serum TSH, prolactin, and dehydroepiandrosterone sulfate (DHEAS) levels are normal, with a slightly elevated serum testosterone level of 80 ng/dL. Which of the following is the most appropriate next step for this patient?

(A) oral contraceptive treatment

(B) endometrial biopsy

(C) GnRH stimulation test

(D) clomiphene citrate

(E) bromocriptine

15. A 24-year-old nulligravid patient presents with complaints of increasing dark coarse hair growth over upper lip and chin, on the abdomen, and on her chest. She denies any change in her voice, balding, or clitoral enlargement. Which of the following is she most likely experiencing?

(A) masculinization

(B) defeminization

(C) virilization

(D) hirsutism

(E) androgenization

16. A 4-year-old girl is brought in by her mother for evaluation of clitoral enlargement. She is tall for her age, with no breast or axillary hair development. There is slight pubic hair growth on examination and an enlarged clitoris with a single perineal opening. Karyotype is 46,XX. The 17-OHP level is 108 ng/mL. What is the most likely diagnosis?

(A) androgen insensitivity syndrome

(B) PCOS

(C) CAH with 21-hydroxylase deficiency

(D) ovarian thecoma

(E) germ cell ovarian tumor

17. Female pseudohermaphroditism refers to individuals who have which of the following?

(A) ovaries, an XX karyotype, and varying degrees of masculinization

(B) testes, an XY karyotype, and varying degrees of masculinization failure

(C) ovaries, an XY karyotype, and varying degrees of masculinization failure

(D) testes, an XX karyotype, and severe masculinization

(E) both ovarian and testicular tissue

18. An infant with ambiguous genitalia is found to have testes and an XY karyotype. Seminal vesicles, ejaculatory ducts, epididymis, and vas deferens (Wolffian duct derivatives) are present. There is no uterus, fallopian tubes, or upper vagina. The ratio of circulating testosterone to dihydrotestosterone (DHT) is elevated compared to normal male infants. What is the most likely diagnosis?

(A) 20,22 desmolase deficiency

(B) 21-hydroxylase deficiency

(C) testicular feminization

(D) 5-alpha-reductase deficiency

(E) embryonic testicular regression

19. A 17-year-old boy presents for delayed sexual development. He is 6 ft 5 in. tall with a weight of 152 lb. There is a reduced amount of pubic hair with a small phallus and small testicles. Endocrine testing reveals increased FSH and LH levels and a low testosterone level. What is the most likely diagnosis?

   (A) Kallmann syndrome
   (B) Klinefelter syndrome
   (C) Savage syndrome
   (D) Beckwith–Wiedemann syndrome
   (E) Turner syndrome

20. During pregnancy, the most likely change in maternal levels of thyroxine-binding globulin (TBG), total thyroxine (T4), and total triiodothyronine (T3) are which of the following?

   (A) TBG levels, total thyroxine (T4), and total triiodothyronine (T3) all rise.
   (B) TBG levels rise, but total thyroxine (T4) and total triiodothyronine (T3) fall.
   (C) TBG levels and total thyroxine (T4) rise while total triiodothyronine (T3) remains unchanged.
   (D) TBG levels fall, while total thyroxine (T4) and total triiodothyronine (T3) both rise.
   (E) TBG levels, total thyroxine (T4), and total triiodothyronine (T3) all remain unchanged

21. Successful lactation is initiated by which of the following?

   (A) estrogen stimulation during pregnancy
   (B) progesterone stimulation during pregnancy
   (C) elevated levels of hCG
   (D) elevated levels of prolactin near term
   (E) the postpartum decline in circulating sex steroid levels

22. Amenorrhea, estrogen deficiency, and elevated circulating gonadotropin levels are noted in a normal-appearing 27-year-old woman. Which of the following conditions is most closely associated with these findings?

   (A) X chromosome abnormalities
   (B) polyglandular autoimmune syndrome
   (C) Kallmann syndrome
   (D) alkylating antineoplastic drugs
   (E) pelvic irradiation

23. A 33-year-old woman who underwent normal puberty describes an 18-month history of secondary amenorrhea and hot flashes. A pregnancy test was negative. A progesterone withdrawal challenge test revealed no bleeding. Her FSH was 94 mIU/mL, and her LH level was 68 mIU/mL. She desires to be pregnant with her current partner. Which of the following is the most appropriate next step in the management of this individual?

   (A) karyotype
   (B) measurement of serum prolactin
   (C) clomiphene citrate therapy
   (D) gonadotropin stimulation therapy
   (E) estrogen replacement therapy

24. What is the principal androgen used for placental estrogen synthesis?

   (A) androstenedione
   (B) testosterone
   (C) DHEAS
   (D) aldosterone
   (E) cortisol

25. What is the principal hormone produced by the maternal zona glomerulosa?

   (A) estriol
   (B) androstenedione
   (C) testosterone
   (D) DHEAS
   (E) aldosterone

26. What is the principal hormone responsible for 1,25-dihydroxy vitamin $D_3$ synthesis?

   (A) aldosterone
   (B) cortisol
   (C) thyroxine
   (D) parathyroid hormone (PTH)
   (E) insulin

27. A patient with hirsutism, ovarian androgen excess, and elevated serum LH levels is most likely to have which of the following?

(A) 11-beta-hydroxylase deficiency

(B) Cushing syndrome

(C) adrenal tumor

(D) polycystic ovarian syndrome (PCOS)

(E) arrhenoblastoma

28. Which of the following is the most common adrenal cause for hirsutism, adrenal androgen excess, and elevated 17-OHP?

(A) 20,22-desmolase deficiency

(B) 3-beta-hydroxysteroid dehydrogenase (3-n HSD) deficiency

(C) 21-hydroxylase deficiency

(D) 11-beta-hydroxylase deficiency

(E) Cushing syndrome

29. Sexual differentiation of the male internal and external genitalia is most dependent on the action of which of the following?

(A) anti-müllerian hormone (AMH)

(B) sex-determining region of the Y chromosome (SRY)

(C) testosterone

(D) DHEAS

(E) cortisol

30. For most girls, the onset of puberty is heralded by which of the following?

(A) growth acceleration

(B) thelarche

(C) pubarche

(D) menarche

(E) ovulation

31. The physical stigmata of Turner syndrome are due to loss of chromosomal material from which chromosome?

(A) chromosome 21

(B) chromosome 18

(C) chromosome 6

(D) the short arm of the X chromosome

(E) the Y chromosome

32. A 14-year-old girl is brought to you for evaluation of lower abdominal pain that has been progressive over the preceding 4 months. History indicates that she experienced a growth spurt at age 11 and has had normal breast and pubic hair growth that began approximately 2 years ago. She appears to be of appropriate height. She has no other medical conditions and takes no medications. She has not had a menstrual period and is not sexually active. What is the most appropriate next step in the evaluation of this patient?

(A) measurement of serum hCG

(B) measurement of serum FSH

(C) imaging of the pituitary and sella turcica

(D) pelvic ultrasonography

(E) pelvic examination

33. A 25-year-old G4P0040 presents for evaluation of recurrent documented pregnancy losses that have occurred between the 10th and 14th weeks of gestation. The patient has no ongoing medical conditions and takes no medications. Pubertal events and menstrual history are unremarkable. A pelvic examination is normal. What is the most appropriate next step in the evaluation of this patient?

(A) measurement of serum FSH on cycle day 3

(B) hysterosalpingography

(C) imaging of the pituitary and sella turcica

(D) pelvic ultrasonography

(E) measurement of mid-cycle LH

34. Which of the following ovarian tumors is most likely to result in virilization of a 35-year-old woman?

(A) Brenner (transitional cell) tumor

(B) dysgerminoma

(C) Sertoli–Leydic cell tumor

(D) mucinous cystademoma

(E) thecoma

# Answers and Explanations

1. **(A)** Pregnancy increases prolactin levels; however, this patient is unlikely to be pregnant because she was taking the oral contraceptive but a urine pregnancy test is still indicated. The oral contraceptive rarely increases prolactin to such high levels. Metoclopramide is a potent dopamine antagonist that can act on the lactotroph to ramp up secretion of prolactin. A prolactin-producing pituitary adenoma is unlikely since most tumors present with serum prolactin levels greater than 100 ng/mL. While athletic nipple stimulation ("jogger's nipples") could cause a modest elevation in serum prolactin, elevations of the level given here are unlikely.

2. **(C)** Maternal serum levels of progesterone rise to term to peak at 190 ng/mL. Maternal prolactin levels continue a steady increase throughout pregnancy to a third-trimester peak level of 200 ng/mL. Maternal hPL levels also increase during the entirety of the pregnancy. However, hCG peaks at 10 weeks and decreases to a lower plateau through the second and third trimesters. This is why trending hCG levels to assess quality of pregnancy is really only useful for the first 6 to 8 weeks of pregnancy. At that point, the rate of increase of hCG is very unpredictable. Estriol, estradiol, and estrone all increase steadily during pregnancy.

3. **(C)** Ovarian cysts and irregular menstrual cycles can both arise from compensated hypothyroidism, which is revealed by this patient's elevated TSH level. Levothyroxine is the treatment of choice. Monophasic or triphasic birth control pills would only mask the underlying problem despite the fact that regular withdrawal bleeding can be achieved. This patient has a normal serum prolactin level, and thus bromocriptine is not indicated.

4. **(E)** Blood often accumulates within a vascularized corpus luteum. A corpus luteum cyst may develop as the blood reabsorbs, causing a physiologic ovarian enlargement. Since progesterone production by the corpus luteum maintains pregnancy until the seventh gestational week, removal of the corpus luteum (luteectomy) before this time will terminate pregnancy. There is a transitional period between the seventh and tenth gestational weeks when the corpus luteum and placenta contribute to circulating progesterone levels. After the tenth week, the placenta is the major source of progesterone. Any ovarian surgery would jeopardize this pregnancy and may decrease subsequent fertility.

5. **(D)** Pituitary infarction (Sheehan syndrome) due to severe intrapartum hemorrhage is associated with low serum prolactin levels and postpartum lactation failure. Other symptoms could include secondary amenorrhea, secondary hypothyroidism, adrenal insufficiency, loss of pubic and axillary hair, and uterine superinvolution. Peripartum women are more at risk for infarction of the pituitary with significant hemorrhage than a nonpregnant population due to increased hypertrophy of the pituitary and the vulnerability to poor perfusion during hypovolemic shock.

6. **(A)** Primary amenorrhea is defined as absence of menarche by age 16 years, or by age 14 years

without appearance of secondary sex characteristics, or within 2 years of the onset of secondary sex changes. A practical approach used by some investigators assigns patients with normal female external genitalia and primary amenorrhea into one of four groups based on physical examination. A series of diagnostic steps unique to each category determines the etiology of amenorrhea. The four groups of patients with primary amenorrhea are (1) no breast development and uterus present, (2) breast development and uterus absent, (3) no breast development and uterus absent, and (4) breast development and uterus present. In the evaluation of a patient from group 1 (as described in this problem), a serum FSH level can distinguish between absence of gonadal function (elevated FSH) such as gonadal dysgenesis and diminished pulsatile GnRH release (suppressed FSH) such as delayed puberty from hypothalamic suppression (Olympic-level gymnast). Further investigation is similar to that of delayed puberty. All individuals with secondary amenorrhea are included in group 4.

7. **(C)** This patient belongs to group 2 (breast development and uterus absent) from answer 6. The two disorders in this group are (1) abnormal müllerian duct development in females and (2) defective androgen action in males. These disorders are distinguished by measuring serum testosterone levels, which are in the female range in women with abnormal müllerian duct development. Mayer–Rokitansky–Küster–Hauser syndrome is a disorder of müllerian duct development in which the uterus and vagina are congenitally absent. Ovarian function is preserved, and ovulation occurs during the reproductive years. In contrast, circulating testosterone levels are in the male range in men with defective androgen action. These individuals commonly have congenital androgen insensitivity syndrome (testicular feminization) due to defective androgen action and should have a karyotype performed to confirm genetic sex.

8. **(C)** Congenital androgen insensitivity syndrome (testicular feminization) occurs in men and is due to defective androgen receptor ac-

tion. It is an X-linked recessive disorder of androgen receptor function and is characterized by lack of masculinization. Androgen insensitivity of target tissues causes failure of male sexual differentiation (female-appearing external genitalia), absence of Wolffian duct development, and lack of pubertal hair growth in the axillary and pubic regions. During puberty, testicular androgen production is normal and provides androgenic precursors for peripheral aromatization to estrogen. Consequently, abundant breast tissue develops at puberty due to estrogen production uninhibited by androgen action. However, müllerian duct regression in response to testicular müllerian inhibitory factor (MIF) during genitalia formation causes the vagina to end as a blind pouch, resulting in primary amenorrhea. The testes are located in the pelvis or within an inguinal hernia and contain immature seminiferous tubules. Gonadectomy is performed to avoid the risk of malignant gonadal degeneration but is delayed until after puberty in order to allow hormone-dependent pubertal changes. These individuals have a female gender identity and should receive postoperative estrogen replacement therapy.

9. **(D)** Genetic males (46,XY) with enzymatic defects in the early pathways of steroidogenesis (20,22 desmolase 17-alpha-hydroxylase, 17,20 desmolase) are extremely rare (group 3 from answer 6). Absence of sex steroid production accounts for elevated gonadotropins, low-circulating testosterone levels, and lack of breast development. Müllerian duct regression due to testicular MIF causes absence of uterine development. Neonates with these disorders often die from cortisol deficiency. Adults with 17-alpha-hydroxylase deficiency have hypertension and hypokalemic alkalosis and should undergo gonadectomy to prevent the risk of developing a malignant gonadal tumor.

10. **(E)** Asherman syndrome refers to the presence of intrauterine scarring (synechiae). The most common cause of this disorder is uterine curettage for postpartum hemorrhage or abortion. It may also accompany myomectomy,

metroplasty, cesarean section, uterine infection due to intrauterine device use, tuberculosis, and schistosomiasis. Intrauterine synechiae are diagnosed either by injecting radiographic dye into the uterus under fluoroscopic view (hysterosalpingography) or by directly visualizing the uterine cavity (hysteroscopy). The latter technique may also be used therapeutically to lyse adhesions. Approximately 70% of patients treated for Asherman syndrome have a subsequent successful pregnancy. Many experience difficulties with placental–uterine separation after birth, leading to an increased risk of postpartum hemorrhage. Gonadal dysgenesis, M–R–K–H syndrome and Kallman are congenital anomalies that would have presented a pregnancy. Sheehan syndrome is rare in the setting of postpartum hemorrhage unless there was hypovolumeic shock that would have been treated with transfusion.

11. **(A)** The first diagnostic step in a reproductive-aged woman with amenorrhea is to exclude pregnancy with a serum hCG determination. After excluding pregnancy, serum prolactin and TSH levels should also be measured, because abnormalities of prolactin secretion and thyroid function disrupt ovulation. Hyperprolactinemia occurs in approximately 20% of amenorrheic individuals without galactorrhea and should be evaluated further if present. Progesterone or LH will not help diagnostically.

12. **(E)** It is not uncommon for a young woman to be anovulatory for the first year or more after menarche. In the absence of androgen and prolactin excess, most anovulatory women with normal circulating gonadotropin levels have hypothalamic dysfunction. This condition may be due to suppression of hypothalamic GnRH release. The resulting decline in circulating estradiol (E2) levels is insufficient to induce the ovulatory LH surge but is able to stimulate endometrial proliferation. Hypothalamic dysfunction may be idiopathic in origin or induced by medication (narcotics), ethanol, stress, excessive physical activity, and weight loss.

13. **(B)** For severe DUB, estrogen therapy inhibits endometrial desquamation and provides prompt but transient relief. Conjugated estrogens may be administered orally (2.5 to 3.75 mg daily) or intravenously (25 mg at 4-hour intervals), depending on the amount of bleeding. Bleeding should be controlled within 24 hours of estrogen therapy. Addition of a progestin after bleeding has ceased allows for withdrawal menstruation when the patient is hemodynamically stable. Administration of estrogen-dominant OCs (containing 50 mg ethinyl estradiol) three times daily for 7 days also controls heavy DUB when gaining cycle control is not urgent. Failure of hormonal management to control DUB requires D&C for therapeutic and diagnostic reasons.

14. **(A)** This patient most likely has PCOS and does not desire to conceive at this time. Thus, clomiphene citrate is not indicated as an ovulation-inducing agent. Since her prolactin level is normal, bromocriptine treatment is not appropriate. An endometrial biopsy might be indicated if she were older or obese with a long period of exposure to unopposed estrogen. A GnRH stimulation test is reserved primarily for patients with hypothalamic disorders. The oral contraceptive is the appropriate therapy for her to reduce androgen levels, provide contraception, and control irregular bleeding.

15. **(D)** Hirsutism is defined as growth of coarse hair in androgen-dependent body regions, such as the sideburn area, chin, upper lip, periareolar area, chest, lower abdominal midline, and thighs. It should be distinguished from masculinization, which refers to development of male secondary sex characteristics (e.g., temporal balding, deepening of the voice, masculinization of body habitus, and clitoromegaly). Defeminization is the loss of female secondary sex characteristics (e.g., decreased breast size). Virilization refers to the combination of defeminization and masculinization. These definitions describe disorders of androgen excess. Since the ovary and adrenal are the major sources of circulating androgens in women, the diagnostic approach to hirsutism and virilization includes investigation of these organs for benign and malignant diseases.

16. **(C)** CAH accounts for the majority of cases of congenital sexual ambiguity with enlarged clitorides. These patients have normal 46,XX karyotypes and elevated adrenal androgens, which are responsible for the external genitalia changes. Androgen insensitivity syndrome (AIS) is associated with the lack of response to androgens and would present as female phenotype with male genotype.

17. **(A)** True hermaphroditism occurs when ovarian and testicular tissue coexist in the same individual. Pseudohermaphroditism is defined as variance between the gonadal and genital sex of an individual. The term male or female denotes the corresponding gonadal and therefore genetic sex. Male pseudohermaphroditism refers to an individual who has testes, an XY karyotype, and varying degrees of masculinization failure. Female pseudohermaphroditism refers to an individual who has ovaries, an XX karyotype, and varying degrees of masculinization.

18. **(D)** Male pseudohermaphrodites generally produce MIF and therefore have no uterus, fallopian tubes, or upper vagina. Inadequate androgen stimulation in males reflects either deficient androgen formation or defective androgen action. The former condition accompanies inheritable enzyme deficiencies in testosterone synthesis. Defective androgen action is caused by either androgen receptor abnormalities or failure of DHT formation in androgen-dependent target tissues. Androgen receptor defects may be total or partial, causing complete absence of testosterone (T) action (testicular feminization) or ambiguous genitalia. Deficiency of 5-alpha-reductase causes failure of T conversion to DHT. Under this condition, structures derived from the urogenital sinus and external genital anlagen are partially masculinized, while those derived from Wolffian ducts are male in character. Ambiguous genitalia occasionally results from embryonic testicular regression at a time in which müllerian duct regression has occurred but masculinization is in progress. The elevated serum T/DHT ratio (combined with the presence of Wolffian duct derivatives) supports the diagnosis of 5-alpha-reductase deficiency in this infant.

19. **(B)** A karyotype should be ordered and most likely will reveal 47,XXY, or Klinefelter syndrome. The phenotype is classic with associated degrees of gynecomastia and azoospermia. They are tall due to the lack of estrogen exposure, leading to appropriate closure of epiphyseal plates. They require testosterone replacement due to the lack of endogenous androgen production from the testicles.

20. **(A)** Both maternal TBG and total T4 and T3 levels rise during pregnancy. The rise in TBG is due to estrogen-induced hepatic glycosylation of TBG with $N$-acetylgalactosamine, which prolongs the metabolic clearance rate of TBG. There is a concomitant rise in total T4 and T3 levels but not free T4 and T3 levels. The secretion of thyroid hormone in the fetus begins at 18 to 20 weeks' gestation. It is important for the provider to appreciate the alteration in common laboratory tests due to pregnancy or they may misdiagnose a pregnant woman's status.

21. **(E)** At puberty, a rise in circulating estrogens, combined with growth hormone, prolactin, and cortisol, stimulates mammary growth and ductal proliferation. Progesterone produced during ovulatory menstrual cycles is also required for alveolar development. These hormonal effects on mammary tissue differentiation play an important role in lactation (milk secretion). Circulating prolactin is the principal hormone that controls lactation. Although it increases in concentration 10-fold during pregnancy, prolactin action on the breast is inhibited by high-circulating sex steroid levels. Therefore, colostrum, a transudate-containing desquamated epithelial cells, is the only product of the gestational mammary gland. As circulating sex steroid levels decline after delivery, the normal postpartum hyperprolactinemia stimulates production of milk protein (casein and alpha-lactalbumin) in the presence of insulin, cortisol, and thyroxine.

22. **(B)** The combination of amenorrhea, estrogen deficiency, and elevated circulating gonadotropin levels confirms ovarian failure (hypergonadotropic hypogonadism). Premature ovarian failure refers to loss of ovarian function before the age of 40. This disorder commonly

reflects early loss of ovarian follicles due to accelerated oocyte atresia or destruction. Approximately 30% to 50% of individuals with premature ovarian failure have autoimmune disorders associated with hypoadrenalism, hypoparathyroidism, mucocutaneous candidiasis, diabetes mellitus, thyroid disease, pernicious anemia, idiopathic thrombocytopenic purpura, vitiligo, myasthenia gravis, and other collagen vascular diseases (polyglandular autoimmune syndrome). Destruction of oocytes can also result from pelvic irradiation, alkylating antineoplastic drugs (e.g., cyclophosphamide), and viral infections. Galactosemia, an autosomal recessive deficiency of galactose-1-phosphate uridyl transferase, leads to ovarian toxicity due to local accumulation of galactose-1-phosphate. All women younger than 30 years should have a karyotype performed to exclude X chromosomal abnormalities and the presence of a Y chromosome. Kallmann syndrome is associated with a tall eunuchoid habitus with a loss of sense of smell.

23. **(E)** This patient has premature menopause with waning ovarian function. This diagnosis is most obvious from her clinical history. Although conventionally performed for all patients with premature ovarian failure, karyotype is generally not necessary in women who present with premature ovarian failure older than the age of 30 as the result is usually 46,XX. Assessment of autoimmune antibodies would be appropriate as they are reported to occur in association with premature ovarian failure and may portend future risk of Addison's disease of hypothyroidism, but this evaluation should be driven by clinical suspicion, rather than routine screening. Estrogen replacement therapy is appropriate, but she will not respond to either clomiphene citrate or gonadotropin stimulation. If she wishes to pursue pregnancy, she must utilize donor egg in vitro fertilization.

24. **(C)** DHEAS, derived primarily from the fetus but also from the mother, is the major androgenic precursor for placental estrogen synthesis.

25. **(E)** Aldosterone plays a role in electrolyte balance by stimulating sodium absorption and potassium secretion in the distal renal tubule. It is produced largely by the zona glomerulosa of the maternal adrenal, with little contribution from the fetal adrenal or placenta. Aldosterone secretion is regulated by the renin–angiotensin system. Renin produced in the kidney converts angiotensinogen (renin substrate) to angiotensin I, which is further metabolized to angiotensin II in order to stimulate aldosterone secretion. During pregnancy, elevated circulating levels of estrogen and progesterone stimulate renin and renin substrate formation, thereby enhancing aldosterone secretion.

26. **(D)** PTH regulates calcium metabolism by stimulating calcium reabsorption from bone, renal tubular calcium reabsorption, and 1-alpha-hydroxylation of 25-hydroxy vitamin $D_3$. The resulting 1,25-dihydroxy vitamin $D_3$ is a potent stimulator of intestinal calcium absorption. An increase in maternal PTH production during pregnancy creates a reservoir of free calcium ions, which are actively transported across the placenta for calcification of the fetal skeleton. The ability of the decidua to synthesize 1,25-dihydroxy vitamin $D_3$ aids in this process.

27. **(D)** Women with PCOS generally have exaggerated release of pulsatile LH secretion. Elevated circulating LH levels enhance ovarian androgen production, inducing hyperplasia of ovarian stroma and thecal cells. Androgen-induced inhibition of folliculogenesis decreases estradiol production and induces multiple small follicular cysts arrested in the early stage of development. Therefore, the ovaries of women with PCOS are classically large and cystic. Because of difficulties in precisely defining PCOS, some investigators use the term *hyperandrogenism/chronic anovulation* (HCA) to define women with hirsutism, ovarian androgen excess, IR, and anovulation. 11-Beta-hydroxylase deficiency will cause a block just prior to cortisol production or corticosterone production. These individuals will have problems with hypertension as a child. An adrenal tumor will typically cause marked virilization not just hirsutism. Cushing syndrome is persistent oversecretion of cortisol that can have a number of etiologies.

28. **(C)** 21-Hydroxylase deficiency is the most common form of CAH. This enzyme is required to convert progesterone to 11-deoxycorticosterone (DOC) and 17-OHP to 11-deoxycortisol (compound S). Circulating levels of 17-OHP, A4, and T are markedly elevated in patients with 21-hydroxylase deficiency. If 21-hydroxylase deficiency occurs at birth, female infants have ambiguous genitalia and may lose large amounts of urinary sodium if aldosterone synthesis is also compromised. A "late-onset" form of this disease causes a peripubertal elevation in circulating androgens, leading to hirsutism. Late-onset CAH occurs in 1% to 5% of hirsute women and exists in high frequency in Ashkenazic Jews (1 in 30), Yugoslavs (1 in 50), and Italians (1 in 300). Two other forms of CAH causing androgen excess in affected females are 3-beta-hydroxysteroid dehydrogenase and 11-beta-hydroxylase deficiencies.

29. **(B)** Sexual differentiation of the male internal and external genitalia is dependent on the action of the sex-determining region of the Y chromosome (SRY) to induce testicular differentiation, production of AMH (or MIH) from Sertoli's cells to induce müllerian regression, production of testosterone from Leydig cells to preserve male internal ductal development, conversion of testosterone to DHT to induce male external genital development, and the presence of androgen receptors in the target tissues to induce end-organ responsiveness. While each of these elements is necessary, they are under the orchestration of the SRY.

30. **(A)** For most girls, the onset of puberty is signaled by an acceleration of growth. Thelarche and pubarche are often synchronous, but when separate, thelarche is more likely to lead the process. Maximal long bone growth is generally achieved approximately 10 to 20 months before menarche and ovulation is often delayed for many months after the start of anovulatory periods.

31. **(D)** The physical stigmata of Turner syndrome include short stature (less than 152 cm), a shield-like chest with hypoplastic areolae, webbing of the neck, a high-arched palate, a low posterior hairline and low set ears. Scoliosis and cubitus valgus are also common. These are the result of loss of genetic material from the short arm of the X chromosome. Several responsible genes from this portion of the chromosome have been identified for various aspects of this syndrome, but approximately 60% of individuals with this syndrome have complete loss of the X chromosome.

32. **(E)** While it is always reasonable to rule out pregnancy in cases of secondary amenorrhea, the likelihood of this being a cause in this case is low. The clinical picture presented is suggestive of an outflow obstruction as the cause of this patient's primary amenorrhea. The most common outflow tract obstruction is an imperforate hymen, with an incidence of between 1 in 1,000 and 1 in 10,000 female births. This and other outflow tract obstructions are initially diagnosed by physical examination, which may obviate the need for any further testing. If the patient does not agree to a pelvic examination, an ultrasound is reasonable as a second choice prior to resorting to doing an examination under anesthesia.

33. **(B)** Between 15% and 25% of women with recurrent late (9–20 weeks' gestation) pregnancy losses have a uterine anomaly, most common of which is a uterine septum. While this might be demonstrated on sonohysterography, routine pelvic ultrasonography would be unlikely to document its presence or absence. There is no indication by history that this patient has any problems with ovulation or conception, making documentation of ovarian reserve by a day 3 FSH, or ovulation by a mid-cycle LH surge unnecessary. Similarly, there is no suggestion of a pituitary abnormality that would support a need for imaging.

34. **(C)** The most frequently encountered androgen-producing tumor found in premenopausal women is the Sertili-Leydig cell type. While thecomas and hilus cell tumors do secrete androgens, their prevalence and biological impact are much less resulting more in hirsuitism and not virilization. Any large ovarian tumor may stimulate androgen production by causing hyperplasia of the adjacent ovarian stroma, which is uncommon and does not have clinical significance.

# CHAPTER 17

# Contraception

## Questions

**DIRECTIONS (Questions 1 through 28): For each of the multiple choice questions in this section, select the lettered answer that is the one _best_ response in each case.**

1. Which of the following is the most direct public health or socioeconomic effect of contraceptive use?

    (A) improved socioeconomic status

    (B) stabilized world population growth

    (C) reduced maternal morbidity

    (D) diminished incidence of fetal abnormalities

    (E) decreased prevalence of sexually transmitted diseases (STDs)

2. A premedical student presents requesting reversible contraception. She is healthy without any problems and a normal examination. As you review her options, she asks which method is most reliable. Which of the following contraceptive methods has the lowest pregnancy rate in 100 women using the method perfectly for 1 year (100 woman-years of use)?

    (A) copper-containing intrauterine contraceptive device (IUCD)

    (B) long-acting progestins (Depo-Provera)

    (C) diaphragm

    (D) oral contraceptives (OCs)

    (E) spermicidal cream

**Questions 3 and 4 apply to the following patient:**

A 23-year-old woman and her husband wish to use natural family planning as their contraceptive method. Her menstrual cycle length is variable, ranging from 26 to 32 days. She does not plan to measure her basal body temperature (BBT).

3. The time of her fertility, with the first day of menses defined as day 1, would be between which cycle days?

    (A) 1 and 14

    (B) 6 and 14

    (C) 6 and 21

    (D) 14 and 21

    (E) 14 and 28

4. You mention that by adding BBT curve, they may be able to determine more effectively when ovulation has occurred. Figure 17–1 on the following page shows the basal temperature graph made by the couple the previous month. Which letter most closely identifies when ovulation may have occurred?

    (A) point A

    (B) point B

    (C) point C

    (D) point D

    (E) point E

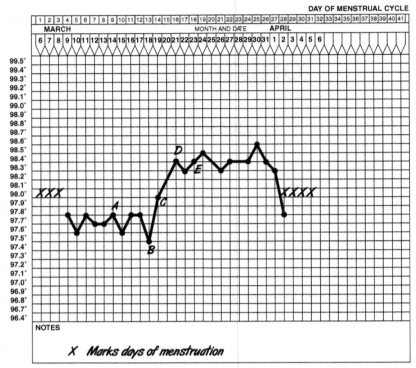

**Figure 17–1.**

5. One of the initial attempts at contraception involved placement of various items in the vagina to prevent sperm from reaching the uterus. Historically, these have included crocodile dung, honey, and preparations with mercury with varying success and complication. Currently available spermicides destroy spermatozoa primarily by which of the following methods?

(A) activating acrosomal enzymes

(B) disrupting cell membranes

(C) inhibiting glucose transport

(D) altering vaginal enzymes

(E) increasing vaginal pH

6. A 19-year-old woman and her boyfriend wish to use condoms as a barrier contraceptive method. This couple should be advised that the most common reason for failure (pregnancy or STD transmission) is which of the following?

(A) breakage

(B) inconsistent use

(C) leakage caused by spermicidal creams

(D) use without concomitant use of a spermicide

(E) spill of condom contents upon withdrawal

7. An 18-year-old woman presents for care because a condom broke during sexual intercourse. Coitus occurred 1 day ago when she was at midcycle. She does not wish to be pregnant and will terminate the pregnancy if menses does not occur. Regarding her fear of pregnancy, which is the most appropriate next step in her management?

(A) advise her that unprotected midcycle coitus has a 5% risk of pregnancy

(B) prescribe intravaginal misoprostol (Cytotec)

(C) advise immediate douching

(D) prescribe a brief course of levonorgestrel

(E) advise her to await her next menses before taking any action

8. A 42-year-old patient (G3P3003) requests a diaphragm for contraception. When fitting the contraceptive diaphragm, it should sit comfortably between which of the following?

   (A) anterior and posterior vaginal fornices
   (B) anterior vaginal fornix and posterior urethrovesical angle
   (C) pubic symphysis and anterior vaginal fornix
   (D) pubic symphysis and posterior vaginal fornix
   (E) pubic symphysis and posterior urethrovesical angle

9. A 23-year-old patient is considering contraceptive methods but is devoutly religious and will not accept a method that may "cause an abortion." What is the primary mechanism by which IUCDs prevent pregnancy?

   (A) creating chronic endometritis
   (B) preventing fertilization
   (C) inhibiting ovulation
   (D) altering tubal motility
   (E) destroying sperm

10. A 35-year-old woman wearing an IUCD complains of amenorrhea of 5 weeks' duration. A serum pregnancy test is positive. Because of the presence of the IUCD, this patient is at significantly increased likelihood of experiencing which of the following?

    (A) ectopic pregnancy
    (B) fetal malformations
    (C) spontaneous abortion
    (D) septic abortion
    (E) placental abruption

11. A patient presents requesting hormonal contraception. She has been researching her options on the Web and has become confused by the large variety of OC pills available, including monophasic, multiphasic, and progesterone only. She asks how the pill prevents pregnancy and why the variety of preparations. Which of the following is the primary mechanism by which OCs prevent pregnancy?

    (A) inhibiting serum follicle-stimulating hormone (FSH) levels
    (B) inhibiting serum luteinizing hormone (LH) levels
    (C) inducing endometrial atrophy
    (D) inducing lymphocytic endometritis
    (E) increasing cervical mucus viscosity

12. Over the years the estrogen component of the oral contraceptive pill has been dramatically decreased. This has in turn minimized certain side effects. Reducing the estrogen content of OCs has resulted in an increase in the rate of which of the following?

    (A) pregnancy
    (B) breakthrough bleeding (BTB)
    (C) thromboembolic complications
    (D) insulin resistance
    (E) premenstrual symptoms

13. A 37-year-old obese woman wishes to use OCs for birth control. Her medical history is remarkable only for a 3-year history of diabetes that is controlled with diet and an oral agent. She smokes one pack of cigarettes daily. Her blood pressure is 140/90. Physical and pelvic examinations are normal. Total serum cholesterol is 275 mg/dL (normal <200 mg/dL). You advise her that combined OCs are primarily contraindicated because of which of the following known factors about her?

    (A) age
    (B) cholesterol
    (C) hypertension
    (D) smoking
    (E) diabetes

**14.** A college student has been "surfing the Web" as she is considering initiating OCP for contraception and cycle control. However, after reading a number of blogs and Web postings, she is frightened that the pill is more dangerous than a pregnancy. You reassure her that the pill has many benefits but can rarely increase the risk of which of the following conditions?

(A) fibrocystic breast disease

(B) hepatic adenoma

(C) salpingitis

(D) ovarian cancer

(E) endometrial cancer

**15.** An 18-year-old woman requests OCs for birth control. She is healthy but occasionally experiences severe migraine headaches. Her menses occur at monthly intervals. Her grandmother has recently been treated for breast cancer. Her brother has juvenile-onset diabetes mellitus. Her physical and pelvic examinations are normal. A serum total cholesterol level is 195 mg/dL (normal, <200 mg/dL). You advise her that based on her history, OC use will increase her risk of which of the following?

(A) breast cancer

(B) migraine headache

(C) diabetes mellitus

(D) stroke

(E) "postpill" amenorrhea

**16.** A 36-year-old obese woman comes to your clinic for an annual examination. She has no complaints and is sexually active with multiple partners. She uses OCs for birth control. There is a strong family history of heart disease. Based on risk factors present in this patient, which of the following is indicated?

(A) prophylactic antibiotic treatment for possible infection by *Chlamydia trachomatis*

(B) fasting serum cholesterol

(C) 3-hour glucose tolerance test

(D) electrocardiogram (ECG)

(E) screening colposcopy

**17.** Compared to users of combination OCs, users of progestin-only OCs (minipills) are less likely to experience which of the following?

(A) intrauterine pregnancy

(B) irregular vaginal bleeding

(C) gonadotropin suppression

(D) ectopic pregnancies

(E) mood swings

**18.** A 36-year-old multiparous woman and her husband request information regarding permanent sterilization. When you advise them about vasectomy in comparison to female sterilization, which of the following is more accurate regarding vasectomy?

(A) has a lower failure (pregnancy) rate

(B) requires a longer stay in the hospital

(C) is effective sooner

(D) carries a higher mortality rate

(E) is less reversible

**19.** The administration of RU-486 (mifepristone) results in which of the following?

(A) abortion when given in early pregnancy

(B) delayed menses when given during the mid-luteal phase

(C) menses when given during the follicular phase

(D) resistance to prostaglandin inhibitors

(E) induction of progesterone receptors in the endometrium

**20.** A 33-year-old woman cannot feel the string of her IUCD. Her last menstrual period was 1 week ago. A serum pregnancy test is negative. The most appropriate next step in the management of this patient is to do which of the following?

(A) obtain an abdominal radiogram

(B) probe the cervical canal gently to pull down the string

(C) obtain a pelvic ultrasound

(D) perform a hysterosalpingogram

(E) insert another IUCD to replace the lost one

21. Toxic shock syndrome has been associated with which of the following contraceptive methods?

    (A) OCs
    (B) progestin-only pill (the minipill)
    (C) male condoms
    (D) cervical cap
    (E) IUCD

22. A 24-year-old G2P2 is requesting contraception 6 weeks postpartum. Her history is unremarkable except for significant primary dysmenorrhea. Which of the following contraceptive methods is most closely associated with an increase in dysmenorrhea?

    (A) OCs
    (B) progestin-only pill (the minipill)
    (C) male condoms
    (D) cervical cap
    (E) copper-containing IUCD

23. A 17-year-old woman with a history of ectopic pregnancy presents for contraceptive counseling. Which of the following contraceptive methods would be relatively or absolutely contraindicated?

    (A) OCs
    (B) progestin-only pill (the minipill)
    (C) male condoms
    (D) cervical cap
    (E) IUCD

24. A 22-year-old woman presents for routine care, having been using depot medroxyprogesterone acetate (DMPA) for contraception for the past 2 years. She has been amenorrheic for the past 6 months and would like to continue the DMPA. Additional history and the physical examination are unremarkable. What is the most appropriate management of this patient at this time?

    (A) change to an alternate contraceptive method
    (B) add cyclic estrogen supplementation
    (C) measure serum calcium concentration

    (D) obtain a dual-energy x-ray absorptiometry (DXA) scan
    (E) continue the current DMPA unchanged for another year

25. A 28-year-old multiparous woman transfers her care to you and presents for an annual examination and contraceptive counseling. She has used OCs in the past but has not been in a sexual relationship for the past 5 years. She would like to restart contraception now. She has no ongoing medical illnesses and takes no medications. Physical examination reveals a 12–14-week, irregular uterus suggestive of uterine leiomyomata. Based on these findings, the most appropriate contraceptive method for this patient would be which of the following?

    (A) monophasic combination OCs
    (B) polyphasic combination OCs
    (C) DMPA
    (D) cervical cap
    (E) IUCD

26. A patient currently on OCs is being scheduled to undergo a laparoscopic tubal ligation. Regarding the perioperative management of her OCs, you should counsel her to do which of the following?

    (A) discontinue her contraceptives at least 30 days prior to surgery
    (B) discontinue her contraceptives 14 days prior to surgery
    (C) discontinue her contraceptives 7 days prior to surgery
    (D) discontinue her contraceptives the day of the surgery
    (E) continue her current use until after the procedure

27. Emergency contraception can be effective if administered up until how long after intercourse?

    (A) 24 hours
    (B) 48 hours
    (C) 72 hours
    (D) 4 days
    (E) 5 days

28. In the United States, what is the most common contraceptive method used by women of reproductive age (15–44 years) and their partners?

    (A) OCs
    (B) male condom
    (C) injectable contraceptives
    (D) IUCD
    (E) sterilization

# Answers and Explanations

1. **(C)** Family planning refers to the use of contraceptive methods to defer or prevent reproduction. The goals of family planning include fertility regulation; reduction in maternal, infant, and childhood morbidity and mortality; decrease in the prevalence of STDs; and stabilization of population growth. Growth of the world population from less than 300 million people at the beginning of the Christian era to nearly 7 billion people today emphasizes the importance of contraception as a worldwide issue. The availability of effective contraception does not directly translate to a stabilization of world populations because of sporadic use and imperfect accessibility. Contraception will have no direct effect on socioeconomic status, though allowing pregnancies to be planned and wanted increases the chance that the birth of an infant will not exceed the family's ability to care for the child. About 3% to 5% of all infants have a birth defect, most of which are multifactorial in origin. The incidence of fetal abnormalities is not affected by the contraceptive method. The availability of reliable contraception may increase the number of sexual partners, thereby potentially increasing the prevalence of STDs.

2. **(B)** Method effectiveness refers to the pregnancy rate of 100 women using a particular contraceptive method correctly for 1 year (100 woman-years of use). Use effectiveness reflects failure due to patient misuse of the contraceptive method and is less than method effectiveness (Table 17-1). The lowest rate of pregnancy is accomplished by the long-acting progestin-based methods such as Depo-Provera, subdermal implants, or progesterone-containing intrauterine contraceptives. These methods actually have failure rates that are comparable to, or lower than, those achieved by sterilization procedures. The copper-containing IUCD, however, is very close and over a 5-year period probably has a better effectiveness rate due to the low-patient compliance needs.

**TABLE 17-1. Contraceptive Failure Rate per 100 Women Using the Method for 1 Year (100 Woman-Years of Use)**

| Type of Birth Control | Method Effectiveness | Use Effectiveness |
|---|---|---|
| Oral contraceptives | 0.1 | 2.5 |
| Intrauterine device | 0.6 | 0.8 |
| Condoms | 2.0 | 15.0 |
| Diaphragm | 6.0 | 18.0 |
| Spermicidal cream | 18.0 | 29.0 |
| Rhythm | 5.0 | 24.0 |

Adapted from *Contraceptive Technology*.

3. **(C)** Natural family planning (the rhythm method) involves abstinence during the periovulatory period. The 1% of women using this birth control method must be able to identify lower abdominal discomfort from the dominant follicle (mittelschmerz); thin, clear, sticky characteristics of estrogenized cervical mucus; and/or the progesterone-induced biphasic shift in BBTs (symptothermal method). The average method and use effectiveness of natural family planning is low. In women with variable cycle lengths (e.g., 26 to 32 days), the time of maximal fertility can be calculated, assuming that (1) ovulation occurs $14 \pm 2$ days before menses, (2) spermatozoa survive in the cervical mucus approximately 2 to 4 days, and (3) the ovulated ovum survives for 1 day. The earliest ovulatory

time is the shortest cycle length (26) minus earliest ovulatory day (14 + 2) minus survival time for sperm (2 to 4 days); or 26 − 16 − 4 = 6. The latest time of fertility is the longest cycle length (32) minus latest ovulation (14 − 2) plus survival of the ovum (+1); or 32 − 12 + 1 = 21.

4.  **(C)** The slight dip in the BBT is correlated ± 1 day with the LH surge. Since the LH surge precedes ovulation by 1 day, point C is probably the better estimate of the day of ovulation. The rise in temperature after ovulation (due to the production of progesterone by the corpus luteum) is an even more reliable indicator of ovulation. The rising temperatures on days C and D, and the maintained elevated temperature by day E, would support the estimate of ovulation on day C. Again BBT curves confirm ovulation has occurred, but they do not effectively predict ovulation. Hence with natural family planning, one should abstain prior to confirmed ovulation in each cycle to maximize effectiveness.

5.  **(B)** Spermicides are surfactant agents that immobilize and destroy sperm by disrupting cell membranes. Nonoxynol-9 and octoxynol-9 are two spermicidal agents that are available in suppositories, creams, foams, and gels. They are placed high in the vagina shortly before coitus (within 20 minutes). Because these agents carry a moderately high failure rate by themselves, they are commonly used in conjunction with barrier methods.

6.  **(B)** Barrier methods (e.g., male and female condoms, cervical caps, vaginal diaphragms, and vaginal sponges) inhibit sperm entry into the uterus. The use of these methods is safe and does not need a prescription but has to be timed with sexual activity. Latex male condoms are placed over the erect penis prior to coitus and are commonly coated on the inner and outer surfaces with a spermicidal cream, though additional spermicide may also be used. Male condoms may be purchased lubricated or nonlubricated. The ability of male condoms to protect against STDs has increased condom use in men from 9% in the early 1980s to 18% in 2002. While no barrier method provides protection from all STDs, the partial protection af-

forded by these methods means that any sexually active couple who are not known to be disease free and mutually monogamous should use condoms for their disease protection alone. Although the incidence of male condom breakage is 1% to 2% or less, inconsistent condom use by men is the major reason for the difference between optimal and actual effectiveness. Spermicidal creams placed within the vagina or male condom provide greater contraceptive effectiveness in the event the condom breaks during intercourse. Men may notice a reduction in sensation with the male condom, and both sexes may experience allergic reactions to the latex or spermicide.

7.  **(D)** Unprotected, midcycle coitus has a 15% to 30% risk of pregnancy. Postcoital contraception may be used after any unprotected coitus. Several emergency contraceptive products are available and offer comparable efficacy. When these progestin-only emergency contraceptives are not available, two OC pills, containing 50 mg ethinyl estradiol (EE2) and 50-mg norgestrel (or equivalent), are given within 3 days (72 hours) of coitus and repeated in 12 hours. The apparent effectiveness of the treatment is ≥70%. Misoprostol (Cytotec) has been used to ripen the cervix in labor and to facilitate medical termination of pregnancy, but would not be indicated in this case.

8.  **(D)** The diaphragm is a latex cup that is stretched across a flat or arching spring. It is available in various sizes and is fitted by a health care provider to cover the cervix. Prior to coitus, a spermicidal agent is placed into the diaphragm, which is then inserted behind the pubic symphysis to fit into the posterior vaginal fornix. The diaphragm is left in place for 6 to 8 hours after ejaculation. Additional spermicide may be inserted vaginally without removing the diaphragm if coitus occurs again within this time. It primarily works by holding the spermicide over the cervical os and not as a barrier. Diaphragm use has been associated with cystitis, vaginal lesions (posing a threat of toxic shock syndrome), and vaginal colonization with *Staphylococcus aureus*, particularly if it is left in place for lengthy intervals. It should not be used

in women with sensitivity to latex or spermicide, and may fit improperly in individuals with significant pelvic relaxation.

9. **(B)** Evidence suggests that the primary mechanism by which the IUCD prevents pregnancy is by altering the sperm's ability to fertilize the ovum. It is true that the IUCD creates a chronic endometritis that could interfere with embryo implantation. The progesterone-releasing IUCD also exerts additional contraceptive effects by altering tubal motility, inducing endometrial atrophy, and altering cervical mucus. The copper-releasing IUCD is detrimental to sperm capacitation and survival but does not destroy sperm per se. The IUCD does not interfere with ovulation.

10. **(C)** Pregnancy must be considered in any IUCD user with amenorrhea. The IUCD is more effective in preventing an intrauterine pregnancy compared to an extrauterine pregnancy. Therefore, IUCD users who become pregnant have a fivefold increase (1 in 20 to 50 pregnancies) in the risk of having an ectopic pregnancy compared to normal women. While this is a significant increase in rate, the greatest probability is that the pregnancy is intrauterine. The IUCD should be removed, if possible, as soon as the patient is found to be pregnant. Pregnant IUCD users have a 25% chance of spontaneous abortion if the IUCD is removed. However, failure to remove the IUCD during pregnancy increases the risk of spontaneous abortion to 50% and also increases the chance of septic abortion and premature birth. IUCD users who are pregnant are not at risk for fetal malformations but must consider pregnancy termination in the event of uterine infection. Patients desiring pregnancy termination can have the IUCD removed at the time of the procedure. If the IUCD remains in place and the pregnancy continues, there is no change in the risk of placental abruption.

11. **(A)** OCs inhibit ovulation through gonadotropin suppression primarily by the progestin agent. While both FSH and LH are suppressed, the suppression of FSH results in the lack of induction of any primordial follicles. As a result, no follicles develop and ovulation does not take place. OCs also induce endometrial atrophy and alter cervical mucus viscosity, making it less penetrable by sperm. These additional mechanisms serve to bolster the efficacy of these medications but are not their primary mechanism of action. The estrogen component is more for cycle control. The variety of pill options are for both lower dosing with good cycle control and contraceptive effectiveness while minimizing side effects.

12. **(B)** In the United States, OCs (birth control pills) are the most common form of temporary contraception. They are used by 20% to 30% of sexually active women. EE2 is the most commonly used estrogen in OCs. (Mestranol is an alternative contraceptive estrogen, which requires hepatic conversion to EE2.) Progestins, derived from 19-carbon androgens (19-nortestosterone derivatives), are also present in OCs. Recognition that hormonal side effects are dose dependent led to development of "low-dose pills" containing 20 to 35 mg (rather than 50 mg) EE2 and lower amounts and new forms of progestins. Multiphasic pills deliver a low estrogen dose and varying progestin amounts over two (biphasic) and three (triphasic) portions of the cycle. Thromboembolic diseases (e.g., venous thrombosis and pulmonary embolism) are related to the dose-dependent effect of estrogen on blood clotting. Estrogen increases blood coagulation factors and decreases circulating levels of antithrombin III. The use of "low-dose pills" has decreased the relative risk of thromboembolic disease from 3 to 11 (70 per 100,000 users) to 2.8 (3 per 100,000 users) times the nonuser rate so that death from OC use is less than that from pregnancy (25 per 100,000 users). The increased risk of these conditions disappears after OCs are discontinued. Carbohydrate metabolism is affected mainly by the progestin component of the pill, which promotes insulin resistance by decreasing insulin receptor number. This is unchanged by reducing the level of estrogen. Low-dose and multiphasic pills have minimal effects on carbohydrate metabolism. The estrogen does help control the amount of BTB so formulations with lower estrogen may have more BTB, but the incidence is still very low. Any preparation seems to decrease premenstrual complaints. The

contraceptive effectiveness of multiphasic and low-dose OCs is similar to that of 50-mg EE2 pills and is used initially whenever possible.

13. **(D)** The risk of myocardial infarction in users of OCs occurs primarily in smokers and in women with other risk factors for coronary heart disease, including hypertension, hypercholesterolemia, obesity, diabetes, and age more than 35 years. Low-dose and multiphasic preparations have little effect on circulating lipid levels and carbohydrate metabolism. Hypertension occurs in less than 5% of current OC users and is mediated by increased circulating angiotensinogen levels. Smoking, which has no positive effects, potentiates all these complications. Thus, using a non–estrogen-containing hormonal preparation such as IUCD or Implanon and encouraging smoking cessation are best. While this patient is at increased risk of cardiovascular disease due to a number of factors, a low-dose OC may still be considered if no other method is an option because the risk of these agents is still significantly less than that associated with pregnancy. Other alternate methods of contraception still should be strongly encouraged as well.

14. **(B)** OCs regulate menses in anovulatory women, decrease dysmenorrhea, improve acne, decreased hirsutism from polycystic ovarian disease, and reduce menstrual bleeding and iron-deficiency anemia. OCs also reduce the risk of benign breast lesions (e.g., fibroadenomas and fibrocystic changes), benign and malignant ovarian tumors, endometrial carcinoma, and pelvic inflammatory disease. OCs increase the risk of hepatic adenoma, especially the mestranol-containing preparations. Estimated annual risk is 3 to 4 per 100,000 women. These benign tumors can rupture, causing severe intraperitoneal hemorrhage and may regress when the OCs are stopped.

15. **(B)** OCs may increase the frequency and intensity of migraine headaches, though this does not always occur. In fact in women with menstrual migraines (severe headaches during mense due to estrogen withdrawal), the use of continuous estrogen preparation may decrease migraine occurrence and severity. Because migraine symptoms may mimic those of stroke, many physicians consider the history of migraine headaches as a relative contraindication to OC use. After discontinuation of OCs, ovulation is usually reestablished within 2 to 3 months. The incidence of amenorrhea for up to 1 year after OC use (mistakenly called "postpill" amenorrhea) is about 0.8%. It usually occurs in women with a history of anovulation. There is no conclusive evidence that OCs significantly increase the risk of breast cancer, even in women with benign breast disease or a family history of breast cancer. OCs reduce the incidence of benign breast disease. Although impaired glucose metabolism may occur (see question 12), OC users with a family history for diabetes mellitus do not alter their risk of developing the disease. Low-dose OCs contain insufficient amounts of progestin to adversely affect circulating lipoprotein levels.

16. **(B)** Young healthy women using OCs are seen annually for exclusion of problems by history, blood pressure measurement, and physical examination. A serum cholesterol and 2-hour postprandial blood glucose should be considered in high-risk individuals (e.g., age more than 35 years, diabetes mellitus, previous gestational diabetes mellitus, obesity, xanthomatosis, strong family history of heart disease, or hyperlipidemia). This patient is at risk for cardiovascular disease by virtue of her age and weight, warranting a screening cholesterol measurement. Without other indications of risk for diabetes, a 3-hour glucose tolerance test is probably not indicated. In the absence of symptoms, an ECG is unlikely to show any abnormality. With a history of multiple sexual partners, a Papanicolaou smear should be performed to rule out cervical pathology, and appropriate cervical cultures and serum tests for STDs should be carried out. Prophylactic or therapeutic antibiotic administrations should be reserved for known exposure or infections confirmed by laboratory testing.

17. **(C)** Progestin therapy may be used for contraception by women who are nursing or unable to take estrogen (e.g., older women who smoke or who have other risk factors). The progestin-only pill (the minipill) contains either

norethindrone (0.35 mg) or norgestrel (0.075 mg). Gonadotropin suppression is not as complete as that associated with OCs and use effectiveness is 2 to 3 pregnancies per 100 woman-years. Ectopic pregnancy is not prevented as effectively as intrauterine pregnancy. Its use is associated with irregular vaginal bleeding, mood change, headache, amenorrhea, and weight gain. Other progestin-only contraception methods include intramuscular medroxyprogesterone acetate, subcutaneous levonorgestrel implants, and progestin-containing intrauterine device.

18. **(A)** Surgical sterilization (permanent contraception) is the most frequently used contraceptive method in the United States. One-third of couples practicing birth control use some type of sterilization procedure. Twice as many females as males undergo surgical sterilization, and the mortality rate from female sterilization is about 3 deaths per 100,000 procedures. Female sterilization has a failure rate of approximately 0.5% and may be performed immediately postpartum (postpartum tubal ligation), or at a time other than after childbirth (interval procedure). The failure rate of tubal occlusion performed puerperally is slightly higher than that of interval procedures. About 1% of women who undergo tubal ligation request a reversal. Successful reversal of tubal ligation is possible if tubal damage is minimal and normal fimbria are present. The ability to reverse either male or female sterilization procedures is poor, and all patients should be counseled that the procedure is considered to be permanent. Male sterilization (vasectomy) is a simple procedure in which a segment of vas deferens is ligated and excised through a scrotal incision. The procedure has a failure rate of less than 0.1%. Since sperm may be stored in the reproductive tract beyond the ligated vas deferens, sterility is not immediate. Semen analysis must be monitored for several months after vasectomy to confirm the absence of sperm in the ejaculate. Because of this monitoring, a failure of the vasectomy can be detected before a pregnancy occurs.

19. **(A)** RU-486 is a 19-norsteroid derivative that acts as an antiprogesterone by binding strongly to progesterone receptors. The major target tissue of RU-486 is the endometrium. RU-486 induces menses within 3 days when given during the mid-luteal phase. It does not induce menses without luteal-phase levels of progesterone (e.g., follicular phase). It induces abortion (abortifacient) with an 85% success rate when given before 6 weeks' gestation. The addition of prostaglandins to RU-486 therapy increases the abortion rate to more than 95%. Although side effects of RU-486 include nausea, vomiting, and gastrointestinal cramping, the major risk accompanying therapy is severe hemorrhage resulting from partial expulsion of products of conception.

20. **(B)** The IUCD string may retract into the cervical canal so that it is not palpable. It may also become displaced because of pregnancy, uterine malposition, expulsion, and perforation. The latter complication accompanies about 1 in 1,000 IUCD insertions and occurs more frequently with insertions performed postpartum when uterine involution is incomplete. The IUCD string can often be found by gently probing the cervical canal. If cervical probing is unsuccessful, further studies, including colposcopy with an endocervical speculum, pelvic ultrasound, abdominal radiography, or hysteroscopy may be necessary (generally in that order).

21. **(D)** The cervical cap is a small diaphragm that is held in place over the cervix by suction. Its prolonged use of 1 to 2 days' duration can cause cervical erosions, which may predispose to toxic shock syndrome. Rare cases of toxic shock syndrome have been reported with the use of the vaginal diaphragm as well.

22. **(E)** About 15% of women discontinue IUCD use during the first year because of dysmenorrhea and abnormal menstrual bleeding. There appears to be a slightly greater incidence of dysmenorrhea in the users of copper-bearing IUCDs compared to those using progesterone-containing devices. OC pills commonly decrease dysmenorrheal. Progestin-only methods, condoms, and cervical caps will not impact dysmenorrhea.

23. **(E)** The IUCD is best suited for older, parous women who wish to use a temporary method of contraception; do not have a history of salpingitis; have a stable, monogamous relationship; and have a normally shaped uterus. IUCD use should be discouraged in women with a history of ectopic pregnancy or a medical condition (e.g., corticosteroid therapy or valvular heart disease) that increases the incidence of infection.

24. **(E)** In 2004, the US Food and Drug Administration issued a black box warning about bone loss with prolonged use of DMPA. This warning stated that prolonged use of DMPA may result in significant loss of BMD, that the loss is greater the longer the drug is used, and that the loss may not be completely reversible after discontinuation. The warning also cautions that the use of DMPA beyond 2 years should be considered only if other contraceptive methods are inadequate. In a letter to physicians, a manufacturer of DMPA suggested DXA monitoring after 2 years of use. This warning was based on intermediate effects on BMD, which may or may not be relevant to increased fracture risk. Because the evidence suggests that the rate of BMD loss may slow with continued DMPA use, and that this bone loss may be reversible, the rationale for restriction to 2 years of use or DXA monitoring is unclear. At the present time, there appears no compelling reasons to limit the duration of use to 2 years to perform any special bone mass screening. The loss of menstrual periods on DMPA is not uncommon, desirable for many, and of no medical concern. It should neither prompt a change in contraceptive methods nor any interventions to try to induce vaginal bleeding. Little of the body's calcium is found free in the serum, and serum calcium levels are not predictive of bone loss.

25. **(C)** Despite earlier worries that OCs might cause growth in uterine leiomyomata, several large epidemiologic studies have shown that OC use does not induce the growth of uterine leiomyomata. As a result, both monophasic and polyphasic contraceptives would be acceptable. The higher failure rates of cervical caps as well as the possibility of cervical changes caused by childbirth may make the cervical cap a less desirable option. Significant distortion of the uterine cavity is a relative contraindication to the use of an IUCD. DMPA is generally associated with less menstrual bleeding, and some epidemiologic studies suggest that the use of DMPA reduces the need for hysterectomy in women with leiomyomata, making DMPA the best option for this patient.

26. **(E)** Because of the low perioperative risk of venous thromboembolism, it is currently not considered necessary to discontinue combination contraceptives before laparoscopic tubal sterilization or other brief surgical procedures. For those patients who are at increased risk of thrombosis by virtue of genetic mutations or the planned procedure, OC-induced procoagulant changes do not substantially resolve until 6 or more weeks after OC discontinuation. As always, for these patients the benefits of stopping combination contraceptives 1 month or more before major surgery should be balanced against the risks of an unintended pregnancy.

27. **(E)** While most published studies have looked at efficacy when given within 72 hours after intercourse, emergency contraception can prevent pregnancy during the 5 or more days between intercourse and implantation of a fertilized egg, but it is ineffective after implantation. The World Health Organization's "Medical Eligibility Criteria for Contraceptive Use" include no conditions in which the risks of emergency contraception use outweigh the benefits; so there is no reason to deny access to this option to women who have had unprotected or inadequately protected intercourse and who do not desire pregnancy.

28. **(E)** Sterilization accounts for 39% of contraceptive method use by U.S. women and their partners. Of those, 28% had tubal sterilization and 11% have partners who had a vasectomy. In comparison, 27% of reproductive age women use OCs, 21% use male condoms, 3% use injectable contraceptives, 2% use diaphragms, and 1% use intrauterine devices.

# CHAPTER 18

# Gynecology: Common Lesions of the Vulva, Vagina, Cervix, and Uterus; Gynecologic Pain Syndromes; Imaging in Obstetrics and Gynecology

## Questions

**DIRECTIONS (Questions 1 through 36): For each of the multiple choice questions in this section, select the lettered answer that is the one *best* response in each case.**

1. A 63-year-old patient is seen for routine examination. An excoriated 2-cm lesion is found on her left labium majus, which, she states, has been present for at least 3 months. What is the next best step in the management of this patient?

   (A) prescribe hydrocortisone cream
   (B) schedule colposcopy
   (C) perform excisional biopsy
   (D) prescribe Burow's solution soaks
   (E) paint the area with toluidine blue stain

2. An 18-year-old woman consults you for a painful swelling of her left labium that has progressively worsened over the past 3 days. She has been treating the discomfort with over-the-counter analgesics and warm sitz baths. On examination, a 6-cm swollen, red, tender, tense cystic mass is present in the base of the left labium majus. What is the most appropriate next step in the care of this patient?

   (A) excision of the mass
   (B) dry heat

   (C) oral antibiotics
   (D) intramuscular or intravenous (IV) antibiotics
   (E) incision and drainage of the mass

3. A 21-year-old G0P0 healthy college student presents to Student Health Center, complaining of severe vulvar puritius. She has a BMI of 24, uses condoms with coitus, and finished her last menses 4 days prior. Last month she was diagnosed with and successfully treated for manila vaginitis. She denies any other symptoms including vaginal discharge. What is the most likely diagnosis?

   (A) vaginal trichomoniasis
   (B) leukemia
   (C) personal hygiene products
   (D) secondary syphilis
   (E) hidradenitis suppurativa

4. A 79-year-old woman presents to your office with a 1-cm fleshy outgrowth from her urethra. It has a slightly infected appearance and bleeds on contact. You perform a biopsy, and the report states "transitional and stratified squamous epithelium with underlying loose connective tissue." Which of the following is the most likely diagnosis?

   (A) urethral leiomyoma
   (B) hidradenitis suppurativa
   (C) senile urethritis
   (D) urethral caruncle
   (E) urethral carcinoma

5. A patient consults you with complaints of recurrent, painful, draining vulvar lesions. Examination shows multiple abscesses and deep scars in the labia. A foul-smelling discharge from the lesions is noted. During the review of systems, the patient reports the occasional appearance of similar lesions in the axilla. Which of the following is the most likely diagnosis?

   (A) herpetic vulvitis
   (B) hidradenitis suppurativa
   (C) lymphogranuloma venereum
   (D) granuloma inguinale
   (E) secondary syphilis

6. A 20-year-old patient complains of painful vulvar ulcers present for 72 hours. Examination reveals three tender, punched-out lesions with a yellow exudate but no induration. Which of the following is the most likely diagnosis?

   (A) chancroid
   (B) granuloma inguinale
   (C) herpes
   (D) lymphogranuloma venereum
   (E) syphilis

7. A 17-year-old girl is seen at a local clinic desiring contraception because she thinks she will soon become sexually active. During her examination, an ulcerative lesion is seen in the vaginal fornix. It has a rolled, irregular edge with a reddish-appearing granular base. The lesion is mildly tender to palpation. This lesion is most likely which of the following?

   (A) vaginal intraepithelial neoplasia
   (B) vulvar carcinoma
   (C) syphilis
   (D) an ulcer caused by the use of tampons
   (E) genital herpes

8. Which of the following is the most common benign neoplasm of the cervix and endocervix?

   (A) polyp
   (B) leiomyoma
   (C) nabothian cyst
   (D) endometriosis
   (E) Gartner's duct cyst

9. A 15-year-old patient has had menstrual bleeding every 2 to 4 weeks since menarche 1 year ago. The bleeding can be both heavy and light. It sometimes lasts as long as 2 weeks. Which of the following is the next best step in the management of her problem?

   (A) obtain a pregnancy test
   (B) perform an endometrial biopsy
   (C) obtain pelvic ultrasonography
   (D) initiate oral contraceptives (OCs)
   (E) initiate cyclic progestin therapy

10. A 47-year-old woman complains of postcoital bleeding, nearly as heavy as menses. Which of the following is the most likely origin of her bleeding?

   (A) cervical polyps
   (B) cervical ectropion
   (C) cervical carcinoma
   (D) cervical nabothian cysts
   (E) cervical infection

11. An obese 63-year-old woman presents with a 3-month history of continuous scanty vaginal bleeding. She denies the use of hormone replacement therapy. Adequate history and physical examination in the office reveal no other abnormalities. A Pap smear is negative. Which of the following is the next most appropriate step in her management?

(A) begin estrogen replacement therapy
(B) sample the endometrium
(C) perform colposcopic evaluation of the cervix
(D) obtain random biopsies of the cervix
(E) obtain serum follicle-stimulating hormone (FSH), luteinizing hormone (LH), estradiol, and prolactin levels

12. A patient being treated for prothrombin deficiency develops abnormal uterine bleeding. An anatomic lesion has been ruled out. Further management to control the bleeding should begin with which of the following?

(A) gonadotropin-releasing hormone (GnRH) antagonists
(B) medroxyprogesterone acetate
(C) conjugated equine estrogens
(D) OC pills
(E) transdermal estradiol

13. A patient complains of heavy but regular menstrual periods. An anatomic cause of the magnitude of her flow has been ruled out. Which of the following has been shown to be most effective in reducing rather than eliminating her menstrual flow?

(A) tranexamic acid
(B) dilation and curettage
(C) depot medroxyprogesterone acetate (DMPA)
(D) misoprostol
(E) ergonovine maleate

14. A patient in her forties presents with dysfunctional bleeding. You want to do an endometrial biopsy. Because she has no insurance, she would prefer not to have the procedure unless it is likely to show important pathology. An endometrial sampling is likely to be reported as showing endometrial hyperplasia in a patient who is which of the following?

(A) obese
(B) postmenopausal
(C) using cyclic combination OCs
(D) using DMPA
(E) using a copper intrauterine contraceptive device (IUCD)

**Questions 15 and 16 apply to the following patient:**

A 35-year-old accountant complains of episodic bloating, breast tenderness, dyspareunia, irritability, and depression, which leave her with "only 1 good week a month." She is currently using condoms and foam for birth control because she "felt terrible" on OCs. Pelvic examination is normal.

15. Which of the following is the best diagnostic course?

(A) begin a prospective diary of symptoms for the next 2 months
(B) obtain a serum progesterone level during the last half of her menstrual cycle
(C) obtain a serum estrogen level during the first half of her menstrual cycle
(D) perform a transvaginal ultrasound examination of the posterior cul-de-sac
(E) begin basal body temperature (BBT) recording

16. She has a normal laboratory and ultrasound evaluation. Her BBT and symptoms calendar are as noted in Figure 18–1 on the following page. Which symptom pattern is most consistent with true premenstrual syndrome (PMS)?

(A) graph A
(B) graph B
(C) graph C
(D) graph D
(E) graph E

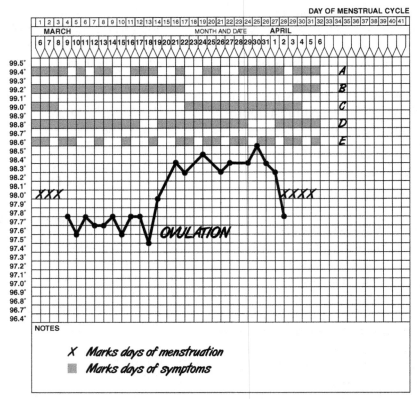

**Figure 18–1.**

**17.** A 33-year-old patient has been diagnosed as having adenomyosis. Which of the following symptoms is most consistent with this diagnosis?

(A) dyspareunia
(B) mood swings
(C) painful defecation
(D) secondary dysmenorrhea
(E) infertility

**18.** A patient has secondary dysmenorrheal and a fixed pelvis. At laparoscopy, lesions are biopsied that are thought to represent endometriosis. The diagnosis of endometriosis is confirmed histologically by identifying extragenital implants containing which of the following?

(A) endometrial glands and stroma
(B) hypertrophic smooth muscle
(C) hemorrhage and iron pigment deposits
(D) fibrosis
(E) stromal decidualization

**19.** Which of the following is the most common indication for treatment of uterine leiomyomata in a 42-year-old woman?

(A) interference with reproductive function
(B) rapid enlargement
(C) pain
(D) excessive uterine bleeding
(E) impingement on another organ

**20.** A 45-year-old patient with uterine leiomyomata found on pelvic examination complains of excessive uterine bleeding. Which of the following should be the next step in the management of this patient?

(A) myomectomy
(B) hysterectomy
(C) ultrasonography
(D) endometrial biopsy
(E) hysterosalpingography

21. A 26-year-old patient is found to have an 8-week size, irregular uterus. She does not complain of pain or excessive menstrual bleeding. Her Pap smear is normal, and a pregnancy test is negative. Which of the following is the best step in the management of this patient?

    (A) continued observation
    (B) endometrial biopsy
    (C) cervical conization
    (D) hysterectomy
    (E) pelvic ultrasonography

22. A 23-year-old woman complains of heavy, painful menstrual periods every 2 weeks. On further questioning, you find that every other episode of bleeding is actually very brief, consisting of only 2 days of spotting. At these times, the pain is also only an occasional twinge. During the heavy bleeding, the pain is crampy, nearly constant, located centrally in the pelvis, and lasts 3 days. She reports that this has been her pattern of menstrual pain since her early teens. A BBT curve is biphasic, compatible with normal ovulatory cycles 28 days in length. Her physical examination is normal. In addition to primary dysmenorrhea, which of the following is the most likely diagnosis?

    (A) anovulatory bleeding
    (B) progressive endometriosis
    (C) chronic constipation
    (D) mittelschmerz
    (E) Halban's disease

23. A 25-year-old patient with her last menstrual period (LMP) 3 weeks ago is being followed for a 5 cm × 4 cm × 4 cm right ovarian cystic mass. She comes to the emergency department complaining of sudden right-sided low abdominal pain and nausea that has been constant for 2 hours. She had intermittent spasms of pain for a week preceding this episode (when you first felt the cyst). All these pain episodes resolved within minutes. The patient denies fever or recent coitus (none in 6 months). Examination demonstrates a 10 cm × 8 cm × 6 cm right pelvic mass that is very tender. White blood cell (WBC) count is 12,500/mL and temperature is 100.2°F. She has had no prior surgery.

    The patient undergoes diagnostic laparoscopy, and a black mass is seen replacing the entire right ovary. Which of the following is the most appropriate management of this patient?

    (A) removal of the ovary
    (B) antibiotic therapy
    (C) *Clostridium* antitoxin
    (D) reverse torsion and oophoropexy
    (E) anticoagulation

24. A 58-year-old G2P2 patient presents with complaints of severe vulvar pruritus. She is 10 years postmenopausal. Her examination is consistent with atrophic vulvitis. Which of the following is the most effective treatment of vulvar pruritus associated with atrophic vulvitis?

    (A) antihistamines
    (B) hydrocortisone
    (C) alcohol injections
    (D) tranquilizers
    (E) topical estrogen therapy

25. A 53-year-old woman is diagnosed with anovulatory dysfunctional bleeding. Which of the following is the most appropriate medical therapy?

    (A) orally administered estrogen for the first 25 days of each month
    (B) vaginal estrogen cream two to three times per week
    (C) orally administered progesterone 5 to 10 mg daily for 10 days each month
    (D) testosterone tablets 10 mg/d
    (E) estrogen 20 mg administered intravenously

**26.** A 63-year-old patient presents with symptoms of vaginal itching, vaginal dryness, and dyspareunia. Which of the following is the most appropriate medical therapy?

    (A) orally administered estrogen for the first 25 days of each month

    (B) vaginal estrogen cream daily

    (C) orally administered progesterone 5 to 10 mg daily for 10 days each month

    (D) testosterone tablets 10 mg/d

    (E) estrogen 20 mg administered intravenously

**27.** A 19-year-old woman is seen in the emergency department with a history of amenorrhea for 8 weeks, 1 week of unilateral adnexal pain. On physical examination, she is found to have an acute abdomen with tenderness and absent bowel sounds. Laboratory evaluations reveal a hematocrit that is 23%, and a positive pregnancy test. Which of the following is the most likely diagnosis?

    (A) ectopic pregnancy

    (B) pelvic inflammatory disease (PID)

    (C) endometriosis

    (D) appendicitis

    (E) ruptured corpus luteum cyst of the ovary

**28.** A 23-year-old G1P1 patient is using barrier contraception and is 1 week past onset of her last mense. She is found to have bilaterally equal adnexal pain; cervical motion tenderness; direct abdominal tenderness; temperature, 101.3°F; and WBC, 12,000/mL. Which of the following is the most likely diagnosis?

    (A) ectopic pregnancy

    (B) PID

    (C) endometriosis

    (D) urinary tract infection (UTI)

    (E) ruptured corpus luteum cyst of the ovary

**29.** A 16-year-old G0P0 patient reports delayed onset of menses, the sudden onset of severe pain, and syncope. A serum pregnancy test is negative. Her CBC reveals an Hct of 42% and a WBC of 8,000. Which of the following is the most likely diagnosis?

    (A) ectopic pregnancy

    (B) PID

    (C) endometriosis

    (D) appendicitis

    (E) ruptured corpus luteum cyst of the ovary

**30.** A 21-year-old patient is seen for a physical examination prior to her return to college. She has been healthy and is using OCs for the past 3 years. On physical examination, you note a 2-mm pigmented flat lesion with irregular margins on the left labia. What is the most appropriate next step in the management of this lesion?

    (A) follow up in 6–12 months

    (B) discontinue OCs

    (C) excisional biopsy of the lesion

    (D) wide local excision of lesion with 5 mm margins

    (E) electrodessication of the lesion

**31.** A 36-year-old patient presents for evaluation of complaints of chronic vaginal infection. She reports little vaginal discharge, but rather a 1-year history of progressively worsening vulvar discomfort that has escalated to pain sufficient to preclude intercourse and tampon use. Inspection of the vulva demonstrates focal inflammation, punctation, and ulceration of the perineal and vaginal epithelium. An attempt to perform a bimanual examination of the pelvic organs reveals intense pain and tenderness at the posterior introitus and vestibule. Which of the following is the most appropriate next step in the management of this lesion?

    (A) topical anesthetics and antidepressant treatment

    (B) reduction of dietary oxylates

    (C) excisional biopsy of the lesions

    (D) interferon injections of the vaginal introitus

    (E) electrodessication of the lesions

32. A 32-year-old G0P0 patient presents complaining of secondary dysmenorrhea that is increasing in severity. The pain is triggered by deep thrusting with coitus. Which of the following is the most common cause of deep-thrust dyspareunia?

    (A) endometriosis
    (B) depression
    (C) vaginismus
    (D) vestibulitis
    (E) atrophic change

33. Treatments of primary dysmenorrhea are directed toward addressing the cause, which is associated with elevations in which of the following?

    (A) estrogen
    (B) progesterone
    (C) FSH
    (D) prostaglandin F2alpha
    (E) prostaglandin E2

34. A 20-year-old woman at 12 weeks' gestation is involved in a serious automobile accident and is brought to the emergency department with multiple traumas. The emergency department physician believes that imaging studies of the abdomen are needed to assess the patient's acute injuries. Regarding this imaging, what should you counsel the managing team?

    (A) Imaging at this stage of pregnancy should not be carried out.
    (B) Imaging should be limited to no more than two views of the abdomen.
    (C) Imaging can only be done if the uterus is shielded during the procedure.
    (D) Only imaging above the level of the uterine fundus should be carried out.
    (E) There are no contraindications to the needed tests.

35. Uterine leiomyomata are thought to arise from which of the following?

    (A) embryonic rests
    (B) vascular smooth muscle cells
    (C) degenerative uterine smooth muscle cells
    (D) pluripotent endometrial epithelium
    (E) placental remnants

36. On pelvic examination of a 28-year-old multiparous patient, several 3–5 mm yellowish translucent or opaque, raised cystic structures are seen on the surface of the cervix. The patient is asymptomatic. What is the most appropriate next step in the management of these findings?

    (A) excisional biopsy
    (B) incision and drainage of cysts
    (C) oral antibiotic therapy
    (D) topical estrogen therapy
    (E) counseling and reassurance

# Answers and Explanations

1. **(C)** Any vulvar ulcer in a woman of this age should be biopsied and, if benign, evaluated at regular intervals for change. If invasive carcinoma is found, radical vulvectomy and inguinal lymphadenectomy are generally the treatment of choice.

2. **(E)** The patient described presents a typical history of a Bartholin's gland abscess. In the acute phase, incision and drainage or by marsupialization is most appropriate. Since the duct of the Bartholin's gland has become obstructed, allowing the formation of an abscess, a neocystostomy must be created. This may be done by placing a short catheter with an inflatable bulb (Word catheter) into the abscess and leaving it there for 10 to 14 days, or constructing a new duct by marsupialization of the abscess wall. Simple incision and drainage is ineffective in creating a long-term cure and allows for reformation of the abscess. The etiology of a Bartholin's duct abscess is unknown. Rest, hot soaks to the area, analgesics, and antibiotics for associated infection may all help speed healing, but these are not definitive. Cystectomy (or excision of the gland) is used to treat only recalcitrant cases or cases suspected of malignancy and can be very difficult surgery.

3. **(C)** An accurate and careful history may yield information that will solve the problem of vulvar pruritus. Obviously, vaginitis, diabetes, and uncleanliness may be contributing factors. A wet prep from the vagina will yield the etiology in many cases. The most common vaginitis to cause vulvar pruritus is *Monilia* infection. Bacterial vaginosis may cause itching, as may trichomoniasis, but itching is not their major symptom. Systemic diseases, including leukemia, may cause vulvar symptoms, but these are rare. Hidradenitis suppurativa causes vulvar pain and suppurative lesions, but generally not itching. The most likely sources of pruritus of those listed are feminine hygiene products. These agents very commonly cause a contact dermatitis that can result in skin changes and itching.

4. **(D)** Small, fleshy, polypoid growths from the urethra are most likely urethral caruncles. They not only are most common in postmenopausal women but also occur in children. Topical estrogen cream will usually allay any symptoms. In postmenopausal women, a biopsy must be done prior to treatment in order to rule out the main differential diagnosis, urethral carcinoma. When these caruncles are found in children, prompt recognition will prevent these lesions from being misinterpreted as evidence of sexual abuse.

5. **(B)** Hidradenitis suppurativa is a refractory infection of the apocrine sweat glands, usually caused by staphylococci or streptococci. Treatment early in the disease consists of drainage and antibiotic therapy. Severe chronic infections may not respond to medical therapy and require extensive surgery. Multiple, recurrent, infected-appearing ulcers occurring bilaterally on the labia should suggest hidradenitis suppurativa. Herpetic vulvitis presents as a maculopapular rash with vesical formation. Lymphogranuloma venereum and granuloma inguinale are both uncommon sexually transmitted diseases

**TABLE 18–1.   Minor Sexually Transmitted Diseases**

| Disease | Causative Agent | Main Symptom | Diagnosis | Treatment |
|---|---|---|---|---|
| Chancroid | *Haemophilus ducreyi* | Painful "soft chancres," adenopathy | Clinical smears, culture | Erythromycin 500 mg qid for 10 days |
| Granuloma inguinale | *Calymmatobacterium granulomatis* | Raised, red lesions | Clinical smears | Tetracyclin 500 mg q6h for 3 weeks |
| Lymphogranuloma venereum (LGV) | *Chlamydia trachomatis* | Vesicle, progressing to bubo | Clinical complement fixation test | Tetracycline 500 mg q6h for 3 weeks |
| Molluscum contagiosum | *Molluscum contagiosum* (DNA virus) | Raised papule with waxy core | Clinical inclusion bodies | Desiccation, cryotherapy, curettage |
| Parasites | *Pediculosis pubis, scabies* | Itching | Inspection | Lindane 1% |
| Enteric infections | *Neisseria gonorrhoeae, Chlamydia trachomatis, Shigella* sp., *Salmonella,* protozoa | Diarrhea | Culture | Based on agent |
| Vaginitis (sexually transmitted)* | *Trichomonas* | Odor, irritation | Microscopic examination of secretions | Metronidazole 500 mg bid for 7 days |

* Debate persists about the sexual transmission of bacterial vaginosis.
From: Beckman CRB, Ling FW, Barzansky BM, et al. (eds.). Sexually Transmitted Disease. *Obstetrics and Gynecology*, 2nd ed. Baltimore, MD: Williams & Wilkins, 1995:309.

(STDs) and present with limited but characteristic ulcers (Table 18–1). Secondary syphilis generally does not present with vulvar symptoms, but rather with a "money spot" rash over the torso, palms, and soles of the feet.

6. **(A)** Very painful punched-out lesions with a yellow exudate but no induration surrounded by an erythematous halo should suggest chancroid. Each of the other conditions listed present with significantly different symptoms and findings (see Table 18–1).

7. **(D)** Tampon ulcers may cause vaginal discharge or spotting but may also be asymptomatic. When seen on examination, they have the characteristic appearance described in the question; rolled-edge ulcers with a granular base. They are found in the vaginal fornices and go away after the discontinuation of tampon use. A herpetic lesion does not have this appearance. A syphilitic lesion is also unlikely if the woman has not been sexually active, but it would be wise to screen with a rapid plasma reagin (RPR) or Venereal Disease Research Laboratory (VDRL) test or a direct treponemum antibody testing. The other diseases mentioned are less likely because they are sexually transmitted or are extremely unlikely in a woman this age.

8. **(A)** Benign endocervical or cervical polyps have been reported in up to 4% of patients in some

series. They are most common in multiparous women in the 40- to 50-year-old age group. The main clinical symptom is intermenstrual bleeding. Though uncertain, their etiology is thought to be some type of inflammation. Nabothian cysts arise at areas of active metaplasia of the cervix, resulting in a squamous cell covering of a mucus-secreting gland. This causes a mucus-filled cyst on the cervix, but they do not involve the endocervical canal. Gartner's duct cysts are lateral on the vaginal wall and represent remnants of the Wolffian duct.

9. **(E)** Reproductive-age bleeding is most likely to be pregnancy-related. Contraceptive-induced bleeding (breakthrough, IUD, etc.) is also common etiology in the reproductive-age woman. Perimenopausal women are most likely to suffer from benign neoplasia in the form of polyps or leiomyomata. Postmenopausal women are at the greatest risk for cancer, especially endometrial cancer—the most common gynecologic malignancy.

10. **(C)** Organic lesions, such as endocervical polyp, cervical ectropion, and infection, may all be the origin of bleeding in a woman of this age. Though rare, the most significant bleeding is generally found with cervical lesions associated with carcinoma. Bleeding from cervical polyps may be heavy, but when sufficient to cause heavy post-coital bleeding, they will generally

cause bleeding at other times as well. In contrast, cervical carcinoma may present with heavy postcoital bleeding alone in the early stages of its growth. Therefore, malignancy must always be ruled out. Nabothian cysts of the cervix are not associated with abnormal bleeding.

11. **(B)** Amenorrhea for at least 6 months establishes the diagnosis of menopause. Uterine bleeding thereafter must be aggressively investigated to rule out neoplasia. Assessment of the endometrium can be accomplished by means of endometrial sampling, for which disposable plastic cannulas are available. Ultrasound evaluation of the endometrial stripe is another method of determining the risk of neoplasia. A stripe of less than 5 mm is very infrequently associated with neoplasia and, with other clinical findings, may be a useful adjunct to patient management. The larger the thickness of the endometrial stripe, the more likely it is that an endometrial neoplasm is present. Given this patient's history, endometrial sampling is indicated, no matter what thickness of endometrium might be found.

12. **(D)** Initially, medical management should be attempted with surgery as a last resort. At times, severe bleeding can be controlled with either OC or cyclic/continuous progestational agents. OC agents offer convenience and a high degree of efficacy in these patients, making them a good first choice unless contraindications to their use exist. They also offer a good method of birth control. In cases in which the endometrium has been denuded, the patient may initially require estrogen to stop her bleeding.

13. **(A)** Epsilon-aminocaproic acid (EACA), tranexamic acid (AMCA), and para-aminomethylbenzoic acid (PAMBA) are potent inhibitors of fibrinolysis. They have been shown to decrease menstrual blood loss by 50% or more in cases of severe menstrual bleeding. Nonsteroidal anti-inflammatory drugs (NSAIDs) such as mefenamic acid (Ponstel) have been shown to provide significant reductions in menstrual blood loss. The reduction caused by these agents is proportional to the severity

of the menorrhagia: the heavier the flow, the greater the reduction. Use of ergot alkaloids to control uterine bleeding is clinically ineffective. Although misoprostol—a PG E analogue used to prevent gastric ulcers in patients taking NSAIDs—has uterotonic effects, it is not recommended for the treatment of menorrhagia. Long-acting progestins should eliminate rather than decrease menstrual blood loss because their inhibitory effect is at the pituitary level. Unopposed estrogen is the cause of much profuse irregular bleeding and seldom offers a cure unless the bleeding is from atrophy, which is unlikely in an ovulatory woman. Progesterone tends to decrease flow in anovulatory patients, if taken cyclically, but evidence is lacking for its effect in the ovulatory patient.

14. **(A)** The obese, diabetic, hypertensive, anovulatory, nulliparous woman is at risk for both endometrial hyperplasia and adenocarcinoma. Progesterone decreases the incidence of, and in some cases can reverse the changes of, endometrial hyperplasia. IUDs are associated with varying degrees of chronic endometritis, but not hyperplasia.

15. **(A)** The patient's symptoms point to PMS as the most likely diagnosis. Because the diagnosis of PMS is based solely on the timing of symptoms, the only way to establish the diagnosis for this, or any other patient, is to begin a prospective symptom diary. Studies have shown that retrospective assessments of symptom timing and severity are consistently inaccurate, making a prospective diary the only reliable method available. No consistent hormonal alterations have been demonstrated to be associated with PMS.

16. **(C)** To establish the existence of a true PMS, the patient must experience distressing symptoms during the luteal phase of the cycle and an absence of symptoms during the follicular phase of the menstrual cycle (Table 18–2). Some patients may experience a worsening of ongoing, cycle-independent symptoms referred to as premenstrual magnification (PMM). Patients with PMM experience variable symptoms that persist throughout the cycle but undergo

**TABLE 18–2.    Diagnostic Criteria for Premenstrual Dysphoric Disorder**

All of the following:
   Symptoms NOT an exacerbation of another underlying
      psychiatric disorder
   Symptoms clustered in luteal phase; absent within first few days
      of the follicular phase
   Symptoms cause significant disability
Plus, five or more of the following:
   At least one:
      Marked affective liability
      Marked anxiety, tension, feelings of being "keyed up" or "on
         edge"
      Markedly depressed mood, feelings of hopelessness, or
         self-deprecating thoughts
      Persistent and marked anger or irritability
One or more of the following:
   Avoidance of social activities
   Decreased interest in usual activities
   Decreased productivity and efficiency
   Increased sensitivity to rejection
   Interpersonal conflicts
   Lethargy, easy fatigability, lack of energy
   Marked change in appetite, cravings
   Physical symptoms (reproducible pattern of complaints)
   Sleep symptoms (hypersomnia, insomnia)
   Subjective sense of being "out of control"
   Subjective sense of being overwhelmed
   Subjective sense of difficulty in concentration

Modified from Reid RL, Yen SSC. Premenstrual syndrome. *Am J Obstet Gynecol* 1981;139:85.

significant worsening just prior to menses. PMS and PMM are part of a continuum of menstrually related symptoms (Figure 18–2).

17.  **(D)** While anyone can have mood swings concurrent with other problems, psychological

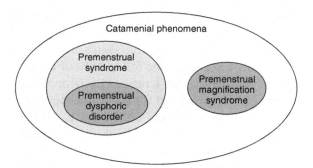

**Figure 18–2.** Summary of menstrually related diagnoses. All menstrually related diagnoses fall into the broad classification of "catamenial" phenomena. Within this grouping are the premenstrual syndromes (PMS and premenstrual dysphoric disorder) and premenstrual magnification syndrome. (Areas shown do not reflect the relative frequency of occurrence.)

(Reproduced with permission from Smith R. *Gynecology in Primary Care.* Baltimore: Williams & Wilkins, 1996, p. 428.)

symptoms are not a characteristic of adenomyosis. Pain and heavy menses are the most common complaints. The pain is typically limited to menses, unlike endometriosis, which begins with menses and often extends to include most or all of the menstrual cycle. Since the definition of adenomyosis is endometrial glandular tissue within the myometrium, there is no pelvic involvement. Pelvic involvement with endometriosis, especially in the posterior cul-de-sac and uterosacral ligaments, may cause pain with intercourse, defecation, and/or pain on examination. Getting rid of or suppressing the endometrial implants is the only way to get rid of the pain in either adenomyosis (endometriosis interna) or endometriosis.

18.  **(A)** Glands and stroma are all that are necessary for the diagnosis, but the other choices are commonly associated findings, though nondiagnostic. Visualization of the lesions alone without biopsy is often an unreliable means to make a diagnosis.

19.  **(D)** Uterine leiomyomata are the most common pelvic tumors and are generally asymptomatic. While the other options offered may be indications for treatment, they are less common. At one time, removal of any uterus greater than 12 weeks' size was recommended, but the ability to evaluate the uterus and adnexa with ultrasonography has militated against this practice.

20.  **(D)** Endometrial biopsy is needed to rule out other etiologies for bleeding. All bleeding from a myomatous uterus is not due to the myomas. Laparoscopy or hysteroscopy allows for better external and internal uterine examination to rule out other causes of bleeding but is not indicated for initial evaluations and can be costly.

21.  **(A)** In the absence of symptoms, the patient should be told of the findings and periodic examinations done to detect any change in uterine size or symptomatology. Therapeutic interventions or further evaluations are not appropriate.

22.  **(D)** Bleeding and pain at midcycle occurs regularly in some women and is associated with ovulation. The bleeding may be due to decreased

estrogen with endometrial sloughing and/or the rupture of the ovarian follicle. The pain associated with ovulation itself is called mittelschmerz (from the German for "middle pain"). The pain at the time of menstrual bleeding is consistent with dysmenorrhea. The patient actually has these problems in combination (which is not unusual). PG inhibitors or OCs are likely to help.

23. **(A)** The severity of symptoms and the black adnexal mass (an infarcted ovary) indicate that excision is imperative. If the ovarian pedicle is twisted tightly so as to completely infarct the ovary, it should be resected without untwisting it to avoid emboli and thromboplastin release with the possibility of resultant disseminated intravascular coagulation (DIC). If the ovary looked viable (not black), it could be untwisted and the cyst removed. This, however, relies solely on the judgment of the surgeon.

24. **(E)** As with most things in medicine, the most effective therapy for any complaint will be tailored to the underlying cause present. Alcohol injections are used only when all else fails, since its use risks the sloughing of vulvar skin. Local testosterone can be very helpful when thinning of the vulvar skin is present, such as in lichen sclerosis. Antihistamines, steroids, and tranquilizers may help decrease symptoms. These approaches are symptomatic only. The most appropriate treatment is estrogen replacement therapy. This can take the form of systemic therapy or local therapy in the form of creams or medicated rings.

25. **(C)** As the patient usually has adequate estrogen, additional estrogen is not indicated. The use of progesterone alone administered in monthly cycles will often stop the bleeding. Ten-day courses have been shown to be the minimum effective dosage required to prevent or reverse hyperplasia. Testosterone can help, but the side effects are significant.

26. **(B)** A local symptom can often be well treated with the local administration of medication. Often, associated urinary symptoms will decrease as well. Systemic estrogen can also be used to relieve these symptoms and provide additional benefits. Since long-term therapy is required, IV therapy is clearly inappropriate.

27. **(A)** Intraperitoneal bleeding may be of a sudden or insidious nature. If pelvic pain exists concomitantly with a falling hematocrit, ectopic pregnancy must be ruled out. Very sensitive, rapid, and specific urine pregnancy tests assist in this diagnostic problem. Still, amenorrhea, pain, bleeding, and an adnexal mass are an ectopic pregnancy until proven otherwise.

28. **(B)** Although pelvic pain will be present in all the diagnoses listed, PID is most likely to produce symmetric, bilateral adnexal pain, abdominal pain, and cervical motion tenderness, along with an elevated temperature and WBC. The others tend to produce pain that is more severe on the affected side. Also, PID may flare as the menses is finishing.

29. **(E)** The sudden, severe pain is often associated with the rupture of a corpus luteum cyst. It may be accompanied by intra-abdominal hemorrhage. Syncope is not uncommon. Observation is generally all that is necessary for the patient. Given the normal hematocrit and white blood count, an appendicitis is unlikely.

30. **(C)** Pigmented lesions on the vulva should always engender suspicion of melanoma. Remember the ABCDs of skin lesions: Asymmetry of the lesion, borders of lesion are irregular, color is varied, and diameter is greater than 5–6 mm. While the vulva accounts for only approximately 1% of the skin's surface area, the vulva accounts for 5% to 10% of all malignant melanomas in women. Excisional biopsy should be carried out for all vulvar nevi or suspicious nevi anywhere on the body. All lesions should be submitted for histologic examination; they never should be removed destructively. If a melanoma is found on histologic examination, further excision to accomplish a 1-cm margin is indicated.

31. **(A)** The clinical picture presented by this patient is typical of vulvar vestibulitis. This is typified by small inflammatory punctate lesions

varying in size from 3 to 10 mm, often with superficial ulceration. The Bartholin gland openings may be inflamed as well. The area involved may be demarcated by light touching with a cotton-tipped applicator, although the level of discomfort is often out of proportion to the physical findings. The management of this condition begins with perineal hygiene, cool baths, moist soaks, or the application of soothing solutions such as Burow's solution. Patients should be advised to wear loose-fitting clothing and keep the area dry and well ventilated. Topical anesthetics and antidepressants (amitriptyline hydrochloride) may reduce pain and itching. While the use of interferon injections has been reported to provide relieve in up to 60% of patients, this and surgical interventions should be reserved until after simple interventions have been tried.

32. **(A)** Deep-thrust dyspareunia suggest intra-abdominal etiologies. Conditions such as vaginismus, vulvar vestibulitis, and atrophic vaginal changes can all cause insertional dyspareunia. Depression can lead to a loss of libido and a subsequent loss of vaginal lubrication (arousal). But this, too, would generally cause insertional pain.

33. **(D)** Primary dysmenorrhea is caused by elevated levels of prostaglandin F2alpha. This prostaglandin not only stimulates strong uterine contractions but is also associated with increased hypermobility of the gut, resulting in the common symptoms of nausea and diarrhea. Elevations in the levels of prostaglandin E2 have been associated with primary menorrhagia. No other hormonal changes have been found in dysmenorrhea.

34. **(E)** The amount of radiation exposure involved with most radiographic imaging is minimal and in cases of the sort presented here, the acute needs of the mother take precedence over any (minimal) concerns about radiation exposure. Imaging that does not involve ionizing radiation, such as MRI and ultrasonography, can be used with even more safety. But the modality that can provide the best answers to the clinical needs of the patient should be employed.

35. **(B)** Uterine leiomyomata are thought to arise from a single smooth muscle cell of vascular origin, resulting in tumors that are each monoclonal. Estrogen, progesterone, and epidermal growth factor all thought to stimulate the growth of these cells. Of uterine fibroids, 70% to 80% are found within the wall of the uterus, with 5% to 10% lying below the endometrium and less than 5% arising in or near the cervix. Multiple fibroids are found in up to 85% of patients. While there is growing evidence that fetal cells can be detected in the maternal circulation even years after pregnancy, there is no evidence that these cells carry any significance in the growth of uterine leiomyomata, as these can often be found in women who have not had children.

36. **(E)** Nabothian cysts are retention cysts of the cervix made up of endocervical columnar cells, resulting from closure of a gland opening, tunnel, or cleft by the process of squamous metaplasia. Chronic or recurrent inflammation can result in a cervical gland opening, tunnel, or cleft that becomes covered by the process of squamous metaplasia. These cysts are common, asymptomatic and require no treatment. Rarely, they may grow to up to 3 cm in diameter when incision and drainage may be justified.

# CHAPTER 19

# Pelvic Floor Dysfunction: Genital Prolapse and Urogynecology

## Questions

**DIRECTIONS (Question 1):** For each of the multiple choice questions in this section, select the lettered answer that is the one *best* response in each case.

1. A 44-year-old woman (gravida 5, para 5) comes in complaining that she has noticed a bulge protruding from her vagina. Her other medical problems include hypertension, diabetes mellitus, and alcoholism. She stands at work as a grocery clerk. She has a family history of genital prolapse. On examination, you notice a uterine prolapse, cystocele, and rectocele. Which of the following is a major risk factor for her pelvic support disorder?

   (A) childbirth
   (B) hypertension
   (C) diabetes mellitus
   (D) positive family history
   (E) environmental factors—job

**DIRECTIONS (Questions 2 through 4):** The following group of questions is preceded by a list of lettered options. For each question, select the one lettered option that is most closely associated with it. Each lettered option may be used once, multiple times, or not at all.

   (A) cystocele
   (B) rectocele
   (C) enterocele
   (D) complete uterine prolapse
   (E) urinary tract infection (UTI)
   (F) hemorrhoid
   (G) vaginal vault prolapse

2. A 49-year-old parous woman comes in complaining that over the last several years, it feels as though "her organs are progressively falling out her vagina." She also complains of losing urine with coughing, occasional urgency, and sometimes a feeling of incomplete emptying of her bladder with voiding. On further examination, which of the above-mentioned options will you likely find?

3. A 56-year-old woman complains that she is "sitting on a ball." She says constipation is a significant problem and that sometimes she needs to push stool out of her rectum by inserting a finger in the vagina and pressing on a bulge. On further examination, which of the above-mentioned options will you most likely find?

4. A 68-year-old woman complains of something falling out of her vagina, and she thinks it causes a constant backache. The backache is least symptomatic when she gets up in the morning and worsens as the day goes on. She says she cannot understand why she has this, because 4 years ago she had an abdominal hysterectomy and urethral suspension (Burch procedure) to correct the "falling out" and some problem with urine loss. Her ability to hold her urine is excellent since the first surgery. Given her history, on examination which of the above-mentioned do you expect to find?

**DIRECTIONS (Questions 5 through 23): For each of the multiple choice questions in this section, select the lettered answer that is the one *best* response in each case.**

5. A 90-year-old woman comes to your office complaining that she feels as though she is "sitting on a ball." On examination, you find that the vagina is essentially turned inside out, and the entire uterus lies outside the vaginal introitus. This condition is known as which of the following?

   (A) first-degree prolapse
   (B) second-degree prolapse
   (C) third-degree prolapse
   (D) fourth-degree prolapse or procidentia
   (E) vaginal evisceration

6. A 54-year-old postmenopausal woman G4P4 presents with complaint of vaginal fullness and pressure. Figure 19–1 depicts a visual drawing of your examination findings on pelvic examination, including split speculum examination. The letter A represents which of the following?

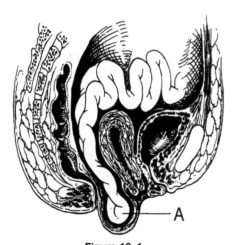

**Figure 19–1.**

   (A) rectocele
   (B) uterine prolapse
   (C) cystocele
   (D) sigmoidocele
   (E) enterocele

7. An 18-year-old nulliparous woman comes into your office, complaining of a 24-hour history of urinary frequency, urgency, and suprapubic pain. She had intercourse for the first time earlier this week. She is using a diaphragm for birth control. Which of the following statements reflects current knowledge about uncomplicated urinary tract infections?

   (A) Cystitis occurs two times more commonly in men than in women.
   (B) In a freshly voided, clean-catch urine specimen, leukocyte esterase and nitrites, in combination have a poor test performance in diagnosing UTI.
   (C) Use of a diaphragm helps prevent the development of UTIs.
   (D) A teenager is more likely to have asymptomatic bacteriuria than is a postmenopausal woman.
   (E) In women who have frequent UTIs related to coitus, infection can be prevented with low-dose postcoital antibiotics.

8. A woman complains of postvoid dribbling of urine when she stands, painful intercourse, and dysuria. She has no other symptoms. Which of the following is she most likely to have?

   (A) a urinary fistula
   (B) detrusor instability
   (C) UTI
   (D) genuine urinary stress incontinence
   (E) a urethral diverticulum

9. A 38-year-old multigravid woman complains of the painless loss of urine, beginning immediately with coughing, laughing, lifting, or straining. Immediate cessation of the activity stops the urine loss after only a few drops. Which of the following is this history most suggestive of?

   (A) fistula
   (B) stress incontinence
   (C) urge incontinence
   (D) urethral diverticulum
   (E) UTI

10. Kegel exercises were designed to do which of the following?

    (A) strengthen the abdominal muscles after childbirth
    (B) increase the blood flow to the perineum to speed the healing of an episiotomy
    (C) improve the tone of the muscles surrounding the bladder base and proximal bladder neck
    (D) prevent denervation of pelvic muscles after childbirth
    (E) decrease the muscle atrophy associated with aging

11. A 10-year-old patient's mother gives a history of the child constantly wetting herself, requiring the continuous use of diapers since birth. The child is otherwise very healthy and happy and does well in school. Which of the following diagnoses would most closely fit this clinical history?

    (A) maternal anxiety
    (B) ectopic ureter with fistula to the vagina
    (C) stress incontinence
    (D) urethral diverticula
    (E) vesicovaginal fistula

12. A 52-year-old postmenopausal woman complains of urinary frequency, urgency, and urge incontinence. She is otherwise healthy. Which of the following should be included in the behavioral treatment you recommend?

    (A) relaxation techniques
    (B) anticholinergic medication
    (C) voiding every hour during the daytime
    (D) bladder retraining
    (E) incontinence pad testing

13. A 35-year-old woman (gravida 4, para 4) complains that she loses urine intermittently and without warning. At other times, she cannot get to the bathroom in time when she first feels the urge to void and also loses urine. She denies dysuria or loss of urine with exercise. Pelvic examination is normal, except for a first-degree cystocele. Postvoid residual is 150 mL. Of the following options, which is the best plan?

    (A) instruct in Kegel exercises
    (B) teach clean intermittent self-catheterization
    (C) do an intravenous pyelogram (IVP) looking for a urinary fistula
    (D) perform urodynamic testing looking for a neurogenic bladder
    (E) give her a trial of anticholinergic medication

14. Which of the following is the most common cause of rectovaginal fistula?

    (A) obstetrical delivery
    (B) irradiation to the pelvis
    (C) carcinoma
    (D) hemorrhoidectomy
    (E) Crohn's disease

15. If a rectovaginal fistula is identified, which of the following should initial treatment include?

    (A) diverting colostomy
    (B) bowel resection
    (C) rectal pull-through operation
    (D) vaginal repair of the fistula
    (E) systemic steroids and antibiotics

16. Fecal incontinence is most likely related to which of the following?

    (A) interplay between the pubococcygeus muscle and rectum
    (B) innervation of the pelvic floor and the anal sphincters
    (C) normal colonic transit time
    (D) nulliparity
    (E) urinary retention

17. When performing a vaginal hysterectomy for any indication, prevention of future enterocele or vaginal vault prolapse is aided by which of the following?

   (A) reattachment of the round ligaments to the vaginal cuff

   (B) closing the vaginal mucosa

   (C) reattachment of the cardinal and uterosacral ligaments to the vaginal cuff

   (D) complete a purse string suture closure of the cul-de-sac peritoneum

   (E) placing a vaginal pack for 24 hours postoperatively

**Questions 18 through 20 apply to the following patient:**

A 30-year-old woman complains of 36 hours of urinary frequency, dysuria, and pelvic pain. She has never had a UTI and has no medical problems.

18. Which of the following is the most likely pathogen?

   (A) *Escherichia coli*

   (B) *Staphylococcus saprophyticus*

   (C) *Klebsiella* pneumonia

   (D) *Proteus mirabilis*

   (E) enterococci

19. Which of the following is the recommended treatment regimen?

   (A) 7-day course of tetracycline

   (B) 3-day course of trimethoprim–sulfamethoxazole (TMP-SMZ)

   (C) 7-day course of ciprofloxacin

   (D) 3-day course of amoxicillin

   (E) 7-day course of erythromycin

20. If the patient is pregnant and in the third trimester, which of the following is the appropriate therapy?

   (A) 3- to 7-day course of ciprofloxacin

   (B) 3- to 7-day course of TMP-SMZ

   (C) 3- to 7-day course of amoxicillin/clavulanic acid (Augmentin)

   (D) 3- to 7-day course of nitrofurantoin

   (E) 1-day course of nitrofurantoin

**Questions 21 and 22 apply to the following patient:**

A 49-year-old woman had a radical hysterectomy and lymph node sampling for stage 1B squamous cell cancer of the cervix. A suprapubic catheter was placed at the time of surgery. She is now 8 weeks postoperative and has not been able to void. She is also leaking urine with activity, coughing, and sneezing.

21. What is the most likely reason for voiding difficulty?

   (A) spasm of the pelvic floor muscles

   (B) outflow obstruction

   (C) postoperative swelling around the bladder

   (D) innervation to the lower urinary tract was transected

   (E) overdistention of the bladder

22. The most likely etiology of her incontinence is which of the following?

   (A) urge incontinence

   (B) stress incontinence

   (C) overflow incontinence

   (D) ureterovaginal fistula

   (E) urethral diverticulum

23. Which of the following is a normal urologic consequence of aging?

   (A) incontinence

   (B) elevated postvoid residual from 50 to 100 mL

   (C) increased daytime diuresis

   (D) increased bladder capacity

   (E) delayed sensation of first desire to void

**DIRECTIONS (Questions 24 through 57): The following groups of questions are preceded by a list of lettered options. For each question, select the one lettered option that is most closely associated with it. Each lettered option may be used once, multiple times, or not at all.**

### Questions 24 through 35

Match the description of the pelvic support abnormality with the correct terminology for that abnormality.

(A) cystocele
(B) direct inguinal hernia
(C) enterocele
(D) femoral hernia
(E) incarcerated hernia
(F) incisional hernia
(G) indirect inguinal hernia
(H) rectocele
(I) Rokitansky's hernia
(J) sliding hernia
(K) Spigelian hernia
(L) strangulated hernia
(M) umbilical hernia
(N) urethrocele

24. Results from injury to the pubourethral ligaments

25. A true hernia into the potential space of the vagina

26. The organ protruding makes up a portion of the wall of the hernia sac

27. Herniation where the vertical linea semilunaris joins the lateral border of the rectus muscle

28. Results from a defect in the posterior levator ani musculofascial attachments

29. The contents of the hernia sac cannot be easily reduced

30. Comes through Hesselbach's triangle

31. Closes during the first 3 years of life in many people

32. Much more common hernia in the female than the male

33. Associated with absorbable suture material

34. Can be closed more tightly in the female than in the male

35. Acute pain, possible surgical emergency

### Questions 36 through 42

Match the type of incontinence with the most appropriate description.

(A) detrusor instability (or overactivity)
(B) genuine stress incontinence (or urodynamic stress incontinence)
(C) incontinence
(D) overflow incontinence
(E) urethral syndrome
(F) urinary urge incontinence
(G) enuresis
(H) sudden onset urinary incontinence, frequency, and urgency

36. Involuntary bladder detrusor contractions leading to urinary loss

37. An inflammatory condition with negative bacterial cultures, sometimes associated with positive chlamydial cultures

38. Involuntary urine loss accompanied by or immediately preceded by a strong desire to void

39. Involuntary loss of urine when intravesical pressure exceeds intraurethral pressure in the absence of a detrusor contraction

40. Incontinence that occurs during sleep

41. Urine loss in association with bladder distention in the absence of bladder contractions

42. All involuntary urine loss

**Questions 43 through 51**

Match the following urodynamic and urologic tests with their intended purpose.

- (A) Bonney or Marshall test
- (B) cystometrogram
- (C) cystoscopy
- (D) IVP
- (E) measurement of residual urine
- (F) pad test
- (G) positive pressure urethrography
- (H) Q-tip test
- (I) urethral pressure profile study
- (J) urinalysis and/or urine culture
- (K) standing cough stress test

**43.** A simple test of urethral hypermobility

**44.** An indirect test of the neurologic function of the bladder

**45.** Screens for infection

**46.** Evaluation of cystocele and overflow incontinence

**47.** Identifies and quantifies incontinence outside the office setting

**48.** Identifies noninfectious inflammation, malignancy, and abnormal anatomy

**49.** A low pressure predicts failure of standard incontinence procedures

**50.** A means of noninvasively confirming the clinical diagnosis of stress incontinence in the office

**Questions 51 through 57**

Select the most likely diagnosis for each patient with a bladder disorder.

- (A) acute cystitis
- (B) acute urethritis (often due to *Chlamydia*)
- (C) interstitial cystitis
- (D) painful bladder syndrome of unknown etiology
- (E) postural diuresis
- (F) sensory urgency
- (G) urethral diverticulum
- (H) urethral syndrome
- (I) vaginitis

**51.** An 18-year-old woman with acute onset frequency, dysuria, suprapubic pain, and a new sexual partner. Office leukocyte esterase dipstick is positive.

**52.** An 18-year-old woman with frequency, urgency, and suprapubic pain. The pain increases with bladder filling and is temporarily relieved with voiding. Multiple urine cultures over 6 months have been negative, and antibiotics have not improved her symptoms. Cystoscopy under anesthesia is negative.

**53.** An 80-year-old woman with nocturia three to five times a night that disrupts her sleep. She voids every 2 to 3 hours during the daytime. Her medical history is complicated by mild congestive heart failure and hypertension.

**54.** An 18-year-old woman with frequency, urgency, nocturia, and suprapubic pain. She voids every 30 minutes, because it temporarily reduces her symptoms. Urine cultures have been negative. Cystoscopy under anesthesia reveals petechial hemorrhages after bladder distention.

**55.** An 80-year-old woman with frequency, urgency, and nocturia. Urine culture is negative, and postvoid residual is 30 mL. Office cystometrics shows no uninhibited detrusor contractions.

**56.** An 18-year-old woman with acute onset frequency, urgency, dysuria, vaginal discharge, and a new sexual partner. Microscopic urine evaluation shows pyuria. Urine culture is negative.

**57.** An 18-year-old woman with acute onset of vaginal discharge, external dysuria, and a new sexual partner. No pyuria is seen on microscopic urine evaluation.

# Answers and Explanations

1. **(A)** Risk factors for pelvic support disorders are increasing parity, increases in intra-abdominal pressure (chronic coughing or straining at stool and possibly obesity), pelvic trauma from radical surgery or pelvic fractures, aging, estrogen deprivation, heredity, or connective tissue disorders. Women who delivered large infants had assisted delivery with either vacuum or forceps, or had lacerations are all at increased risk of future support disorders and incontinence.

2. **(A)** The sensation of pressure, fullness, or falling out is probably the most common symptom of anterior vaginal prolapse or cystocele formation. Mild urine loss with coughing, sneezing, straining (urinary stress incontinence), some urinary urgency, and incomplete emptying are also common complaints. Rectocele will be associated with complaints of difficulty voiding.

3. **(B)** The sensation of pressure, fullness, or falling out is probably the most common symptom of any uterovaginal prolapse. The rectal symptoms that she has with defecation, however, are pathognomonic for a rectocele. When symptoms are this severe, the treatment of choice is surgical repair.

4. **(C)** The sensation of pressure, fullness, or falling out is probably the most common symptom of any uterovaginal prolapse, as we have seen in the preceding examples. The point to be made here is that this patient has supposedly had a repair of her prolapse and incontinence. Two things contribute to the development of an enterocele: (1) she has had a prior hysterectomy and (2) she has had a transabdominal urethral suspension, which contributes to enterocele formation in approximately one in six to seven patients. The history of symptoms worsening throughout the day and getting better with rest is characteristic for genital prolapse and especially so for any enterocele. The most common treatment for enterocele is surgical repair. Pessaries or exercises are of little value with severe prolapse. The pessary is unlikely to be retained in the vagina.

5. **(D)** Uterovaginal prolapse describes the position of the cystocele, rectocele, enterocele, or uterus. It is usually described as a "degree" of prolapse. First-degree prolapse is when the leading edge of the prolapsed organ (cervix or vagina) extends below the ischial spines (or into the distal one-third of the vagina); second-degree prolapse is just to the vaginal introitus; third-degree prolapse is when the organ readily passes through the introitus; and fourth-degree (or total procidentia) is when the entire body of the pro-lapsing organ (uterus or vagina) lies outside the vaginal introitus. The more advanced the prolapse, the more difficult is the therapeutic task of restoring comfort and/or function.

6. **(E)** The marked prolapse in Figure 19–1 shows an enterocele protruding posterior to the uterus. The figure also shows a uterine prolapse. Enterocele is definitively diagnosed by observing and palpating small bowel peristalsis behind the vaginal wall. A recotvaginal examination is critical for confirmation. A sigmoidocele is not seen as no sigmoid colon is depicted in the picture; instead, small bowel is depicted.

7. **(E)** Low-dose postcoital antibiotic use has been shown to be effective at reducing frequency of postcoital UTIs. UTIs are rare in men less than 50 years of age. In contrast, 40% to 50% of women will have a UTI in their lifetime. The use of diaphragms and spermicides has been associated with recurrence of UTIs. The vaginal flora is altered by the spermicide. Older women, particularly elderly with chronic neurologic illness or functional impairments, will often have asymptomatic bacteriuria. The presence of both leukocyte esterase, a surrogate for the WBC count, and nitrates, a metabolic product of bacteria have a very high predictive value for a positive UTI.

8. **(E)** A small outpouching of the urethra can contain enough urine to dribble after voiding. Such a diverticulum may be very difficult to demonstrate. A specialized urethrogram, urethroscopy, magnetic resonance imaging (MRI), or examination by a very experienced examiner may allow diagnosis to be made. If suspicion is strong enough, surgical exploration is indicated. The classic history is dribbling, dysuria, and dyspareunia. A urinary fistula usually leads to continuous incontinence. Detrusor instability is a urodynamic diagnosis with incontinence symptoms associated with a strong urge to void. UTIs usually also have symptoms of frequency and dysuria.

9. **(B)** Stress incontinence is precipitated by anything that increases intra-abdominal pressure. The patient is able to suppress this loss after a few drops in most cases. Patients with mild stress incontinence lose only a small spurt of urine that stops when not straining.

10. **(C)** Kegel first described these isometric exercises to improve the strength of the levator ani and pubococcygeus muscles after childbirth. These exercises can improve the condition in many women with mild stress incontinence. The exercises may work better to prevent stress incontinence, if done regularly and properly, than to cure it. The addition of pelvic floor physical therapy with biofeedback can help women strengthen these muscles, particularly those having trouble contracting these muscles.

11. **(B)** With any congenital incontinence, anatomic defects must be considered. If the child is neurologically normal, an ectopic ureter (one that opens into the vagina) is the most likely cause. A congenital vesicovaginal fistula is unlikely. A test that would help delineate the etiology of this problem would be an intravenous dye (indigo carmine or methylene blue) study with follow-up examination to see where the dye is extruded. An IVP might also be helpful.

12. **(D)** Behavioral therapy benefits many patients and encompasses bladder retraining, pelvic muscle rehabilitation, and timed/prompted voiding. Bladder retraining involves increasing the time between voiding episodes gradually so that the patient relearns to suppress the micturition reflex. Eventually, this leads to a larger functional bladder capacity and fewer incontinence episodes. Medications could be helpful for this patient, but that is not a behavioral treatment. Timed voiding is a behavioral treatment, but it is generally used for neurologically impaired patients, and voiding every hour would not be appropriate for treating this patient.

13. **(D)** The urgency and unheralded loss of urine are classic symptoms of a neurologically abnormal bladder. The different types of incontinence that could cause this problem must be distinguished from one another, as the treatments are different. Standard urodynamic testing should be performed.

14. **(A)** The most common cause of rectovaginal fistula is obstetrical delivery. This is mainly due to a breakdown of a repaired third- or fourth-degree laceration. Fistulas can occur after complicated gynecologic surgery, pelvic radiation, and inflammatory conditions such as Crohn's disease. Symptoms include passing flatus per vagina with or without fecal passage. Air can enter the vagina under other circumstances and be passed later, such as when a patient gets up from a knee–chest position. Some patients will also present with recurrent bladder or vaginal infections, bleeding, or pain. Spontaneous fistulization has not been reported.

15. **(D)** Fistula repair should be postponed until all inflammatory reaction around the fistula has resolved (8–12 weeks in most cases). The initial repair should be definitive; feeble attempts at repair, because the hole is small, are apt to result in a larger defect. A complete bowel preparation before surgery is mandatory. More extensive surgery, including diverting colostomy, may be necessary in complicated cases, failed initial repair, after pelvic irradiation.

16. **(B)** Fecal continence requires normal stool consistency and volume, intact innervation of the pelvic floor and anal sphincters, and coordination of the puborectalis muscle, rectum, and anal sphincters. Increased colonic transit time can lead to fecal incontinence. More than 30% of women reporting urinary incontinence also report fecal incontinence. Vaginal delivery is the most common cause of fecal incontinence.

17. **(C)** Isolating the uterosacral and cardinal ligaments during the hysterectomy is important; so they can be used in the support of the vaginal vault. Many people suture the uterosacral ligaments together to decrease the opening in the pouch of Douglas. The vaginal mucosa has no inherent strength, but it is important to close the pubocervical and rectovaginal fascia underlying the vaginal mucosa. The round ligaments are not considered a major support structure to the vaginal vault. While the peritoneum is often closed and is described in enterocele repairs, it is not the best procedure for reducing later prolapse.

18. **(A)** In acute uncomplicated cystitis, *E. coli* is seen 80% of the time, *S. saprophyticus* 5% to 15% of the time, and occasionally *Klebsiella* or *Proteus* species are seen. This is a predictable and narrow group of pathogens, which helps determine the antibiotic choice.

19. **(B)** Because the pathogens and antimicrobial susceptibilities are so predictable in acute uncomplicated cystitis, therapy has been evaluated extensively. Approximately a third of strains are resistant to amoxicillin and sulfonamides. Resistance to trimethoprim–sulfamethoxazole is 5% to 15% and may be rising. Three-day regimens are optimal. In fact, longer treatment courses are associated with more adverse events, are more costly, and have higher rates of noncompliance. In areas of low resistance for *E. coli*, Trimethoprim-sulfamethoxazole double strength twice daily for 3 days is recommended. Alternatives include ciprofloxacin, in high resistance areas. Single-dose therapy can be used, although lower cure rates are seen. A 3-day course of a fluoroquinolone would also be acceptable, and resistance is closer to 5%. Tetracycline and erythromycin are not appropriate regimens.

20. **(D)** Recent data and review of the Cochrane Database reveal that a 3-day course of antibiotics is adequate in most cases of asymptomatic bacteriuria and acute cystitis in pregnancy. Nitrofurantoin, amoxicillin, and cephalexin are all reasonable choices. Fluoroquinolones should be avoided in pregnancy. Sulfonamides (TMP-SMZ) cross the placenta and can displace bilirubin from plasma-binding sites in the newborn, with the theoretical concern of increased risk for kernicterus. Augmentin should be reserved for resistant infection due to its high cost.

21. **(D)** Transaction of the nerves supplying the lower urinary tract can result in a denervated, atonic bladder. Some women can learn to void by Valsalva or pelvic floor muscle relaxation, while others will require clean, intermittent self-catheterization. Spasm of the pelvic floor muscles can cause voiding difficulty after pelvic operations or even pelvic infections, but would not usually persist for 8 weeks. Outflow obstruction is usually seen after anti-incontinence procedures. Overdistention would cause voiding difficulty, but she has had a catheter in place.

22. **(B)** If she has denervation injury to her bladder, she most likely would not have urge incontinence. She may have denervation to the urethra and reduced urethral pressure, leading to stress incontinence. Overflow would be unlikely while catheterized. A ureterovaginal fistula is a well-documented risk in radical pelvic surgery, but she would usually have continuous leakage.

23. **(B)** There are many normal changes in the lower urinary tract with aging—increased nocturnal diuresis, nocturia one to two times per night, urogenital atrophy, increased postvoid residual, decreased capacity, earlier first desire to void, and decreased urine flow rates. However, incontinence is not a normal part of aging!

24. **(N)** A urethrocele probably never exists without some component of cystocele. It results from detachment, attenuation, or atrophy of the pubocervical fascia known as the pubourethral ligaments. The primary symptom involved is urinary incontinence in the presence of increased intra-abdominal pressure (urinary stress incontinence).

25. **(C)** An enterocele is a true hernia into the potential space of the vagina with bowel pushing peritoneum between the uterosacral ligaments and down the plane dividing the rectovaginal septum. It is most common after hysterectomy. Its main symptom is an uncomfortable, pressure-like sensation. The associated "bulge" emanates from the vaginal apex.

26. **(J)** In a sliding hernia, the organ protruding makes up a portion of the wall of the hernia sac.

27. **(K)** In this rare type of hernia (Spigelian), the herniation occurs where the vertical linea semilunaris joins the lateral border of the rectus muscle. This is also called a lateral ventral hernia.

28. **(H)** A rectocele is not a true hernia but rather results from a defect in the posterior levator ani musculofascial attachments or covering of the rectum. It allows the rectum to bulge into and sometimes out of the vagina. It is associated with the symptoms of a falling-out feeling, retention of stool in the rectal reservoir, and sometimes pushing stool out the rectum by applying posterior, transvaginal pressure with the finger (splinting).

29. **(E)** In an incarcerated hernia, the contents of the hernia sac cannot be easily reduced but are not strangulated. This condition can be acute or chronic, asymptomatic, or very painful.

30. **(B)** In a direct inguinal hernia, the hernia sac comes through the area known as Hesselbach's triangle (with borders formed by the lateral margin of the rectus muscle, the inguinal ligament, and the lateral epigastric artery).

31. **(M)** A large percentage of infants are born with umbilical hernias (more African American than Caucasian infants). Most infants will have a spontaneous resolution of small umbilical hernias. Pregnancy also predisposes to the formation of umbilical hernia.

32. **(D)** Femoral hernias occur more frequently in women. They often pass beneath the inguinal ligament and require division of this ligament, with later repair of the ligament in order to mobilize structures sufficiently to correct the hernia.

33. **(F)** Incisional hernias are those that occur after surgery. While the patient may have inherently weak fascia, many experts feel that the use of absorbable suture of low tensile strength and short half-life may predispose to incisional hernia formation. Several operations through the same wound, as well as diabetes, steroid use, and malignancy all contribute to the formation of incisional hernias.

34. **(G)** An indirect hernia passes through the inguinal ring. In the male, the inguinal ring is the passage for the spermatic cord. If repaired too tightly, damage to the spermatic cord and pain will result. This hernia can be repaired more tightly in women because only the round ligament passes through the canal, and it is not easily damaged.

35. **(L)** A strangulated hernia is generally a surgical emergency. The blood supply becomes compromised by the neck of the hernia sac, and without relief, the involved organ may undergo necrosis.

36. **(A)** Involuntary bladder contractions with or without incontinence are called detrusor instability. The bladder with involuntary contractions is neurologically impaired, but the etiology of the impairment is seldom known. It is the second most common cause of incontinence

in women. Involuntary contractions are also a common cause of urgency without incontinence.

37. **(E)** Urethral syndrome, an inflammatory condition with negative bacterial cultures, most often has no known etiology but sometimes is associated with positive chlamydial cultures. The urethra has a reddened, inflamed appearance on cystoscopy.

38. **(F)** Involuntary urine loss associated with a strong desire to void is a symptom called urinary urge incontinence. The diagnosis of detrusor instability or detrusor overactivity requires urodynamic testing to show involuntary detrusor contractions.

39. **(B)** Involuntary loss of urine when intravesical pressure exceeds intraurethral pressure in the absence of a detrusor contraction is called genuine stress incontinence. This is a physical problem in which the proximal urethra and bladder base are not adequately supported anatomically. To treat it, intraurethral pressure must be increased, usually by performing Kegel exercises or by stabilizing the urethra surgically.

40. **(G)** Incontinence during sleep is enuresis. The proper term is *nocturnal enuresis*. This may be a form of bladder instability. Adults with this problem often report a history of childhood bedwetting.

41. **(D)** Urine loss in association with bladder distention in the absence of bladder contractions is called overflow incontinence. The underlying problem is urinary retention. It can have neurologic causes, such as diabetes or lower motor neuron disease; pharmacologic causes, such as anticholinergic or antipsychotic drugs; obstructive causes, such as massive prolapse; or may even be psychogenic.

42. **(C)** All involuntary urine loss is referred to as incontinence. Incontinence, however, is the symptom, not the disease; an underlying cause must be sought.

43. **(H)** The Q-tip test is abnormal in the great majority of patients with urinary stress incontinence. It demonstrates urethral hypermobility. Simply, a sterile cotton-tipped applicator lubricated with anesthetic jelly is placed into the urethra to the level of the vesical junction. When the patient strains, if the wooden tail portends an arc of more than 30° when measured from the horizontal, hypermobility is present.

44. **(B)** A cystometrogram is an indirect test of the neurologic function of the bladder. It evaluates bladder sensation, identifies any evidence of detrusor instability (involuntary contraction), and measures capacity.

45. **(J)** Urinalysis and urine culture are both tests for infection. When infection of the bladder is present, function can be greatly altered. Testing or instrumenting the infected bladder is inaccurate and may be harmful to the patient.

46. **(E)** Measurement of residual urine helps in the evaluation of cystocele and overflow incontinence. The patient voids, and then a catheter is inserted in the bladder to see if urine remains. Under normal circumstances, at least 150 mL should be voided and less than 50 mL remain. Ultrasound scanning is now readily available and can be used as a noninvasive means to determine residual urine volume.

47. **(F)** Some women lose urine quite readily in their normal settings, but in clinical settings they may lose none. The pad test is performed to identify incontinence outside the office setting, or it may be used to objectify amounts of urine loss. The patient puts on a menstrual pad that has been weighed. After normal activity the pad is removed and may be checked to make sure urine is present and weighed to determine the amount of urine loss. This test may also be combined with administration of a urinary dye to check for small amounts of loss.

48. **(C)** Cystoscopy of the urethra and bladder identifies noninfectious inflammation, malignancy, and abnormal anatomy. It also allows the examiner to observe anatomic changes with strain, cough, Valsalva, and so on.

49. **(I)** Urethral pressure profile testing is used to measure pressures within the urethra and may demonstrate a low pressure in the condition of intrinsic urethral sphincter deficiency. A low-pressure urethra, in the opinion of many authorities, predicts failure when standard incontinence procedures are performed. Many feel a suburethral sling is the only correct choice of operation for these patients.

50. **(K)** The standing cough stress test is a simple, inexpensive way to confirm stress incontinence. The patient is asked to come to clinic with a full bladder. She stands with legs apart and is asked to cough. An immediate loss of urine confirms stress incontinence. Delayed leakage might signify cough-induced detrusor instability.

51. **(A)** Leukocyte esterase dipstick rapidly identifies pyuria and has a sensitivity of 75 to 96%. Women with acute, uncomplicated cystitis symptoms can be safely treated on the basis of detection of pyuria on leukocyte esterase dipstick or on microscopy.

52. **(D)** This patient has an unexplained painful bladder syndrome. Her symptoms are distinguished from sensory urgency due to the pain component. Treatment might include bladder training, fluid management, avoidance of dietary irritants, or medications.

53. **(E)** A normal consequence of aging is increased nighttime diuresis. Additive to her problem may be dependent fluid excretion at night when supine because of her congestive heart failure. Treatment might include altering her fluid consumption time to avoid drinking fluids in the evening, avoiding diuretic use at bedtime, or trying medications like desmopressin or anticholinergics.

54. **(C)** The symptoms mentioned for interstitial cystitis are often severe, and the pain may be varied in location. Complete remissions are rare and the symptoms may be quite disabling. The etiology is not known, and the diagnosis is generally by history and at cystoscopy with distention. The classic findings are Hunner's ulcers, fissures and linear scars, small bladder capacity, and glomerulations (petechial hemorrhages).

55. **(F)** Sensory urgency is defined as a strong desire to void in the absence of a detrusor contraction. In an elderly woman, especially if a smoker, bladder cancer must be ruled out with urine cytology and cystoscopy. If the workup is negative, treatment with bladder retraining, fluid management, and avoidance of dietary irritants can be useful.

56. **(B)** Differentiating infectious causes of acute dysuria in women is best done by evaluating for pyuria and hematuria, performing a wet mount and obtaining urine culture if needed and sexually transmitted disease (STD) cultures when appropriate. Acute urethritis with chlamydia, gonorrhea, or herpes usually causes pyuria, rarely hematuria and negative urine culture. Cervicitis or herpetic lesions may be seen.

57. **(I)** Vaginitis symptoms may include external dysuria and discomfort, but rarely frequency or urgency. Vaginal wet mount preparation often is most helpful in making the diagnosis in the absence of pyuria and hematuria. STD cultures should be obtained as well.

# CHAPTER 20

# The Pelvic Mass

## Questions

**DIRECTIONS (Questions 1 through 21): For each of the multiple choice questions in this section, select the lettered answer that is the one *best* response in each case.**

1. Examination of an asymptomatic 2-day-old infant girl shows a distended abdomen. The urinary bladder and rectal ampulla are empty. A solitary unilocular cyst is visualized with ultrasonography. Which of the following is the best next step in the management of this patient?

   (A) observation
   (B) intravenous pyelogram (IVP)
   (C) cystoscopy
   (D) barium enema
   (E) exploratory surgery

2. You are called to the operating room to evaluate a pelvic mass in an infant girl. Laparoscopy shows a 3-cm cystic mass in the broad ligament between the fallopian tube and ovarian hilum. Which of the following is the best next step?

   (A) observation
   (B) cyst aspiration
   (C) cystectomy
   (D) adnexectomy
   (E) hysterectomy

3. A young girl presents with abdominal distention and a mass. Ultrasound and serum tumor markers confirm a neoplastic origin to her ovarian mass. Childhood neoplastic ovarian masses most commonly originate from which of the following?

   (A) gonadal epithelium
   (B) gonadal stroma
   (C) germ cells
   (D) sex cords
   (E) metastatic disease

4. A 6-year-old girl has a history of 2 weeks of abdominal pain. She is significantly taller than her peers. Physical examination shows early breast development and abdominal distention. Blood is present at the introitus, and pelvic examination is attempted but cannot be accomplished. Serum gonadotropin levels are in the prepubertal range and do not change after gonadotropin-releasing hormone (GnRH) administration. Abdominal sonography shows a 6-cm solid right adnexal mass. Which of the following is the most likely diagnosis?

   (A) epoöphoron
   (B) granulosa cell tumor
   (C) corpus luteum cyst
   (D) endometrioma
   (E) fibroma

5. A colleague asks you to evaluate a 5-year-old Caucasian girl with sexual precocity. Areas of mucocutaneous pigmentation are present. Rectal examination demonstrates a 4-cm pelvic mass. Prepubertal levels of serum gonadotropins do not change after GnRH administration. In addition to the findings noted above, the patient is most likely to have which of the following?

   (A) dextrocardia
   (B) renal agenesis
   (C) gastrointestinal polyps
   (D) skeletal anomalies
   (E) Müllerian anomalies

6. An 8-year-old girl has acute right lower abdominal pain. The pain began last night in the periumbilical area and shifted this morning to the right lower abdomen. She noted a loss of appetite over the past day and has vomited three times since yesterday. She has not had a bowel movement today. Vital signs are blood pressure, 120/60 mm Hg; pulse, 90 bpm; and temperature, 101.8°F. Abdominal examination demonstrates tenderness halfway between the umbilicus and the right anterior superior iliac spine. Bowel sounds are absent. Rectal examination shows a fluctuant, fixed, ill-defined right pelvic mass. A hematocrit is 34% (normal, 35% to 45%); white blood count, 23,000/mL (normal, 3–10,000/mL). Stool guaiac is negative for occult blood. Abdominal radiogram shows a calcified fecalith in the right lower quadrant. What is the most likely diagnosis in this patient?

   (A) regional enteritis
   (B) ulcerative colitis
   (C) Meckel's diverticulum
   (D) appendicitis
   (E) ovarian torsion

7. A 22-year-old female patient presents with 3 months of amenorrhea and some gastrointestinal complaints. On examination, she is bloated with a masses appreciated in the lower pelvis approximately 12 cm in diameter and cystic feeling. Which is the most probable diagnosis?

   (A) follicular cyst
   (B) corpus luteum cyst
   (C) benign cystic teratoma
   (D) leiomyoma
   (E) pregnancy

8. A 14-year-old girl has had progressively increasing cyclic left pelvic pain since menarche. She is not sexually active. Menses occur at monthly intervals. Pelvic examination demonstrates a uterus deviated to the right. An elongated left adnexal structure is palpable above a left-sided vaginal mass. You should suspect the presence of which of the following?

   (A) an ovarian cyst
   (B) a uterine anomaly
   (C) cervical stenosis
   (D) vaginal adenosis
   (E) a pelvic kidney

9. A 23-year-old woman desiring conception has amenorrhea of 5 weeks' duration. She noticed a persistent elevation in her basal body temperatures (BBTs) since unprotected coitus 3 weeks ago. Her vital signs are blood pressure, 120/80 mm Hg; pulse, 80 bpm; and temperature, 98.6°F. Physical examination is normal with the exception of the pelvic examination, which demonstrates a tender 3-cm right adnexal mass. A hematocrit is 38% (normal, 35% to 45%). A serum pregnancy test is negative. What is the best next step?

   (A) observation
   (B) estrogen therapy
   (C) progesterone therapy
   (D) RU-486 therapy
   (E) laparoscopy

10. You are asked to evaluate a 28-year-old unconscious woman involved in a motor vehicle accident. An abdominal radiogram shows two teeth in the right pelvis. Pelvic examination demonstrates a 7-cm semisolid mass in the right adnexa. Which of the following is the most likely diagnosis?

(A) severe head and facial trauma

(B) fetal demise

(C) fetus papyraceus

(D) calcified leiomyoma

(E) mature teratoma

11. A 39-year-old woman with acute right lower abdominal pain is seen in the emergency department. She is nauseated and has vomited four times today. She is monogamous and uses a diaphragm for contraception. Vital signs are blood pressure, 90/40 mm Hg; pulse, 110 bpm; and temperature, 102.4°F. Physical examination demonstrates a rigid abdomen with rebound tenderness. Pelvic examination shows a fluctuant 3-cm right adnexal mass. A hematocrit is 35% (normal, 35% to 45%); white blood cell (WBC) count, 28,000/mL (normal, 3000–10,000/mL). At laparotomy, you find a pelvic abscess and a ruptured fingerlike pouch arising 40 cm proximal to the ileocecal junction. Which of the following is the most likely diagnosis?

(A) regional enteritis

(B) diverticulitis

(C) Meckel's diverticulum

(D) chronic appendicitis

(E) Walthard rest

12. You are asked to see a 34-year-old woman with intermittent abdominal pain and bloody diarrhea. She has experienced similar symptoms previously but has always recovered. She is married and uses a diaphragm for contraception. Vital signs are blood pressure, 130/80 mm Hg; pulse, 90 bpm; and temperature, 101.0°F. A localized area of tenderness is present in the right lower abdominal quadrant. Pelvic examination shows a fluctuant 4-cm right adnexal mass. A hematocrit is 35% (normal, 35% to 45%); WBC count, 27,000/mL (normal, 3–10,000/mL). Stool testing shows blood intermixed with WBC. Gastrointestinal imaging studies show mucosal changes and narrowing of the terminal ileum. Which of the following is the best next step?

(A) corticosteroid therapy

(B) estrogen therapy

(C) appendectomy

(D) colectomy

(E) salpingo-oophorectomy

13. A 23-year-old woman has left lower abdominal pain of 1 week's duration. Her last menstrual period (LMP) was 8 weeks ago. Vital signs are blood pressure, 130/72 mm Hg; pulse, 76 bpm; and temperature, 98.6°F. Abdominal examination is unremarkable. Pelvic examination demonstrates an enlarged uterus and a tender 4.5-cm left adnexal mass. A serum human chorionic gonadotropin (hCG) level is 3,500 mIU/mL. Transvaginal sonography shows a single viable intrauterine pregnancy and a left echogenic adnexal mass. The cyst most likely represents which of the following?

(A) heterotopic ectopic pregnancy

(B) follicular cyst

(C) hemorrhagic corpus luteum

(D) cystic teratoma

(E) degenerated leiomyoma

14. A 21-year-old woman has amenorrhea, mild vaginal spotting, pelvic pain, and left shoulder pain. Her vital signs are blood pressure, 90/50 mm Hg; pulse, 110 bpm; and temperature, 98.6°F. Abdominal examination shows left lower quadrant tenderness with rebound. Pelvic examination demonstrates a painful 4-cm left adnexal mass. A serum pregnancy test is positive. A hematocrit is 22% (normal, 35% to 45%). Which of the following is the best next step?

(A) observation

(B) estrogen therapy

(C) progesterone therapy

(D) methotrexate therapy

(E) surgery

15. A 38-year-old healthy woman comes for prenatal care. Her medical history is unremarkable. General physical and pelvic examinations before conception were normal. She undergoes chorionic villus sampling, which shows a 46,XX karyotype. She has noticed progressive hirsutism during pregnancy. She eventually delivers an infant with ambiguous genitalia. A maternal pelvic examination in the delivery room confirms a 6-cm left adnexal mass. Which of the following is the most likely diagnosis?

   (A) luteoma
   (B) theca lutein cyst
   (C) persistent corpus luteum
   (D) luteinized unruptured follicle
   (E) luteinized endometrioma

16. A 8-cm cystic ovarian tumor is detected during routine prenatal examination. Which of the following is the most common complication of such a tumor during the first trimester of pregnancy?

   (A) torsion
   (B) rupture
   (C) intracystic hemorrhage
   (D) solid degeneration
   (E) luteinization

17. Which of the following is the most common pelvic mass in a postmenopausal woman?

   (A) follicular cyst
   (B) corpus luteum cyst
   (C) germ-cell tumor
   (D) leiomyoma
   (E) endometrioma

18. The cell line that produces a neoplastic ovarian mass will influence imaging modalities and which, if any, serum tumor markers will be of help. Most neoplastic ovarian masses in postmenopausal women originate from which of the following?

   (A) ovarian epithelium
   (B) ovarian stroma
   (C) ovarian germ cells
   (D) ovarian sex cords
   (E) metastatic disease

19. A large adnexal/ovarian mass is removed in a perimenopausal patient. Prognosis of cure depends on the origin of the tumor. Signet ring cells are characteristic findings in which tumor of the ovary?

   (A) Brenner tumor
   (B) Krukenberg's tumor
   (C) dermoid cyst
   (D) endometrioid carcinoma
   (E) dysgerminoma

20. A 1-year-old girl has an abdominal mass. Rectal examination demonstrates a mass extending into the right pelvis. The cervix is not palpable. Abdominal sonography shows that the uterus and vagina are absent. Both ovaries appear normal. Which of the following is the most likely origin of the mass?

   (A) gastrointestinal
   (B) renal
   (C) musculoskeletal
   (D) hepatic
   (E) pancreatic

21. A 23-year-old woman with right-sided lower abdominal pain and chills is seen in the emergency department. The pain began 3 days ago and is associated with a vaginal discharge. Her LMP was 5 days ago. She uses an intrauterine device for contraception and had coitus 1 week ago with her new boyfriend. There is no history of nausea, vomiting, or diarrhea. Her vital signs are blood pressure, 120/80 mm Hg; pulse, 100 bpm; and temperature, 101.4°F. Abdominal examination shows bilateral lower quadrant guarding with rebound tenderness on the right side. Pelvic examination shows pus at the cervical os and a tender 6-cm right adnexal mass. Laboratory data are hematocrit, 38% (normal, 35% to 45%); WBC count, 25,000/mL (normal, 3–10,000/mL); and serum pregnancy test, negative. Transvaginal sonography shows a 6-cm complex right adnexal mass. The uterus and left adnexa are normal. Which of the following is the most likely diagnosis?

(A) appendicitis

(B) adnexal torsion

(C) pyosalpinx

(D) hydrosalpinx

(E) endometritis

**DIRECTIONS (Questions 22 through 31): The following groups of questions are preceded by a list of lettered options. For each question, select the one lettered option that is most closely associated with it. Each lettered option may be used once, multiple times, or not at all.**

**Questions 22 through 28**

(A) follicular cyst

(B) adnexal torsion

(C) benign cystic teratoma

(D) leiomyomata

(E) endometrioma

(F) corpus luteum cyst

(G) ovarian fibroma

(H) theca lutein cysts

(I) distended bladder

22. A 35-year-old woman complains of constant, deep, pelvic pain that is increasing in intensity over the past few years. It worsens during menstruation, sexual intercourse, and bowel movements. Her LMP was 1 week ago. Vital signs are blood pressure, 110/70 mm Hg; pulse, 80 bpm; and temperature, 98.6°F. Abdominal examination elicits bilateral lower quadrant tenderness without rebound. Pelvic examination demonstrates a tender 6-cm left adnexal mass and fixation of the uterus and uterosacral ligaments. Laboratory data are hematocrit, 40% (normal, 35% to 45%); WBC count, 7,000/mL (normal, 3–10,000/mL); and serum pregnancy test, negative. Transvaginal sonography shows a 6-cm echogenic left adnexal mass. The uterus and right adnexa are normal. Which of the aforementioned options is the most likely diagnosis?

23. A 25-year-old woman has had intense right lower abdominal pain and nausea since jogging yesterday afternoon. Intermittent episodes of similar pain have occurred over the past sev-

eral days. She has vomited twice today, but her bowel movements are normal. Her vital signs are blood pressure, 108/60; pulse, 90 bpm; and temperature, 100.4°F. Abdominal examination shows right lower quadrant tenderness. Pelvic examination demonstrates a tender 5-cm right adnexal mass anterior to the uterus. The uterus and left adnexa are normal. Laboratory data are hematocrit, 39% (normal, 35% to 45%); WBC count, 11,000/mL (normal, 3–10,000/mL); and serum pregnancy test, negative. Which of the aforementioned options is the most likely diagnosis?

24. A 35-year-old woman is seen for annual examination. Her LMP was 1 week ago. Menses occur at 30-day intervals but are heavier than they were 5 years ago. She has experienced three spontaneous abortions over the past 5 years. Abdominal examination is normal. Pelvic examination demonstrates an enlarged, firm, irregular uterus and a 4-cm left adnexal mass fixed to the uterus. A complete blood cell (CBC) count is normal, and a serum pregnancy test is negative. Which of the aforementioned options is the most likely diagnosis?

25. A 7-year-old child is referred for evaluation of sexual precocity, cystic bone lesions, and café au lait spots. Right adnexal fullness is noted on rectal examination. Which of the aforementioned options is the most likely diagnosis?

26. A 28-year-old woman with a twin gestation is found to have bilateral adnexal masses at 26 weeks' gestational age. Which of the aforementioned options is the most likely diagnosis?

27. You are called to evaluate a 1-day-old female neonate with a palpable anterior abdominal mass. The baby was born by vaginal breech delivery. Which of the aforementioned options is the most likely diagnosis?

28. A 45-year-old woman is found to have a 4-cm adnexal mass, ascites, and bilateral pleural effusions. Which of the aforementioned options is the most likely diagnosis?

**Questions 29 through 31**

    (A) fallopian tube carcinoma

    (B) ovarian carcinoma

    (C) endometrial hyperplasia

    (D) uterine sarcoma

    (E) endometrial carcinoma

    (F) uterine leiomyoma

    (G) fallopian tube cancer

    (H) cervical carcinoma

29. A 58-year-old postmenopausal woman has pelvic pain of 3 months' duration. She has recently noticed irregular vaginal bleeding, urinary frequency, and rectal pressure. Last year a physician remarked that her uterus was 12 gestational weeks in size. Physical and pelvic examination shows a firm, irregular, midline abdominal mass approximately 20 gestational weeks in size. Stool guaiac is negative for occult blood. Which of the aforementioned options is the most likely diagnosis?

30. A 63-year-old woman has bloating associated with tightening of her clothing around her abdomen. She recently has developed dyspepsia and has lost 15 pounds unintentionally. She is short of breath. Pulmonary auscultation shows loss of breath sound. Abdominal percussion causes a wavelike movement of fluid around a central tympanitic area. Pelvic examination demonstrates a fixed, irregular nodular adnexal mass with cul-de-sac nodularity. A chest radiogram shows bilateral pleural effusions. Which of the aforementioned options is the most likely diagnosis?

31. A 51-year-old woman is hospitalized for treatment of right pyelonephritis. An IVP shows right-sided hydronephrosis and a dilated ureter. Physical examination is unremarkable. During pelvic examination, you observe a malodorous vaginal discharge. A firm, irregular right adnexal mass extends to the pelvic sidewall. The patient experiences vaginal bleeding after examination. Which of the aforementioned options is the most likely diagnosis?

**DIRECTIONS (Questions 32 through 41): For each of the multiple choice questions in this section, select the lettered answer that is the one *best* response in each case.**

32. A 75-year-old woman has long-standing, self-limited episodes of left lower abdominal pain. An episode of pain occurred yesterday and has progressed to severe left lower abdominal pain. She vomited once this morning. Vital signs are blood pressure, 150/90 mm Hg; pulse, 90 bpm; and temperature, 102.4°F. Abdominal examination demonstrates guarding over the left lower quadrant. There is no rebound tenderness. Pelvic examination shows a fluctuant, fixed, ill-defined left adnexal mass. A hematocrit is 38% (normal, 35% to 45%); WBC, 15,000/mL (normal 3–10,000/mL). Stool guaiac is positive for occult blood. Which of the following is the most likely diagnosis?

    (A) regional enteritis

    (B) ulcerative colitis

    (C) Meckel's diverticulum

    (D) appendicitis

    (E) diverticulitis

33. A 69-year-old woman noticed a reduction in the size of her stool over 6 months. Abdominal examination elicits left-sided abdominal tenderness. Pelvic examination shows a hard, tubular mass with a transverse orientation behind the left adnexa. The patient is afebrile, and her vital signs are normal. A CBC count is unremarkable. Stool guaiac is positive for occult blood. Which of the following is the most likely diagnosis?

    (A) regional enteritis

    (B) ulcerative colitis

    (C) ovarian carcinoma

    (D) colorectal carcinoma

    (E) diverticulitis

34. A 26-year-old woman undergoes a laparoscopic tubal ligation using Falope rings. Approximately 8 hours after the procedure, she presents to the emergency department, complaining of increasing lower abdominal pain, nausea, but no vomiting. Examination finds a diffusely tender abdomen with an ill-defined midline

fullness rising to 4 cm below the umbilical incision. Which of the following is the most like cause of this patient's symptoms?

(A) abdominal wall hematoma
(B) broad ligament hematoma
(C) urinary retention
(D) ovarian ischemia
(E) normal postoperative pain

35. A 62-year-old woman undergoes a computed tomography examination for left hip pain and a 4-cm simple adnexal mass is seen on the patient's right side. The patient went through natural menopause at age 51 and has had no other complaints. Which of the following is the most appropriate management of this radiographic finding?

(A) exploratory laparotomy
(B) diagnostic laparoscopy
(C) measurement of serum CA-125
(D) BRCA-1/2 testing
(E) ultrasonographic evaluation in 3 months

36. A 27-year-old woman is undergoing ovulation induction for assisted reproductive treatment of infertility. On an ultrasonographic evaluation of follicular maturation, bilateral 4-cm solid ovarian tumors and moderate collections of peritoneal fluid are found. Which of the following is the most appropriate management of these findings ?

(A) exploratory laparotomy
(B) diagnostic laparoscopy
(C) measurement of serum CA-125
(D) human menopausal gonadotropin therapy
(E) delay conception for at least 1 month

37. An 18-year-old patient is seen for a school physical examination. Mild right lower abdominal tenderness is noted, and on pelvic examination, a smooth, mobile, mildly tender 4-cm cystic mass is found in the right adnexa. The patient has had regular periods since her menarche at age 12. She is not sexually active. What is the most appropriate next step in the management of this lesion?

(A) exploratory laparotomy
(B) diagnostic laparoscopy
(C) measurement of serum CA-125
(D) oral contraceptive therapy
(E) reexamination in 1 to 2 months

38. A 38-year-old multiparous patient transfers her care from another city and presents for an annual health-maintenance examination. The patient is married and sexually active and underwent a sterilization procedure a year after the birth of her last child. She has been healthy, takes no medications, and has not sought care for several years. A review of symptoms is negative. Her menstrual periods are regular, though they have become somewhat heavier over the past year. On bimanual examination, the uterus is found to be firm, irregular, nontender, mobile, and the size of a 14-week gestation. A cervical cytologic specimen is obtained. Which of the following is the most appropriate next step in this patient's management?

(A) diagnostic laparoscopy
(B) pelvic ultrasonography
(C) measurement of serum CA-125
(D) reexamination in one month
(E) reexamination in 1 year

39. Cancer antigen 125 (CA-125) is expressed by approximately what percentage of ovarian epithelial carcinomas?

(A) 20
(B) 40
(C) 60
(D) 80
(E) 100

40. When compared to age-matched women, those with higher parity are at lower risk for uterine leiomyomata due to which of the following?

(A) reduced estrogen exposure
(B) myometrial stretch
(C) inhibition of cellular growth hormones
(D) lower levels of sex hormone–binding globulin
(E) reduced number of lifetime ovulations

**41.** A 42-year-old woman with a uterus the size of a 16-week gestation undergoes bilateral uterine artery embolization for the treatment of suspected uterine leiomyomata. Five days after the procedure she presents to the emergency department with pelvic pain and cramping, nausea and vomiting, a low-grade fever, and malaise, which have been getting progressively worse over the past 48 hours. What is the most appropriate next step in the management of this condition ?

(A) intravenous antibiotic therapy

(B) exploratory laparotomy

(C) exploratory laparoscopy

(D) computed tomography of the pelvis and abdomen

(E) analgesics and reassurance

# Answers and Explanations

1. **(A)** Age is one of the best predictors of the etiology of an adnexal mass. During infancy, the most common adnexal mass is an ovarian cyst. It arises in response to a transient elevation in circulating gonadotropins after birth. Unilocular ovarian cysts usually regress as serum gonadotropin levels decline. The other options are invasive and are not indicated in an asymptomatic 2-day old with an ultrasound that is only remarkable for ovarian enlargement

2. **(B)** Mesonephric (wolffian) duct remnants may persist after fetal life as cystic structures adjacent to the fallopian tube, uterus, or cervix. Parovarian cysts develop from the cranial portion of the mesonephric duct and are found in the broad ligament between the fallopian tube and ovarian hilum (Figure 20–1). Gartner's duct cysts develop from the caudal portion of the mesonephric duct and are located lateral to the uterus or vagina. While these cysts are benign and could be merely followed, in the situation given with the patient already in the midst of an operation, most would aspirate and decompress the cyst.

3. **(C)** Most childhood pelvic masses in females are either neoplastic or endocrinologic in origin. Two to five percent of malignant pediatric tumors involve the female reproductive organs, most commonly the ovary. Childhood neoplastic ovarian masses originate from the germ-cell component in approximately 80% of cases. This means that tumor markers AFP and hCG are commonly positive and can be trended for success of intervention.

4. **(B)** Abdominal distention with signs of pseudosexual precocity is suggestive of an endocrinologically active tumor. Estrogen-producing ovarian neoplasms are most commonly granulosa cell tumors. These low-grade malignant tumors are usually solid and unilateral. They are capable of recurring 15 to 20 years after initial diagnosis and apparently successful treatment.

5. **(C)** Peutz–Jeghers syndrome is characterized by the presence of an estrogen-secreting ovarian tumor (causing pseudoprecocious puberty), gastrointestinal polyposis, and mucocutaneous pigmentation. The ovarian tumor is composed of sex cord and stromal elements, which are arranged in annular tubules. Granulosa–theca cell tumors are also associated with this syndrome.

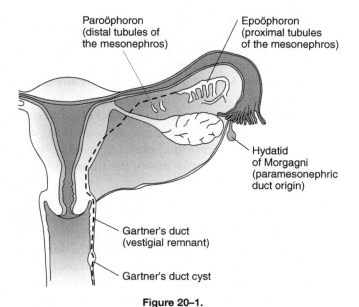

Paroöphoron
(distal tubules of
the mesonephros)

Epoöphoron
(proximal tubules
of the mesonephros)

Hydatid
of Morgagni
(paramesonephric
duct origin)

Gartner's duct
(vestigial remnant)

Gartner's duct cyst

**Figure 20–1.**

6. **(D)** Appendicitis occurs in 10% of the general population, most commonly during childhood. Nausea, vomiting, and loss of appetite occur early in the disease process. The abdominal pain often begins in the periumbilical area and shifts to the right lower abdomen, halfway between the umbilicus and the right anterior superior iliac spine (McBurney's point). Several intestinal disorders, including periappendiceal abscess, regional enteritis, colitis, and diverticulitis, may produce a local inflammatory mass (phlegmon) that is palpable on pelvic examination. Torsion of an ovarian mass causes acute pain but is not associated with a fever or the laboratory findings present in this case.

7. **(E)** In reproductive-age women, pregnancy is the most common cause of a pelvic mass associated with amenorrhea. Any reproductive-age woman who experiences amenorrhea must be considered pregnant until proven otherwise. If the pregnancy test is negative, then other diagnoses are more feasible and can be evaluated by pelvic ultrasound and a detailed history.

8. **(B)** Defective Müllerian duct fusion causes varying degrees of uterine duplication. Fusion failure involving the entire Müllerian duct results in a double uterus and cervix (uterine didelphys), occasionally accompanied by a longitudinal septum of the upper vagina (double vagina). If one of the reproductive tracts does not communicate with the outside (obstructive anomaly), menstrual blood accumulates in the portion of the tract preceding the obstruction (e.g., vagina and uterus), causing abdominal pain and a pelvic mass. Surgery is required to drain blood from the obstruction site. Endometriosis, secondary to retrograde seeding from these obstructed structures, is common. Uterus didelphys, with one of two vaginas ending in a blind pouch, is associated with renal agenesis on the side of the pouch.

9. **(A)** A corpus luteum cyst may occur as a result of hemorrhage or cyst formation. Delayed involution of the corpus luteum cyst (Halban's syndrome) causes prolonged progesterone secretion, leading to persistently elevated BBTs, amenorrhea, and pelvic pain. Luteolysis is even-

tually accompanied by the onset of spontaneous menses. Symptoms of Halban syndrome are similar to those of ectopic pregnancy but are distinguished from the latter by a negative serum pregnancy test. Treatment unless concerns for ongoing hemorrhage and anemia is observation.

10. **(E)** The mature teratoma, or dermoid cyst, is the most common germ-cell tumor. It is composed of three germ-cell layers: ectoderm, mesoderm, and endoderm. It commonly occurs in young women and has a bilaterality rate of 15% to 25%. Ectodermal derivatives (e.g., hair and skin elements) predominate, causing accumulation of a greasy, sebaceous fluid within the cyst. Bone fragments, teeth, and gastrointestinal mucosa are often present and located adjacent to projections within the cyst cavity, referred to as Rokitansky's protuberances. These protuberances are the sites from which 1% to 3% of benign cystic teratomas undergo malignant transformation in postmenopausal women, most commonly a squamous carcinoma. However, if any of the teeth have a dental filling, then facial trauma is more likely,

11. **(C)** During human development, the midgut communicates with the yolk sac via the yolk stalk or vitelline duct. The intra-abdominal portion of the yolk stalk connecting the umbilicus to the intestine usually atrophies but may persist as a Meckel's diverticulum in 2% to 4% of persons, more commonly in males. It appears as a 3- to 6-cm-long fingerlike pouch arising 40 to 50 cm from the ileocecal junction. It may be attached to the umbilicus by a fibrous cord or fistula. Twenty percent of Meckel's diverticula contain secretory gastric mucosa that may ulcerate, leading to intra-abdominal bleeding. Meckel's diverticulum also may cause symptoms mimicking appendicitis and intestinal obstruction (due to intussusception or volvulus of the diverticulum).

12. **(A)** Inflammatory bowel disease commonly occurs during reproductive life and includes ulcerative colitis and regional enteritis (Crohn's disease). The former refers to inflammation confined to the colon, whereas the latter is characterized by multiple sites of small bowel or colonic inflammation. The symptoms of regional

enteritis mimic those of appendicitis but often can be distinguished from the latter by the presence of bloody diarrhea, blood and WBCs in stool specimens, and bowel mucosal changes on gastrointestinal studies. Acute inflammatory bowel disease generally responds to corticosteroid therapy and is associated with poor healing and fistula formation after surgery.

13. **(C)** A hemorrhagic corpus luteum may accompany an intrauterine pregnancy. It may cause pelvic pain indistinguishable from that of an ectopic pregnancy. The corpus luteum cyst generally persists for the first 8 to 12 gestational weeks and then regresses spontaneously as progesterone production is shifted to the placenta. A heterotopic ectopic pregnancy refers to the coexistence of an ectopic pregnancy and an intrauterine pregnancy. Heterotopic ectopic pregnancies occur in approximately 1 in 7,000 pregnancies and increase in frequency to 1 in 900 pregnancies after ovulation induction therapies. While degenerated leiomyomata may have cystic areas, their overall appearance on ultrasonographic studies is that of a solid tumor.

14. **(E)** This woman has a ruptured ectopic pregnancy until proven otherwise. She clearly has a surgical abdomen with diaphragmatic irritation. The intra-abdominal bleeding is potentially life-threatening and requires immediate surgery. Methotrexate is only an option for a stable patient.

15. **(A)** A luteoma results from extensive luteinization of ovarian thecal cells during normal pregnancy. The benign tumor is solid, occurs bilaterally in 45% of cases, and produces significant amounts of androgens. It is associated with a 25% risk of maternal virilization with concurrent, female, and fetal masculinization in many of the newborns. Luteomas regress spontaneously after delivery.

16. **(A)** Most ovarian tumors detected during pregnancy are cystic. The most common complication of ovarian tumors during pregnancy is adnexal torsion during the first trimester. Cystic ovarian tumors may rupture, causing intra-abdominal hemorrhage and extrusion of cyst

contents into the peritoneal cavity. A large tumor also may obstruct labor.

17. **(D)** Uterine leiomyomas are the most common pelvic masses in postmenopausal women. Most authors report a prevalence of up to 45% for postmenopausal women. Uterine leiomyomata are also the most common indication for major surgery in women. Follicular or corpus luteum cysts would be very rare in this age group because they would require functional follicles. Germ-cell tumors are also rare at this age. Endometrioma would require elevated estrogen levels to still be symptomatic which is uncommon at this age.

18. **(A)** Ovarian tumors derived from capsular epithelium are the most common neoplastic ovarian tumors in reproductive- and postreproductive-age women. Ca 125 may be useful.

19. **(B)** Signet ring cells are characteristic findings in Krukenberg's tumors. These tumors arise in the gastrointestinal tract (most often the stomach) and spread to the ovary. It is characterized by areas of mucoid degeneration and the presence of signet ring cells.

20. **(B)** Forty percent of abdominal masses in children younger than 2 years are renal in origin. An ectopic pelvic kidney occurs in up to 15% of girls without a uterus or vagina. The pelvic kidney may be palpable abdominally or rectally.

21. **(C)** In reproductive-age women, infections of the adnexa may result from sexually transmitted diseases. The patient commonly gives a history of recent sexual activity, multiple sexual partners, or a new sexual partner. She usually experiences fever, chills, low bilateral abdominal pain, and vaginal discharge. During acute salpingitis, the tube becomes distended with purulent material, causing a tender tubal abscess (pyosalpinx). As chronic salpingitis develops, peritubal adhesions obstruct the fimbriated ends of the fallopian tubes, leading to hydrosalpinges and infertility. In contrast to most cases, pelvic infection associated with intrauterine contraceptive

device (IUCD) use may involve only one adnexa. In the setting of acute PID, many would recommend removal of the IUCD until infection resolves and the patient is reevaluated for continued IUCD use.

22. **(E)** Endometriosis should be suspected when pelvic examination in a reproductive-age woman shows tenderness, an ovarian mass, or fixation of the uterus with nodularity of the uterosacral ligaments. An ovarian collection of endometriosis large enough to form a tumor is called an endometrioma. Endometriomas contain hemorrhagic debris, which gives them an echogenic appearance by ultrasound. They are often called "chocolate cysts" because their contents have a chocolate-like appearance.

23. **(B)** Adnexal torsion results from twisting of the fallopian tube and ovary around their long axes. Torsion commonly occurs in reproductive-age women and often is precipitated by abrupt pelvic movement. The right adnexa have a greater tendency to twist than the left adnexa (perhaps because the sigmoid colon fills the left pelvis). The most frequent findings of torsion are lower abdominal pain and a tender adnexal mass located anterior to the uterus. Two-thirds of patients with adnexal torsion have nausea, vomiting, and episodes of previous intermittent abdominal pain (presumably due to incomplete torsion). Conditions associated with an increased risk of adnexal torsion are pregnancy and ovarian tumors, particularly benign cystic teratomas. During early torsion, venous and lymphatic obstruction causes ovarian cyanosis and edema. The adnexa can be untwisted, and the ovarian tumor can be removed if necessary. Prolonged adnexal torsion interrupts the arterial blood supply to the ovary, causing necrosis, low-grade fever, and temperature elevation. Salpingo-oophorectomy removes necrotic tissue and avoids the risks of infection, intraabdominal hemorrhage, and embolization of necrotic tissue into the circulation.

24. **(D)** Uterine leiomyomas, also called "fibroids" and myomas, are benign smooth muscle tumors (Figure 20–2). They are the most common solid pelvic tumors, occurring in at least

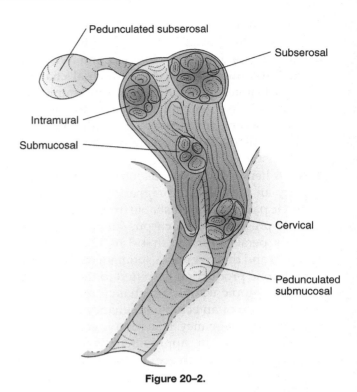

**Figure 20–2.**

20% of all women by age 40 years, 50% of Black women, and 25% of Caucasian women. Myomas are round, firm, myometrial tumors and may extend from the uterine wall into the broad ligament (intraligamentous leiomyoma), giving the impression of an adnexal mass. Although most women with uterine leiomyomas are asymptomatic, some women experience abnormal vaginal bleeding (metrorrhagia and/or menorrhagia). Distortion of the uterine cavity may interfere with embryo implantation, leading to spontaneous abortion. Leiomyomata may undergo degeneration, infarction, or infection, causing abdominal pain. Rarely sarcomatous changes within the leiomyomata cause rapid enlargement of the uterus.

25. **(A)** The McCune–Albright syndrome is a rare disease in which pseudosexual precocity results from an estrogen-secreting ovarian follicular cyst. Multiple cystic bone lesions (polyostotic fibrous dysplasia), and café au lait spots are also present in these children.

26. **(H)** Theca lutein cysts occur in response to high-circulating hCG levels (e.g., gestational trophoblastic disease, multifetal pregnancy)

and ovulation-inducing medication. Bilateral, smooth, thin-walled cysts contain clear, straw-colored fluid and are surrounded by extensively luteinized stroma. The cysts generally disappear after termination of pregnancy or discontinuation of medication.

27. **(I)** Voiding usually occurs shortly after birth but may be delayed until the second day of life. A female infant delivered in a breech presentation may develop swelling of periurethral soft tissues. Inability to void causes bladder distention that is alleviated by catheterization.

28. **(G)** Fibromas are benign ovarian tumors derived from stromal mesenchyme. They are solid, irregular, and mobile (ranging in size from small to several thousand grams). Fibromas contain spindle cells that form collagen but do not produce hormones. Meigs syndrome refers to the findings of ascites and pleural effusions in combination with an ovarian fibroma. Peritoneal fluid accumulates intra-abdominally and traverses diaphragmatic lymphatics into the pleural cavities.

29. **(D)** Leiomyomas enlarging after menopause are suspicious for malignancy, most commonly sarcoma. Leiomyosarcomas consist of malignant mesenchymal (sarcomatous) tissue originating from stromal components of the uterus (e.g., endometrial stroma, myometrium, or connective tissue). The risk of a uterine leiomyoma transforming to a malignant leiomyosarcoma is 0.1% to 0.5%. Less than 10% of leiomyosarcomas originate in a leiomyoma. Most women with a leiomyosarcoma experience symptoms of short-term duration. Symptoms commonly include abdominal bloating. Pressure on adjacent organs may cause urinary symptoms (e.g., urinary frequency, retention, and incontinence), backache (due to ureteral obstruction with hydronephrosis), and rectal pressure (e.g., constipation and/or tenesmus).

30. **(B)** Most women with ovarian carcinoma have a palpable abdominal or pelvic mass. Twenty to thirty percent of these individuals have clinically detectable malignant ascites, defined as accumulation of serous fluid-containing cancer-

ous cells within the abdominal cavity. Abdominal percussion of ascites causes a wave-like movement of fluid around a central tympanitic area of bowel. Malignant pleural effusions may be detected as a loss of breath sounds by pulmonary auscultation. The pelvic examination remains the cornerstone for detection of ovarian neoplasia, and the presence of a fixed, irregular nodular adnexal mass with cul-de-sac nodularity or a palpable postmenopausal ovary should be considered an ovarian carcinoma until proven otherwise.

31. **(E)** The most common symptoms of cervical cancer are abnormal vaginal bleeding and vaginal discharge. The cervix is friable and may bleed with examination. The discharge may be serous, mucoid, or purulent. The tumor usually spreads by direct extension through the parametrium. Approximately 30% to 50% of women with advanced disease suffer ureteral obstruction, with death occurring by uremia.

32. **(H)** Colonic diverticula, formed by herniation of bowel mucosa through weaknesses in the colonic muscularis, occur in up to one-third of postmenopausal women. Disruption of the mucosa may lead to episode bleeding and local infection (diverticulitis), causing self-limited left lower abdominal pain. The pain usually subsides as the mucosa heals. Severe diverticulitis causes intense left lower abdominal pain, fever, and leukocytosis. The local inflammatory process may produce a palpable adnexal phlegmon.

33. **(D)** In the United States, colorectal cancer is the second most common malignancy in women of all ages. Colorectal carcinoma should be suspected when a hard, tubular, pelvic mass with a transverse orientation is palpable in an elderly patient or in any individual with a family history of colorectal cancer or polyposis.

34. **(C)** This patient's symptoms and findings are most compatible with acute urinary retention. This can be easily confirmed by history and the placement of a catheter. Hematomas near the site of abdominal wall punctures should be centered at or very near to surgical site and generally are not large or extremely painful. Most

sterilization procedures are not associated with acute disruptions of ovarian blood flow, and hematomas of the broad ligament would not explain the findings present here.

35. **(E)** Small, asymptomatic, simple ovarian cysts found incidentally in postmenopausal women can safely be followed. While the incidence of ovarian cancer rise dramatically in postmenopausal women, small simple cysts that appear benign on imaging have a very small chance of malignancy. Serum CA-125 measurements have very poor positive and negative predictive value and have little place in establishing a preoperative diagnosis. While women with BRCA-1/2 abnormalities have an increased risk of ovarian cancer, without other reasons for such testing, such assessments would be of little value in the evaluation of this incidental finding. Diagnostic laparoscopy might be justified if there were an increased suspicion of malignancy, but in the absence of other indications such an investigation may be unjustifiably invasive.

36. **(E)** Theca lutein cysts are uncommon but are a not infrequent complication of iatrogenic stimulation of the ovaries. Almost always bilateral and frequently associated with ascites, these tumors are benign and self-limited. Conception should be delayed because the persistent stimulation by hCG could cause further growth. Spontaneous regression should be expected.

37. **(E)** In women below the age of 40, more than 60% of ovarian tumors are benign cystic teratomas. Follicular cysts are usually thin walled and may achieve sizes up to 10 cm and generally regress over a period of 1–3 months. The overwhelming probability that the findings presented represent one of these two tumors, suggests that reevaluation in 4 to 6 weeks would be appropriate. Oral contraceptive therapy to suppress ovarian function and speed cyst regression has been shown to be ineffective, so in the absence of other indications for oral contraceptives, this option is not appropriate.

38. **(E)** The diagnosis of uterine leiomyomata is a clinical one and does not require imaging or other testing. Since the patient is experiencing minimal symptoms, routine well-woman examinations are all that are necessary.

39. **(D)** First described in the 1980s, cancer antigen 125 (CA-125) is expressed by approximately 80% of ovarian epithelial carcinomas, though less often by mucinous tumors. CA-125 is increased in endometrial and tubal carcinoma, in addition to ovarian carcinoma, and in other malignancies, including those originating in the lung, breast, and pancreas. A level higher than 35 U/mL is generally considered increased. Unfortunately, any process that results in peritoneal irritation, such as PID or endometriosis, may also result in elevations of this marker, making its utility as a diagnostic tool in premenopausal women limited.

40. **(A)** Uterine leiomyomata are sensitive to both estrogen and progesterone, but the exact mechanism of their initiation and growth is unclear. Through several mechanisms, uterine leiomyomata are more sensitive to estrogen and are even able to increase the estrogen levels of their environment by reduced conversion of estradiol to estrone, and a greater degree of aromatization of androgens to estrogens within the tissue. While these tumors appear to be sensitive to a number of cellular growth hormones, the levels of these hormones would not be materially affected by pregnancy or birth. Women of higher parity are thought to be at reduced risk because of the relative interlude from estrogen exposure brought on by the high progesterone state of pregnancy.

41. **(E)** What has been termed postembolization syndrome consists of pelvic pain and cramping, nausea and vomiting, a low-grade fever and malaise occurring 2 to 7 days after the procedure. These symptoms are due to necrosis and involution of the uterine leiomyomata and are generally self-limited. Hospitalization may be required if the symptoms of pain are severe or if the patient is unable to maintain oral hydration. When leiomyomata are intracavitary or contact the endometrial surface, passage of necrotic tissue or a copious discharge may occur.

# CHAPTER 21

# Gynecologic Oncology: Premalignant and Malignant Diseases of the Lower Genital Tract—Vulva, Vagina, and Cervix

## Questions

**DIRECTIONS (Questions 1 through 46): For each of the multiple choice questions in this section, select the lettered answer that is the one *best* response in each case.**

1. A 65-year-old woman returns for the results of her vulvar biopsy. Which of the following is the etiologic agent (or immediate precursor lesion) for vulvar cancer?

    (A) squamous cell hyperplasia
    (B) atrophic dystrophy
    (C) chronic granulomatous diseases
    (D) chronic irritation
    (E) unknown

2. A 56-year-old woman has a biopsy-proven vulvar intraepithelial neoplasia (VIN III). She undergoes a wide excision and returns 3 months later with vulvar pruritus. What should you advise the patient?

    (A) Steroid cream on the vulva will reduce the itching.
    (B) She may need a repeat biopsy.
    (C) There is minimal chance of cancer.
    (D) There is minimal chance of recurrence.
    (E) If there is a recurrence, it will regress spontaneously.

3. A 65-year-old woman presents with complaints of vulvar redness, pruritus, and occasional weeping from the skin. Examination reveals erythematous, eczematoid of the labia minora, and periclitoral area. This is consistent with Paget's disease of the vulva. Which of the following characterizes Paget's disease of the vulva?

    (A) recurrences are infrequent after treatment
    (B) frequent association with other invasive carcinomas
    (C) appears as a solitary hypopigmented lesion
    (D) is treated with laser vaporization
    (E) occurs predominantly in premenopausal women

4. Which of the following types of vulvar cancer occurs most commonly?

    (A) Paget's
    (B) squamous
    (C) melanoma
    (D) adenocarcinoma
    (E) basal cell

5. A 48-year-old woman presents with a large verrucous lesion of her vulva. It is not particularly painful, but the appearance is worrisome to the patient. Such a lesion is most likely which of the following?

   (A) clear cell carcinoma
   (B) condyloma acuminata
   (C) adenocarcinoma
   (D) hidradenoma
   (E) urethral caruncles

6. Which of the following is the most common symptom of vulvar carcinoma in elderly women?

   (A) abnormal bleeding
   (B) a foul smell
   (C) pruritus
   (D) vulvar atrophy
   (E) painful intercourse

7. A 1-cm vulvar carcinoma with tumor-positive unilateral nodes and no distant spread would be in which FIGO (International Federation of Gynecology and Obstetrics) stage?

   (A) I
   (B) II
   (C) III
   (D) IV
   (E) cannot be staged without further information

**Questions 8 through 10 apply to the following patient:**

A 58-year-old woman has a 1-cm vulvar ulcer. A biopsy shows invasive squamous cell carcinoma with more than 1 mm of stromal invasion.

8. Which of the following is the preferred treatment?

   (A) Burow's soaks
   (B) 5-fluorouracil (5-FU) cream
   (C) radiotherapy

   (D) radical local excision and ipsilateral inguinofemoral lymph node dissection
   (E) radical hysterectomy and node dissection

9. If the lymph nodes in this case are negative, the 5-year survival should be approximately what percentage?

   (A) 12
   (B) 25
   (C) 52
   (D) 78
   (E) 90

10. This patient undergoes radical vulvectomy. Which of the following is the most common complication of radical vulvectomy?

    (A) debilitating edema of the lower extremities
    (B) pulmonary embolism
    (C) necrotizing fasciitis
    (D) breakdown of the surgical wound
    (E) urinary and rectal incontinence

11. A 72-year-old woman has had a radical vulvectomy for stage II squamous cell vulvar cancer. She wants to know the most likely site of recurrence if the tumor comes back. Where would the tumor most likely appear?

    (A) at the site of tumor resection
    (B) in the bladder or rectum
    (C) in the scalene lymph nodes
    (D) the chest
    (E) the upper leg

12. Which of the following tumors of the vulva has the best prognosis?

    (A) stage I verrucous carcinoma
    (B) melanoma
    (C) stage I squamous cell cancer of vulva
    (D) basal cell carcinoma
    (E) rhabdomyosarcoma

13. A 56-year-old woman presents with painless mild vaginal spotting. She had a hysterectomy at age 40 for persistent cervical dysplasia. She is otherwise healthy and takes no medications. On further review of symptoms, she has occasional urgency and dysuria. On pelvic examination, a 0.5-cm lesion is felt and visualized in the anterior vagina. What is the next step in the evaluation or treatment of this lesion?

(A) refer to gynecologic oncologist
(B) perform directed punch biopsy of the lesion
(C) perform Papanicolaou (Pap) smear of the vagina and vaginoscopy
(D) perform laser ablation therapy
(E) order ultrasound of the pelvis

14. A 30-year-old woman presents for her annual examination. On history, she reports that her mother was prescribed diethylstilbestrol (DES) during the pregnancy with her. Which of the following conditions is she most at risk for as a result?

(A) endometrial adenocarcinoma
(B) ovarian adenocarcinoma
(C) clear cell adenocarcinoma of the vagina
(D) ovarian cysts
(E) fallopian tube adenocarcinoma

15. Which of the following is a malignant tumor of the vagina of young children that appears clinically as a mass of grape-like edematous polyps?

(A) emphysematous vaginitis
(B) squamous cell carcinoma
(C) sarcoma botryoides
(D) adenocarcinoma
(E) choriocarcinoma

**Questions 16 through 18 apply to the following patient:**

A 72-year-old woman complains of vaginal bleeding. On evaluation, a 2-cm vaginal lesion is found in the upper third of the anterior vagina. On bimanual and rectovaginal examination, the mass extends to the lateral pelvic wall. On biopsy, vaginal carcinoma is confirmed.

16. What stage cancer does this patient most likely have?

(A) 0
(B) I
(C) II
(D) III
(E) IV

17. Which of the following is the most likely histology of vaginal carcinoma in this woman?

(A) melanoma
(B) verrucous
(C) clear cell
(D) adenocarcinoma
(E) squamous cell

18. Which of the following is the best treatment for her?

(A) total vaginectomy
(B) upper vaginectomy
(C) chemotherapy
(D) combination radiation and chemotherapy
(E) exenteration

19. Which of the following is the most common method used to diagnose cervical intraepithelial neoplasia (CIN)?

(A) complaints of abnormal discharge
(B) postcoital bleeding
(C) chronic pelvic pain
(D) vaginal wet preparation
(E) abnormal Pap smears

20. Which of the following reflects the etiology of cervical dysplasia and cervical cancer?

(A) Human papillomavirus (HPV) is the major causal agent.
(B) They are associated with obesity.
(C) They are associated with nulliparity.
(D) There is a strong genetic component to the development of cervical cancer.
(E) They are the direct result of cigarette smoking.

**21.** Which of the following reflects HPV?

  (A)  Only 20% of sexually experienced women will be infected with HPV.

  (B)  The virus is transient for most women.

  (C)  Most women with HPV will go on to develop warts, CIN, or cancer.

  (D)  Other cofactors such as cigarette smoking and altered immune response have not been shown to be related to the development of cervical neoplasia.

  (E)  There are only 10 subtypes of HPV identified to date.

**Questions 22 through 26 apply to the following patient:**

A 40-year-old woman is seen for a routine examination. Her menses have been regular, and she has no complaints. Findings, including those on pelvic examination, are normal. Ten days later, her Pap smear is returned as "high-grade squamous intraepithelial lesion."

**22.** Which of the following options is the best course of action?

  (A)  immediate wide-cuff hysterectomy

  (B)  repeated Pap smears at 3-month intervals

  (C)  fractional dilation and curettage (D&C)

  (D)  punch biopsy of anterior cervical lip

  (E)  colposcopy with biopsy

**23.** The colposcope permits one to do which of the following?

  (A)  view the cervix at 1–4 power magnification

  (B)  see the entire transition zone in all patients

  (C)  choose the most suspicious areas on the cervical portio to biopsy

  (D)  treat invasive cancer with a biopsy

  (E)  make the diagnosis of cancer

**24.** Under colposcopic examination, a distinct area of acetowhite change is noted with associated coarse pattern vessels and punctation. This is consistent with what histologic finding on directed biopsy?

  (A)  CIN I

  (B)  atrophy

  (C)  squamous cell cancer

  (D)  CIN II–III

  (E)  a nabothian cyst

**25.** Conization of the cervix would be inappropriate in which of the following instances?

  (A)  when there is disparity between Pap smear and biopsy results

  (B)  when colposcopy is inadequate

  (C)  when microinvasion is diagnosed by biopsy

  (D)  when deeply invasive cancer is shown on a biopsy

  (E)  for treatment of biopsy-proven CIN III

**26.** This patient has biopsy-proven CIN III. She requests cryotherapy for treatment. Cryotherapy is appropriate to consider in which clinical circumstance?

  (A)  CIN III

  (B)  a patient with well-circumscribed, small lesion of mild dysplasia (CIN 1)

  (C)  invasive carcinoma

  (D)  a patient who wishes to preserve fertility

  (E)  an HIV-positive patient

**27.** A 25-year-old woman presents with irregular vaginal bleeding. She is otherwise healthy and uses condoms for contraception. She smokes occasionally and takes no medications. Her aunt had cervical cancer and she is worried that she may also have cervical cancer. What is the most common symptom associated with cervical cancer?

  (A)  no symptom

  (B)  pain with intercourse

  (C)  vaginal bleeding

  (D)  weight loss

  (E)  vulvar pruritus

28. When sampling the cervix for a Pap smear, it is critical to sample which area since it is the most likely source of cervical cancer. Where do most cervical cancers arise?

   (A) on the portio vaginalis
   (B) at the internal os
   (C) in the endocervix
   (D) at the squamocolumnar junction
   (E) at the external os

29. What percentage of clinical stage I carcinomas of the cervix will have lymphatic spread?

   (A) 0–1
   (B) up to 7
   (C) 15
   (D) 25
   (E) 40

30. If a nonhealing ulcer is seen on the cervix, it is best evaluated by which of the following?

   (A) repeat examination
   (B) Pap smear
   (C) punch biopsy
   (D) cone biopsy
   (E) vaginal steroid cream

**Questions 31 and 32 apply to the following patient:**

A 48-year-old woman presents for her routine annual examination. Her last Pap smear was more than 10 years ago. She has had occasional abnormal Pap smear during her lifetime, but no treatments were recommended. Otherwise, she has mild hypertension and is on a beta-blocker. On examination, she has a normal pelvic examination, but her Pap smear reveals high-grade squamous intraepithelial lesion (SIL). A colposcopically directed biopsy reveals invasive squamous cell carcinoma.

31. Which of the following should be the most appropriate next step in the care of the patient?

   (A) metastatic evaluation
   (B) conization
   (C) radical hysterectomy

   (D) radiation therapy
   (E) both irradiation and radical hysterectomy

32. The woman had a negative metastatic workup. Her clinical examination shows cancer growth shown in Figure 21–1. Her preliminary clinical stage is which of the following?

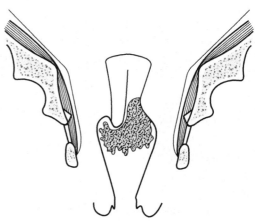

**Figure 21–1.**

   (A) IA
   (B) IB
   (C) IIA
   (D) IIB
   (E) III

33. The majority of deaths from cervical carcinoma are due to which of the following?

   (A) local spread obstructing the ureters, causing renal failure
   (B) brain metastasis with resultant cerebral hemorrhage
   (C) hemorrhage into the pelvis from erosion of vessels by the tumor
   (D) pulmonary failure secondary to metastatic disease filling the lungs
   (E) bone metastasis causing crush injuries to the central nervous system

**34.** The 5-year survival rate for stage IV invasive cervical cancer is approximately what percentage?

(A) >1

(B) 15

(C) 30

(D) 50

(E) 80

**35.** Which of the following is the best term for a bulky, friable, papillary tumor mass growing from the cervix?

(A) exophytic

(B) endophytic

(C) nodular

(D) ulcerating

(E) edematous

**36.** A 34-year-old woman G1 is 16 weeks pregnant and has a Pap smear suspicious for cancer. How do you advise her?

(A) have colposcopy with biopsy

(B) have colposcopy, but biopsy is too risky in pregnancy

(C) have a repeat Pap smear in 3 months

(D) undergo a termination of pregnancy and then undergo complete evaluation

(E) have cervical conization

**37.** A 65-year-old woman presents with vaginal discharge and rare mild bleeding. She had a cone of the cervix for CIN III 20 years ago. She has since had a complete hysterectomy for uterine fibroids. You perform a pelvic examination and see an irregular area in the vagina. Vaginal colposcopy and directed biopsy reveal vaginal intraepithelial neoplasia (VAIN). VAIN is most commonly found in which part of the vagina?

(A) the upper one-third

(B) the mid-vagina

(C) the distal vagina

(D) at the hymenal ring

(E) the posterior fourchette

**38.** The preferred treatment for a 1.5-cm stage I vaginal carcinoma confined to the upper one-third of the lateral vagina in a 29-year-old woman would be which of the following?

(A) intravaginal 5-FU

(B) upper vaginectomy

(C) simple hysterectomy and upper vaginectomy

(D) radical hysterectomy, bilateral pelvic lymphadenectomy, and upper vaginectomy

(E) anterior exenteration

**39.** A 42-year-old presents with a history of postcoital spotting. Examination of the cervix reveals a raised/reddened well-circumscribed lesion next to the os. Which of the following is the most likely diagnosis?

(A) carcinoma

(B) condyloma lata

(C) ectropion

(D) cervical polyp

(E) nabothian cyst

**40.** The treatment of carcinoma of the cervix during pregnancy should depend on all except which of the following?

(A) the recommendation of the oncologist

(B) the religious and moral beliefs of the patient

(C) the trimester of the pregnancy

(D) the stage of the lesion

(E) the length of the cervix

41. A 42-year-old woman with cervical cancer undergoes a radical hysterectomy and requires postoperative radiation. During the radiation therapy she returns complaining of watery vaginal discharge and recurrent urinary tract infections. Which of the following would be the first test to perform to evaluate the most likely cause of the discharge?

    (A) intravenous pyelogram (IVP)
    (B) cystoscopy
    (C) wet mount
    (D) sigmoidoscopy
    (E) inject diluted methylene blue in sterile water into the bladder and examine the vagina

42. A 35-year-old woman with stage IIB squamous cell carcinoma of the cervix will receive radiation. Regarding reproductive changes, how should you advise her?

    (A) Ovaries are radioresistant.
    (B) Fertility is maintained.
    (C) Radiation will likely result in endometrial ablation.
    (D) Younger patients are more susceptible to radiation-induced castration.
    (E) There is no change in vaginal function.

43. A 46-year-old obese woman smokes two packs of cigarettes a day. She had a radical hysterectomy with a para-aortic and pelvic lymphadenectomy for stage IB squamous cell carcinoma of the cervix. At surgery she was found to have dense pelvic small-bowel adhesions from a prior ruptured appendix and appendectomy. Lymph nodes were positive for cancer cells. In discussing postoperative radiation, you counsel her that she has an increased rate of radiation-related complication because of which of the following?

    (A) obesity
    (B) excision of lymph nodes
    (C) decreased bowel motility from adhesions
    (D) age
    (E) stage of the cancer

44. A 24-year-old healthy woman has her routine examination and Pap smear. Her Pap smear is atypical squamous cells of undetermined significance (ASCUS). Which of the following reflects our current knowledge about ASCUS?

    (A) the risk of CIN II or III on biopsy is 1%
    (B) the risk of invasive cervical cancer is 0.1%
    (C) represent a minority of abnormal Pap smears per year in U.S. women
    (D) requires immediate colposcopy
    (E) is not associated with high-risk HPV subtypes

45. A 48-year-old postmenopausal woman presents for routine gynecologic examination. The examination is normal; however, the Pap smear returns atypical glandular cells (AGCs). What would be the most appropriate management for this patient?

    (A) repeat Pap smear in 4 to 6 months
    (B) treat with intravaginal estrogen and repeat Pap smear
    (C) perform cone biopsy of the cervix
    (D) perform colposcopy, cervical and endometrial biopsies
    (E) refer to Gynecologic Oncology

46. A 30-year-old woman presents for her annual examination. She inquires whether she should receive the HPV vaccine. For which patient population is the HPV vaccine FDA approved?

    (A) women of all ages
    (B) only women who are virginal and have never had an abnormal Pap smear
    (C) men, for the prevention of female cervical dysplasias and cancer
    (D) girls and women aged 9 to 26 years
    (E) for pregnant or lactating women

# Answers and Explanations

1. **(E)** The etiologic agent for vulvar carcinoma is unknown. Vulvar diseases (squamous cell hyperplasia, previously known as hyperplastic dystrophy, sexually transmitted diseases, granulomatosis diseases) are all associated with an increased incidence of vulvar cancer, but none are considered the cause. The majority arise within squamous epithelium. For squamous cell carcinoma, high-risk HPV infection is found in 40% of cases.

2. **(B)** VIN can certainly recur, although it has a much longer transition time than CIN. Some VINs may regress spontaneously, but this is not guaranteed. VIN can be multifocal, and approximately 20% of patients with an initial biopsy of VIN III have been reported to have microinvasive cancer in the resected specimen. Steroid cream is the treatment of choice for pruritus from vulvar dystrophies, but this woman needs a vulvar examination and possible biopsy to rule out recurrence.

3. **(B)** Paget's disease may be identified by the typical vacuolated, large, pale, mucin-containing cells infiltrating the epidermis, often in a serpiginous manner (Paget cells). It presents typically with pruritus and appears as diffuse erythematous eczematous change of the vulva. The gynecologist must be vigilant to evaluate the rest of the vulva and cervix, as well as the breast and GI track as frequently other carcinomas coexist. Treatment consists of full-thickness wide excision with a 1-cm margin around the visible lesion. Recurrences are common and require regular surveillance examinations. This disease typically affects women aged 60–70 years.

4. **(B)** Cancer of the vulva makes up approximately 5% of all gynecologic malignancies, and approximately 90% of vulvar cancer is squamous cell. Paget's disease is an intraepithelial lesion derived from an undifferentiated glandular cell. Extramammary Paget's disease is most often an intraepithelial lesion that may spread over the perineum. Adenocarcinoma probably arises from glandular structures of the vulva and comprises <1% of all vulvar carcinomas. Malignant melanoma can occur over any skin area but is relatively rare in the vulva (approximately 5% of cases).

5. **(B)** At age 48, this lesion is most likely condyloma acuminate or genital wart. These are due to HPV and typically range from flat papules to raised irregular verrucous exophytic lesions. However, it could be verrucous carcinoma, which is a locally invasive tumor that does not tend to metastasize via the lymphatics. Clear cell carcinoma and adenocarcinoma are much less likely and carcinoma in general presents with erythema, pruritus. If any doubt exists, adequate biopsy should be done. Hidradenomas typically start as a nodule and can form an abscess. They are often uncomfortable and can be found within intertriginous areas. Urethral caruncles originate from the urethral meatus, not on the vulva

6. **(C)** Pruritus is the presenting complaint in over one-half of patients. Twenty percent are asymptomatic, and the remainder may have pain, bleeding, or a foul smell from tumor necrosis. Atrophy is not usually a complaint.

7. **(C)** The tumor could be of any size, but the positive unilateral nodes place the lesion in stage III. In the Tumor, Node, Metastasis (TNM) staging, T1N1M0. The TNM system seems to be more prognostic than the FIGO system.

8. **(D)** This patient has a stage IB vulvar carcinoma (if the invasion is >1 mm, the stage is IB instead of IA). In IB, there is an 8% incidence of positive ipsilateral nodes. Deep pelvic nodes are excised only if the others are positive, and there is little salvage demonstrated by removing these deep pelvic lymph nodes. If the lesion was central in the vulva or crossed the midline, bilateral lymph node dissection would be warranted.

9. **(E)** If multiple inguinal nodes are positive, the cure rate drops to less than 15%, and if the deep nodes are involved, the cure rate is very low. This illustrates the importance of the lymphatic route of spread in this disease and the importance of extirpative surgery in treating the disease. Before radical surgery, almost no one survived this disease. Survival for stage II is 67%, stage III is 40%, and stage IV is 22%.

10. **(D)** While all of the choices may be complications of radical vulvectomy, approximately 50% of the patients experience significant problems with wound healing. This is because of the large amount of tissue removed and the poor blood supply of the remaining tissues. Patients often spend 2 or more weeks in the hospital just for the postoperative care of their wounds. Leg edema is also common, and incontinence of urine is not unusual (likely due to resection of the distal third of the urethra), but neither is as frequent as wound problems.

11. **(A)** The most common site of recurrence is the site of the primary surgical resection or the groin area where nodes were positive (if not previously resected). The tumor occurs centrally and seldom as distant metastases.

12. **(D)** Pure basal cell tumors can be cured by wide excision. The other tumors are all treated as invasive carcinomas with radical surgery. Rhabdomyosarcomas are found in young patients,

are extremely malignant, and, fortunately, are very rare.

13. **(B)** Vaginal bleeding is the most common complaint in women diagnosed with vaginal cancer however, most vaginal cancers are asymptomatic and not visible to the unaided eye on routine examination nor palpable to the average examiner. If a lesion is seen or palpated on examination, immediate directed biopsy is indicated to make a diagnosis. If no lesion is apparent, Papanicolaou screening and vaginoscopy are useful for further evaluation of the vagina. Ablative therapy, like laser, would not be appropriate until a diagnosis is established and no malignancy is found. A referral to Gynecologic Oncology would follow once a diagnosis of cancer is made.

14. **(C)** Epithelial endometrial, ovarian, and fallopian tube cancers are not linked to DES exposure. Vaginal clear cell or adenocarcinoma is quite rare, but it is increased in the offspring of women who took DES (incidence estimated at 1 per 1,000 exposed female fetuses). In addition, cervical SILs and squamous cell cancer are also increased in DES-exposed women. Other reproductive tract abnormalities associated with DES include adenosis (columnar irregular cells in the vagina), T-shaped uterus, endometrial adhesions, and transverse vaginal septum.

15. **(C)** This highly malignant tumor of the vagina is fortunately rare but must be thought of whenever vaginal bleeding or discharge occurs in a young female patient. A small scope or examination under anesthesia may be used for diagnostic purposes. Sarcoma botryoides, so called because of its sometimes grape-like gross appearance. This is a highly aggressive tumor but multimodal therapy with surgery, chemotherapy, and radiation has increased survival to 75%.

16. **(D)** Vaginal cancer staging criteria are similar to the criteria used in cervical cancer. Carcinoma of the vagina does not respond as well to treatment as carcinoma of the cervix.

A clinical classification that describes the extent of spread of vaginal carcinoma.

Stage I: Limited to the vaginal wall
Stage II: Extends to the subvaginal tissue
Stage III: Reaches to pelvic wall
Stage IV: Extends beyond the true pelvis or into the mucosa of the bladder or rectum

17. **(E)** Vaginal carcinoma is primarily squamous cell (80% to 90%), followed by adenocarcinoma (5%), melanoma (3%), and less frequent yet, verrucous, and clear cell.

18. **(D)** In advanced vaginal cancer, a combination of chemotherapy with radiation is superior to either alone. Some women will benefit from both external beam and brachytherapy. Platinum chemotherapy is the agent of choice. Surgery is not likely to completely debulk all the tumor burden. Pelvic exenteration is a morbid procedure limited to appropriately selected women with recurrences.

19. **(E)** CIN is an asymptomatic disease generally found on Pap smear. In the United States, 3.5 million women have an abnormal Pap smear per year. Two million will be ASCUS and the other 1.5 million, any CIN.

20. **(A)** HPV has been found to be the causal agent in the majority of cervical dysplasias and cancers. Studies reveal that 75% of women with CIN I have HPV; 85% with CIN II/III, and 95% of women with squamous cell cervical cancer have HPV. This is a sexually transmitted virus. Genetics, obesity, and parity probably play little, if any, role. Cigarette smoking is a risk factor for cervical dysplasia but the mechanism is unclear.

21. **(B)** Up to 80% of sexually experienced women will be positive for HPV during their reproductive lifetime. Most infections are asymptomatic and transient. Only approximately 10% of HPV infections persist. The prevalence of genital warts is 1% and cytologic abnormalities is 4% to 5%. The annual infection rate for HPV is ~1,000× higher than an annual incidence of CIN. Other cofactors are believed to affect the development of CIN, including cigarette smoking and altered host defenses (i.e., women with HIV, or on chemotherapy, or pregnant). To date, there are more than 100 types of HPV that have been identified.

22. **(E)** The type and extent of the lesions must be determined before treatment. The most appropriate next step is colposcopy. Colposcopically directed cervical biopsy will provide information necessary to determine treatment.

23. **(C)** The colposcope permits 6 to 40× power magnification and the addition of a bright light source. If one cannot see the entire cervical transition zone, the colposcopic examination is unsatisfactory, and other diagnostic methods must be used. One should have a tissue diagnosis before instituting treatment for invasive cancer. The greatest advantage of colposcopy is in allowing directed biopsies for diagnosis, not for making the diagnosis. Histologic confirmation is needed, and more than one biopsy should be taken if the suspicious area is large or more than one suspicious area is present.

24. **(D)** On colposcopy, certain visual patterns raise suspicion for pathology. Acetowhite refers to the pale color of cervical dysplasia after application of dilute acetic acid. Vascular patterns include punctate and mosaic patterns, as well as atypical vessels. The more coarse, thick, or irregular the vascular pattern, the more likely the lesion is of a higher grade. Nabothian cysts are normal variants that will often have benign surface vessels.

25. **(D)** If invasive cancer is diagnosed by the biopsy, you have all the necessary information. The next step is staging. One must always carefully examine a microinvasive lesion to rule out frank invasion, as the treatments are quite different. Patients with invasive cervical cancer are badly compromised by treatment for the lesser disease. If a possible invasive cancer cannot be adequately evaluated by colposcopic biopsy, a cone biopsy is indicated.

26. **(B)** Cryotherapy allows for cryonecrosis of cells by crystallizing intracellular water. It may be

considered for small lesions, where the entire lesion is visualized and the histology is CIN I–II. However, in advanced abnormalities, the recurrence rate is high (10% to 20%), and therefore, it is not recommended for CIN III. HIV-positive women with CIN have a higher failure rate with this treatment and should be offered excisional treatments. Patients with cancer need to be clinically staged and then recommended appropriate surgery or chemo/radiation. Although excisional treatments, such as loop electrosurgical excision procedure and cold-knife conization can increase the risk of cervical incompetence or scarring, they are not contraindicated in a women who wishes to preserve fertility. These treatments do not increase infertility.

27. **(A)** Most women with cervical cancer will be asymptomatic. However, women may have watery, bloody discharge or intermittent vaginal bleeding. Other symptoms include postcoital bleeding, lower extremity edema, and back and leg pain (can occur with advanced disease that extends to the pelvic sidewall).

28. **(D)** If the entire squamocolumnar junction is not seen on a colposcopic examination, that examination is inadequate. It is believed that abnormal change begins here because this is the site of metaplastic cells (junction between endocervical columnar cells and ectocervical squamous cells) that are more capable of transformation.

29. **(C)** Such lymphatic spread is often undetected during clinical staging of early cervical cancer. For clinical stage IA1, there is a 1% risk of nodal metastasis and for stage IA2, there is a 7% risk of lymph node involvement. For bulky stage IB, there is up to a 15% nodal involvement. Five-year survival is 100% for IA and 88% for IB

30. **(C)** Any unexplained lesion on the cervix that does not heal must be biopsied. Treatment with creams does not replace adequate diagnosis. Infectious etiologies, such as syphilis and herpes, must also be considered as the cause of the ulcer.

31. **(A)** This patient is already known to have invasive cancer. Proper staging and evaluation for surgery or irradiation is the next step. Cervical cancer is staged clinically: Pelvic and rectovaginal examination, chest radiograph, blood work, such as liver function tests, cystoscopy, and proctoscopy. Once a clinical stage is determined, treatment can be recommended.

32. **(C)** Stage IIA with carcinoma extending beyond the cervix and uterus with left vaginal vault involvement but no parametrial spread.

33. **(A)** Urinary or intestinal obstruction and simple wasting away (cachexia) cause the majority of deaths from cervical cancer. If the recurrence is totally central in the pelvis, exenteration may be indicated.

34. **(B)** Five-year survival for stage I is 80% to 93%, stage II is 58% to 63%, stage III is 32% to 35%, and stage IV is 15% to 16%. Most cervical cancers are diagnosed as either stage I or II.

35. **(A)** Descriptive terms should mean the same thing to everyone using them. Exophytic lesions are seen and biopsied, while endophytic lesions may be quite large before they become visible. Exophytic lesions project outward from the cervix, like condylomata.

36. **(A)** The pregnant patient with a suspicious Pap smear needs colposcopy with directed ectocervical biopsy to rule out invasive cancer. Endocervical curettage is not performed as there is an increased risk of significant bleeding and other pregnancy complications. If CIN or carcinoma in situ is found, the patient can be observed and delivered at term, and then have a final evaluation and therapy 6 weeks postpartum. Cervical conization can be considered in the second trimester if needed to rule out invasive cancer, but colposcopy and biopsy would be appropriate initial evaluation. The majority of even high-grade dysplasias will resolve after the pregnancy.

37. **(A)** The majority of vaginal neoplasias are found in the upper one-third of the vagina and represent in extension of CIN. It is thought that HPV may enter the vaginal mucosa through abrasions in that tissue.

**38. (D)** An early stage of vaginal carcinoma in a young woman would be treated in a manner that would allow you to remove the lesion but preserve as much of her normal functions as possible. In this case, the cancer must be removed, but ovarian preservation and conservation of a functional vagina are the other great concerns. The 5-FU would not cure an invasive cancer. The upper vaginectomy is also likely to fail because approximately 20% of the stage I patients will have pelvic lymph node metastases; therefore, the simple hysterectomy and vaginectomy will also fail in too high a percentage of patients. Radical hysterectomy with nodal extirpation and wide removal of the vagina will likely cure the cancer and preserve ovarian function, and a graft could be used to restore vaginal length, if necessary. Anterior exenteration (removal of all pelvic tissue in the anterior pelvis, including the bladder) is likely to be too much surgery. Radiotherapy is also an option but some studies indicate a lower 5-year survival as compared to surgery.

**39. (D)** The purpose of this question is to reemphasize the point that a cervical lesion can be any number of abnormal findings, and the only way to be certain is to adequately sample the tissue by biopsy and microscopic evaluation. However in a 42-year-old women, the leading diagnosis is a cervical polyp. A Pap smear or colposcopic examination is not a substitute for evaluation of a gross cervical lesion. Biopsy is necessary. A nabothian cyst is usually a clear cystic lesion that is not tender, does not bleed, and is an incidental finding.

**40. (E)** This question is designed to point out two things. The major medical concerns should be (1) the trimester of the pregnancy and (2) the stage of the lesion involved. Patients in the first and early second trimesters should not wait to begin treatment; the delay is too long. In the third trimester, treatment often can be postponed until a viable fetus can be delivered. Treatment with radiation versus surgery depends on the stage, size, and type (histologic differentiation) of the lesion involved. Treatment must be individualized, with decisions being made by an informed patient and a physician. Two commonly held fallacies—(1) cancer of the cervix grows more rapidly during pregnancy and (2) delivery of an infant through a cancerous cervix spreads the disease—should be ignored; they do not appear to be true. The desires of the patient are also important and must be respected even though they might be contrary to current medical opinions. Neither the age of the patient nor the length of the cervix is an important factor.

**41. (E)** A vesicovaginal fistula can occur after radiation therapy or hysterectomy (even a hysterectomy for benign disease). The classic symptoms are described in the case. Methylene blue–stained saline in the bladder can help make the diagnosis by visualizing blue dye in the vagina or by instilling the fluid in the bladder and placing a tampon in the vagina, which becomes stained. Cystoscopy can help in visualizing the lesion and assessing the size, location, and number of fistulas. An IVP is useful for diagnosing ureterovaginal fistula, which is a rare complication but could present with watery vaginal discharge. A wet mount is useful for diagnosing vaginitis, which might occur, but the amount of discharge is likely to be much less with vaginitis than with a fistula. Sigmoidoscopy would not be helpful.

**42. (C)** Ovaries are very radiosensitive organs. Radiation-induced castration can occur with doses as low as 500 rad (or less) in women older than 40 years. Younger women are more resistant to radiation effects on the ovaries, but at doses of 1,000 to 1,500 rad, virtually all women will become postmenopausal from ovarian failure. The typical dose for cervical cancer is in the range of 6,000 to 6,500 rad, so she will lose her reproductive capacity, because of both ovarian failure and endometrial ablation. She will also have loss of vaginal elasticity. Vaginal stenosis can be a major problem if not addressed early.

**43. (C)** After previous surgery where marked adhesions were found, it is likely that adhesions will reform and lead to bowel being fixed in place. These fixed loops of bowel will receive a higher-than-normal dose of radiation. There may also be decreased vascularity after surgery, which can make the bowel more susceptible to radiation damage. Other factors that may increase the risk of radiation injury include concomitant chemotherapy, superimposed infection, presence of malnutrition, and use of tobacco. She should be advised to stop smoking.

44. **(B)** ASCUS represents the majority (2 million of the 3.5 million abnormal Pap smears per year in the United States) of Pap smear abnormalities. It is associated with concurrent cervical dysplasia in 5% to 15% of cases. The incidence of concurrent invasive cancer is 1 per 1,000. When HPV (high-risk subtype) is detected in women with ASCUS, there is a higher incidence of dysplasia found at the time of colposcopy and biopsy. The current recommended triage for ASCUS Pap smear is to check HPV. If the high-risk subtype HPV is negative, the risk of concurrent dysplasia is essentially 0% and patients should be seen in 1 year for repeat Pap smear. If there is HPV, those patients should undergo colposcopy as there is a significant rate of dysplasia (up to 17%).

45. **(D)** AGC is associated with a substantially higher risk for neoplasia than either ASCUS or low-grade SILs. Between 9% and 54% will have biopsy-confirmed CIN, 0% to 8% will have adenocarcinoma in situ, and up to 9% will have invasive carcinoma. Initial workup includes colposcopy, cervical biopsy, endocervical curetting, and endometrial sampling in woman >35 years old or any premenopausal woman with abnormal bleeding. Cone biopsy would be performed as a diagnostic tool if the initial colposcopy is negative.

46. **(D)** Currently the HPV vaccine is approved for girls and women aged 9 to 26 years. In addition, the FDA and Advisory Committee on Immunization Practices approved HPV for boys and men aged 9 to 26 years for the prevention of genital warts, but not specifically to reduce the frequency of cervical dysplasias in their female partners (10/2009). The recommendation for HPV is regardless of sexual activity, abnormal Pap smears, history of HPV, and sexually transmitted infections. At the present time, pregnancy and lactation are contraindications for the administration of HPV vaccine; however, an ongoing registry of exposures and adverse events is underway.

# CHAPTER 22

# Gynecologic Oncology: Upper Genital Tract Benign and Malignant Conditions

## Questions

DIRECTIONS (Questions 1 through 55): For each of the multiple choice questions in this section, select the lettered answer that is the one *best* response in each case.

**Questions 1 through 3 apply to the following patient:**

A 44-year-old multiparous obese woman complains of abnormal vaginal bleeding of 5 months' duration. Pelvic examination demonstrates a small, anteverted uterus and a normal-appearing cervix. No adnexal masses are present. A serum pregnancy test is negative, and a cervical Papanicolaou (Pap) smear is normal. Prolactin and thyroid-stimulating hormone (TSH) levels are normal.

1. Which of the following is the most efficient next step in the evaluation of this patient?

    (A) dilation and curettage (D&C)
    (B) endometrial biopsy
    (C) endometrial cytology
    (D) transvaginal sonography
    (E) hysteroscopy

2. Tissue sampling in this patient reveals endometrial hyperplasia. What is the most common symptom associated with this condition?

    (A) vaginal discharge
    (B) vaginal bleeding
    (C) amenorrhea

    (D) pelvic pain
    (E) abdominal distention

3. Which of the following factors is protective against endometrial hyperplasias?

    (A) obesity
    (B) tamoxifen
    (C) oral contraceptive pills (OCPs).
    (D) early menarche or late menopause
    (E) unopposed exogenous estrogen therapy

4. A 49-year-old woman experiences irregular vaginal bleeding of 3 months' duration. You perform an endometrial biopsy, which obtains copious tissue with a velvety, lobulated texture. The pathologist report shows proliferation of glandular and stromal elements with dilated endometrial glands, consistent with simple hyperplasia. Cytologic atypia is absent. Which of the following is the best way to advise the patient?

    (A) She should be treated to estrogen and progestin hormone therapy.
    (B) The tissue will progress to cancer in approximately 10% of cases.
    (C) The tissue may be weakly premalignant and progresses to cancer in approximately 1% of cases.
    (D) She requires a hysterectomy.
    (E) No further therapy is needed.

5. A 48-year-old woman is referred to you for irregular vaginal bleeding of 6 months' duration. Her referring physician removed tissue protruding through the cervix 3 months ago. Microscopic examination of the tissue shows a mass with cystic hyperplasia and a central vascular channel surrounded on three sides by epithelium. The vaginal bleeding has continued. Which of the following is the best way to advise the patient?

(A) Risk of developing endometrial cancer is increased 10-fold.

(B) Bleeding is from an endometrial polyp.

(C) Histology of the tissue may not reflect the source of the bleeding.

(D) Uterus should be probed with a forceps to remove more tissue.

(E) Patient should receive cyclic progestin therapy.

6. A 58-year-old woman on combined estrogen and progesterone hormone replacement has postmenopausal bleeding. You obtain a pelvic ultrasound that shows an endometrial stripe thickness of 12 mm. Which of the following is most correct?

(A) If the endometrial stripe thickness had been less than 5 mm, you would have told the patient that no further evaluation was needed.

(B) An endometrial stripe thickness of 5 to 10 mm confers no risk of endometrial cancer.

(C) She has a greater than 50% risk of having adenocarcinoma of the endometrium.

(D) The endometrial stripe thickness in premenopausal women is interpreted similar to the endometrial stripe thickness dimensions in postmenopausal women.

(E) Hysterectomy should be performed.

7. An internist calls you for consultation regarding a 55-year-old postmenopausal woman with some vaginal spotting. On examination, a small, round, bright red mass was noted to protrude through the cervical os. It bled during the Pap smear. The Pap smear result was normal. You should advise the internist to do which of the following?

(A) Recheck the mass in 6 months and refer if it enlarges.

(B) Refer the patient for probable polyp removal.

(C) Refer the patient for cone biopsy.

(D) Tell the patient not to worry since the Pap smear is negative.

(E) Tell the patient polyps are never cancerous and refer for removal.

8. A 44-year-old female biochemist has complex hyperplasia without atypia on endometrial biopsy. You prescribe 40-mg megestrol acetate daily. She inquires about the mechanism of action and regression rate. Which of the following explanations is most correct?

(A) The regression of endometrial hyperplasia takes at least 12 months.

(B) Progestins oppose estrogen action in endometrial tissue by reducing the amount of estrogen receptors.

(C) Hyperplastic endometrium has few progesterone receptors so a large dose of progestin is needed.

(D) If regression of endometrial hyperplasia occurs within 3 months, it will recur if she stops the medication.

(E) Progestins bind to progesterone receptors in the endometrium and convert the histology to proliferative endometrium.

9. A 45-year-old woman complains of pelvic pressure and abnormal uterine bleeding. Ultrasound reveals an enlarged uterus with an intramural 4 cm mass. Which of the following is the most common uterine neoplasm?

(A) sarcoma

(B) adenocarcinoma

(C) adenomyosis

(D) choriocarcinoma

(E) leiomyoma

10. During a presentation to a group on women's health a discussion of gynecologic/reproductive cancers including their etiology, risk factors, and normal clinical course is presented. Which of the following types of cancer is the leading cause of gynecologic/reproductive cancer death in women?

   (A) cervical
   (B) uterine
   (C) ovarian
   (D) breast
   (E) vulva

11. A 69-year-old postmenopausal woman is being admitted for surgical treatment of endometrial cancer. She has no health insurance and would like to know which is the most important preoperative screening test to look for metastasis?

   (A) chest X-ray
   (B) hysterosalpingogram
   (C) pelvic ultrasound
   (D) intravenous pyelogram (IVP)
   (E) barium enema

12. A 58-year-old woman develops postmenopausal bleeding. An endometrial biopsy shows adenocarcinoma. She undergoes a total abdominal hysterectomy with pelvic lymph node sampling. The final pathology shows tumor extending from the uterus into the cervix but no other invasion (see Figure 22–1). Lymph nodes were negative for metastasis. The cancer is classified as which stage?

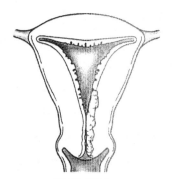

**Figure 22–1.**

   (A) 0
   (B) I
   (C) II
   (D) III
   (E) IV

13. A patient has just been diagnosed with endometrial cancer by endometrial biopsy. During her counseling regarding the disease, staging, management, and prognosis the patient is told that most endometrial cancers are diagnosed as which of the following stages

   (A) I
   (B) II
   (C) III
   (D) IV
   (E) recurrent

**Questions 14 through 16 apply to the following patient:**

A healthy 65-year-old woman is seen for postmenopausal bleeding. The pelvic examination is normal. A fractional D&C demonstrates adenocarcinoma of the endometrium. Histologically, endometrial glands are confluent without solid areas of tumor cells. The endocervical curettage shows normal endocervical cells. The cervical Pap smear and other preoperative investigations are normal.

14. Which of the following statements most likely reflects this patient's endometrial carcinoma stage or treatment.

   (A) Invasion of tumor through most of the myometrium will not be found.
   (B) Invasion of tumor into pelvic lymph nodes will not occur.
   (C) Steroid hormone receptors will not be present in tumor tissue.
   (D) Radical hysterectomy and bilateral salpingo-oophorectomy is the primary treatment modality.
   (E) Therapy depends on surgical and histologic evaluation of pelvic viscera, peritoneal cavity, and retroperitoneal lymph nodes.

15. Exploratory laparotomy is negative for metastatic disease. The uterus is opened in the operating room and found to have tumor invasion into the myometrium. Histologic examination of the uterus confirms tumor invasion beyond the inner half of the myometrium. Peritoneal washings and pelvic and para-aortic nodes are negative for malignancy. What should you advise this patient?

    (A) no further therapy
    (B) radiation therapy
    (C) hormonal therapy
    (D) single-agent chemotherapy
    (E) multiple-agent chemotherapy

16. This patient underwent postoperative radiation. During radiation therapy she develops nausea, anorexia, diarrhea, and mild abdominal pain. Which of the following is the most likely diagnosis?

    (A) radiation cystitis
    (B) radiation enteritis
    (C) radiation proctitis
    (D) enterovaginal fistula
    (E) vaginal ulceration

17. A pulmonary nodule is discovered on the chest radiogram of a healthy 82-year-old woman. Four years ago, she was treated for endometrial adenocarcinoma. Excision of the nodule shows moderately differentiated endometrial adenocarcinoma-containing progesterone receptors. There is no other evidence of metastatic disease. What should you advise this patient?

    (A) exploratory laparotomy
    (B) lobectomy
    (C) radiation therapy
    (D) brachytherapy
    (E) progestin therapy

18. A 52-year-old patient undergoes a hysterectomy for a rapidly growing uterine mass. At surgery the frozen biopsy is reported as a sarcoma. What is the most common uterine sarcoma?

    (A) leiomyosarcoma
    (B) endometrial stromal sarcoma
    (C) endolymphatic stromal myosis
    (D) malignant mixed müllerian tumor
    (E) lymphoma

19. A 55-year-old woman undergoes a total abdominal hysterectomy and bilateral salpingo-oophorectomy for a rapidly enlarging pelvic mass. A frozen section is sent, although the pathologist tells you he cannot distinguish leiomyosarcomas very well on frozen section. Nonetheless, the specimen looks very suspicious. You still have her abdomen open in the operating room. Which of the following statements describes the optimal next step in the evaluation and management for this patient?

    (A) Radical parametrectomy should be performed.
    (B) Lymphadenectomy should be performed.
    (C) Radiation to the pelvis has no effect on pelvic recurrence of sarcoma.
    (D) There are no additional benefits from intraoperative radiation, radical surgery, or optimal cytoreduction.
    (E) Intraperitoneal radioactive phosphorus ($^{32}$P) should be considered for treatment.

20. A 40-year-old woman is found on pelvic examination to have an enlarged uterus. Ultrasound reveals a well-circumscribed intramural mass consistent with the leiomyoma. The patient asks: what is the incidence of sarcomatous degeneration in a uterine leiomyoma?

    (A) <1%
    (B) 3%
    (C) 10%
    (D) 15%
    (E) 30%

21. Which of the following is a factor predisposing to the development of malignant mixed müllerian tumors?

    (A) prenatal exposure to diethylstilbestrol (DES)
    (B) exposure to mumps virus
    (C) family history of ovarian cancer
    (D) previous pelvic irradiation
    (E) perineal use of talc

22. A 38-year-old nulliparous woman presents requesting a bilateral salpingo-oophorectomy. Her mother died of ovarian cancer at the age 64, and her sister at the age 48. There is no family history of other cancers. You advise her that her risk of developing ovarian cancer is what percentage?

    (A) 1–2%
    (B) 7%
    (C) 20%
    (D) 30–40%
    (E) >50%

23. The same patient gets on the Internet and returns asking about the hereditary types of epithelial ovarian cancer. Which of the following statements is true?

    (A) A site-specific defect transmitting the trait for only ovarian carcinoma is common.
    (B) A *BRCA1* gene mutation increases her lifetime risk of ovarian cancer to 10%.
    (C) Lynch type II cancer syndrome includes ovarian malignancy.
    (D) Fifty percent of ovarian cancer is hereditary.
    (E) A *BRCA2* mutation increases the risk of ovarian cancer by 70%.

24. A 56-year-old healthy woman develops vague complaints and presents to her primary care physician. Which of the following accurately describes symptoms that could be associated with a diagnosis of ovarian cancer?

    (A) there are no identifiable symptoms in women with ovarian cancer
    (B) symptoms are usually present for years prior to a diagnosis
    (C) shortness of breath and cough
    (D) diarrhea
    (E) urinary urgency and bloating

25. Which of the following is a cornerstone for detection of ovarian neoplasia?

    (A) CA-125
    (B) human chorionic gonadotropin (hCG)
    (C) pelvic examination
    (D) pelvic ultrasound
    (E) alpha-fetoprotein

26. Ovarian neoplasms most commonly arise from which of the following cell lines?

    (A) ovarian epithelium
    (B) ovarian stroma
    (C) ovarian germ cells
    (D) ovarian sex cords
    (E) metastatic disease

27. Which of the following postmenopausal women is most protected from ovarian epithelial carcinoma?

    (A) a married woman using perineal talc powder
    (B) an unmarried woman with a history of breast cancer
    (C) a nun with a history of late menopause
    (D) a nulliparous woman with a history of regular menses
    (E) a multiparous woman who used OCPs and now postmenopausal

28. Which of the following statements accurately reflects the natural history of ovarian epithelial carcinoma?

   (A) The incidence of ovarian carcinoma increases with age until the seventh decade of life.

   (B) Elderly women are less likely than younger women to have disease diagnosed at an advanced stage.

   (C) Most women with ovarian cancer do not have any symptoms prior to dissemination of disease.

   (D) Seventy-five percent of all ovarian tumors in women older than 50 years are malignant.

   (E) Twenty-five percent of all ovarian tumors in women between 20 and 40 years of age are malignant.

**Questions 29 and 30 apply to the following patient:**

A 35-year-old woman desiring fertility undergoes exploratory laparotomy for a 12-cm pelvic mass. At surgery, a large, lobulated, right ovarian mass is observed. It has a smooth external capsule and a bluish-gray appearance. The uterus, fallopian tubes, and left ovary appear normal. Abdominal exploration is negative for metastatic disease. A right salpingo-oophorectomy is performed. The tumor is opened intraoperatively and found to be divided by septa into lobules. Frozen section of the tumor shows a mucinous cystadenoma of low malignant potential.

29. One would base the remainder of the surgical intervention at this time on which of the following statements regarding mucinous cystadenoma of low malignant potential?

   (A) Spread of the tumor outside the ovary occurs 30–40% of the time in the form of intraperitoneal growth of mucin-producing cells.

   (B) It has 1–2% incidence of bilaterality.

   (C) It has a 5-year survival rate of 60%.

   (D) It typically occurs in postmenopausal women.

   (E) It comprises atypical epithelial proliferation without stromal invasion.

30. Two days after surgery, you receive the pathology report of the ovarian tumor. It is a mucinous cystadenoma of low malignant potential mixed with well-differentiated carcinoma. The tumor has not invaded the ovarian capsule, lymphatics, or mesovarium. Omental and retroperitoneal lymph node biopsies and peritoneal washings are negative for tumor cells. How do you advise this patient?

   (A) biopsy of the contralateral ovary

   (B) removal of the uterus and contralateral adnexum

   (C) postoperative chemotherapy

   (D) postoperative radiation therapy

   (E) no further therapy

31. A 54-year-old healthy woman comes for an annual examination. Her last menstrual period (LMP) was 4 years ago. The physical examination is normal. Pelvic examination shows vaginal atrophy and a small, mobile uterus. The right ovary is 2.5 × 4.5 cm in diameter. The left ovary is nonpalpable. Vaginal ultrasonography shows that the right ovary is similar in size to that of a premenopausal ovary. What should you advise this patient?

   (A) The ovaries of a postmenopausal woman are usually palpable.

   (B) The right ovary of a postmenopausal woman is usually palpable by right-handed examiners.

   (C) A palpable ovary in a postmenopausal woman is suspicious for malignancy.

   (D) The right ovary is still producing significant amounts of estrogen.

   (E) The vaginal ultrasound is an unnecessary diagnostic test.

**Questions 32 through 41 apply to the following patient:**

A 65-year-old woman has abdominal distention of 3 months' duration. Abdominal percussion causes a wavelike movement of fluid around a central tympanitic area. Pelvic examination shows a right adnexal mass. It is 8 cm in size, nodular, and fixed in the pelvis. The left ovary is nonpalpable. Blood chemistries, urinalysis, cervical Pap smear, mammography, and chest X-ray are normal. Stool guaiac examination and gastrointestinal studies are also normal. A serum CA-125 level is 250 U/mL (normal, <35 U/mL).

32. Which of the following statements reflects CA-125?

    (A) It is a circulating antigenic marker for germ cell ovarian carcinoma.

    (B) It is found in normal fetal and adult ovaries.

    (C) It is secreted by mesothelial cells of the pleura, pericardium, and peritoneum.

    (D) It is not useful in monitoring tumor progression.

    (E) It is never elevated in the sera of women with benign diseases.

33. Which of the following is the most likely diagnosis?

    (A) gonadoblastoma

    (B) Meigs' syndrome

    (C) Krukenberg's tumors

    (D) serous cystadenocarcinoma

    (E) endodermal sinus tumor

34. Her surgical treatment should do which of the following?

    (A) remove all gross disease if the risk of fatal complications is minimal

    (B) avoid resection of bowel

    (C) be done through a Pfannenstiel incision

    (D) be done laparoscopically

    (E) be done without a bowel preparation

35. Exploratory laparotomy shows a tumor involving the right ovary. The left ovary appears normal. Several tumor implants are present on the peritoneal surfaces of small bowel and omentum. Biopsies of the peritoneal implants and ovarian tumor show moderately differentiated serous cystadenocarcinoma. There are no distant metastases, and the liver appears normal (see Figure 22–2). What is the initial intraoperative assessment of stage of the tumor?

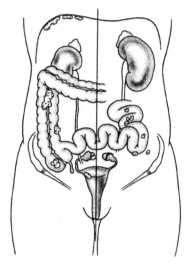

**Figure 22–2.**

    (A) 0

    (B) I

    (C) II

    (D) III

    (E) IV

36. The primary tumor and all metastases are surgically removed. You meet with the patient postoperatively to discuss her prognosis. How do you advise this patient?

    (A) The 5-year survival rate with no postoperative chemotherapy is approximately 70%.
    (B) The response to chemotherapy is related to the amount of residual disease after surgery.
    (C) Older patients achieve results from postoperative chemotherapy superior to those of younger patients.
    (D) A second-look operation is performed in patients with incomplete response to chemotherapy.
    (E) Few women thought to be free of disease after therapy have disease present at second-look operation.

37. You are called to the operating room by the general surgeons at a local children's hospital. A 4-year-old girl with acute abdominal pain was thought to have appendicitis; instead, she has a large right ovary. What is the most likely diagnosis?

    (A) germ cell tumor
    (B) epithelial stromal tumor
    (C) sex cord–stromal tumor
    (D) nonneoplastic follicle or theca lutein cyst
    (E) metastatic tumor

38. An 18-year-old woman with a history of pelvic inflammatory disease (PID) undergoes a laparoscopic ovarian cystectomy for a 5-cm ovarian mass containing a tooth. The contents of the cyst spill during removal and contain thick sebaceous material and hair. Copious irrigation was used to remove this material. She is noted to have marked bowel adhesions in the pelvis, which require dissection to reach the ovarian cyst. Four days postoperatively she returns to the emergency department with a temperature of 101.1°F, abdominal pain, nausea, and vomiting. White blood cell (WBC) count is 15.0. What is the most likely diagnosis?

    (A) ileus
    (B) narcotic-induced constipation
    (C) chemical peritonitis
    (D) influenza
    (E) bowel perforation

39. An 11-year-old girl presents with abdominal pain, and a right 5-cm solid ovarian mass is found. The alpha-fetoprotein level is elevated. In which of the following ways should you counsel the girl and parents?

    (A) Seventy percent of cases are stage I.
    (B) The tumor is common and accounts for half of all germ cell tumors.
    (C) Bilateral salpingo-oophorectomy is indicated since bilateral tumors are common.
    (D) No surgery is indicated until after puberty.
    (E) If the tumor is stage I, no further therapy is needed.

40. A 10-year-old girl presents with abdominal pain. During the emergency department workup, an adnexal mass is found. You suspect a germ cell tumor. In preoperative discussion, her parents are told that the most common germ cell tumor is which of the following?

    (A) dysgerminoma
    (B) endodermal sinus tumor
    (C) embryonal carcinoma
    (D) choriocarcinoma
    (E) mature teratoma

41. A 19-year-old woman with an ovarian mass is thought to have a dermoid or teratoma based on ultrasound findings and gross examination at removal by laparoscopy. At her postoperative visit the pathology returns with the finding of an immature teratoma. Which of the following statements reflects current knowledge about immature teratomas?

    (A) They are the most common malignant germ cell tumor.
    (B) They are commonly bilateral.
    (C) They produce alpha-fetoprotein.

(D) They commonly occur during the first two decades of life.

(E) They contain malignant squamous cell elements.

**Questions 42 and 43 apply to the following patient:**

A 26-year-old nulliparous woman is seen in the emergency department for acute abdominal pain. Her vital signs are blood pressure, 90/50 mm Hg; pulse, 120 bpm; and temperature, afebrile. Abdominal examination shows right lower quadrant tenderness with rebound. Pelvic examination demonstrates a painful 10-cm right adnexal mass. A serum pregnancy test is negative. A hematocrit is 24% (normal, 35–45%). Exploratory laparotomy confirms a hemoperitoneum. A smooth right ovarian tumor is bleeding from its ruptured capsule. Inspection of the uterus, fallopian tubes, and left ovary is normal. A right salpingo-oophorectomy is performed. Frozen section of the tumor shows primitive germ cells with intervening connective tissue infiltrated by lymphocytes.

42. The tumor is most likely which of the following?

(A) dysgerminoma

(B) endodermal sinus tumor

(C) choriocarcinoma

(D) embryonal carcinoma

(E) mature teratoma

43. Which of the following statements reflects current understanding about the above tumor?

(A) It occurs in women of all ages with equal frequency.

(B) It has a bilaterality rate of less than 1%.

(C) It is usually resistant to radiotherapy.

(D) It can occur in combination with other germ cell elements.

(E) It has a poor survival rate following unilateral adnexectomy for stage I disease.

**Questions 44 and 45 apply to the following patient:**

An 18-year-old woman with primary amenorrhea complains of a right inguinal mass. Physical examination demonstrates a normal-appearing female. Bilateral breast development is present. Axillary and pubic hair are sparse. The vulva appears normal, but the vagina ends in a blind pouch. The uterus is nonpalpable by rectal examination.

44. The right inguinal mass is most likely which of the following?

(A) lymph node

(B) gonad

(C) endometrioma

(D) cyst of Nuck's canal

(E) inguinal hernia

45. Which of the following tumors is most likely to occur in the right inguinal mass?

(A) endodermal sinus tumor

(B) dysgerminoma

(C) choriocarcinoma

(D) gonadoblastoma

(E) Sertoli–Leydig cell tumor

46. Malignant changes occur in what percentage of streak ovaries when a Y chromosome is present?

(A) 5

(B) 25

(C) 45

(D) 65

(E) 85

47. A 5-year-old girl experiences early breast development. She is taller than her peers. Her mother has noticed blood at the girl's introitus. Serum gonadotropin levels are low and are unchanged after intravenous administration of gonadotropin-releasing hormone (GnRH). Which of the following is the most likely diagnosis?

(A) Sertoli–Leydig cell tumor

(B) granulosa cell tumor

(C) hilar cell tumor

(D) lipid tumor

(E) fibroma

**48.** A 48-year-old woman is taken to surgery for a solid pelvic mass of 6×7 cm and marked ascites. At laparotomy the adnexa is removed and sent for frozen section examination. The report returns as metastic adenocarcinoma to the ovary. Although uncommon, metastatic tumors to the ovary most often originate from which of the following?

(A) breast

(B) stomach

(C) large intestine

(D) uterus

(E) vagina

**49.** A hormonally active neoplasm is likely to cause clinical signs through the hormonal effect that would prompt earlier evaluation and hence diagnosis. Which one of the following tumors is likely to be found primarily based on physical size and location of the neoplasm?

(A) Sertoli–Leydig cell tumor

(B) granulosa cell tumor

(C) hilar cell tumor

(D) fibroma

(E) thecoma

**Questions 50 and 51 apply to the following patient:**

An 18-year-old G1P0 patient presents with vaginal bleeding at 10 weeks estimated gestational age. She has not received any prenatal care. You find the uterine size more consistent with 12–14 weeks and no fetal heart tones are found. Ultrasound is consistent with a molar pregnancy.

**50.** Which of the following accurately reflects current knowledge regarding gestational trophoblastic disease?

(A) occurs in 1 per 10,000 pregnancies

(B) high incidence of malignant sequelae after primary treatment for partial mole

(C) correlates with lower than expected serum hCG levels

(D) treatment is primarily with D&C, alone

(E) fetal tissue found in presence of complete mole

**51.** Pathology returns as choriocarcinoma. During counseling of the patient regarding the disease, treatment and prognosis, which of the following statements is accurate?

(A) It is generally effectively treated only with surgery.

(B) Chemotherapy has allowed a salvage rate for this disease of approximately 25%.

(C) Up to 90% of patients with choriocarcinoma can achieve a normal life expectancy.

(D) Choriocarcinoma is 100% curable in all cases with combination chemotherapy.

(E) Occurs in approximately 1 per 10,000 pregnancies.

**52.** Tumors grow exponentially due to which of the following?

(A) rapid proliferation

(B) gompertzian growth

(C) rapid doubling time

(D) disruption in the regulation of programmed cell death (apoptosis)

(E) lack of regulatory proteins to control cell growth

**53.** Which of the following does the stem cell theory state?

(A) All malignant changes begin in the primitive cells of the hematopoietic system.

(B) Malignancies are actually formed at the time of embryonic development and lie dormant until activated.

(C) Any cell has the capability to become malignant under the influence of releaser cells called "stems."

(D) Only certain undifferentiated cells (stem cells) are able to divide to reproduce a tissue.

(E) Malignancy results from a disruption of a major organ system—by background radiation, constant irritation, or other mechanism.

54. As a general rule, drugs used in multiagent chemotherapeutic regimens should be which of the following?

   (A) effective as individual agents if they are to be effective together
   (B) less effective than large-dose single agents, but also less toxic
   (C) used in smaller doses to prevent tumor resistance
   (D) most effective on slow-growing tumors
   (E) be in the same class of agents (i.e., all alkylating agents)

55. A 43-year-old woman has stage III epithelial ovarian carcinoma. She had surgical debulking and has received five courses of carboplatin and paclitaxel. She is now due for her sixth course. She comes to clinic complaining of fatigue and myalgias. She has a temperature of 101.3°F. On examination, you find no obvious source of the fever. WBC count is $1,000/mm^3$ (normal 4,500 to $11,000/mm^3$). Your next course of action is to do which of the following?

   (A) send home and instruct to check temperature twice a day
   (B) give a broad-spectrum antibiotic as outpatient
   (C) admit to hospital and observe
   (D) admit to hospital and start antibiotics
   (E) admit to hospital and give sixth course of chemotherapy

**DIRECTIONS (Questions 56 through 71): The following groups of questions are preceded by a list of lettered options. For each question, select the one lettered option that is most closely associated with it. Each lettered option may be used once, multiple times, or not at all.**

**Questions 56 and 57**

Match the single best therapy for the case described.

   (A) danazol
   (B) progestin
   (C) clomiphene citrate
   (D) hysterectomy
   (E) radical hysterectomy

   (F) radiation
   (G) no further treatment

56. A 37-year-old woman has a D&C for irregular bleeding. The pathology shows simple hyperplasia without atypia.

57. A 48-year-old nulliparous woman has a 20-year history of oligomenorrhea and hirsutism. She recently had an episode of menorrhagia. Office endometrial biopsy shows complex hyperplasia with severe atypia.

**Questions 58 through 60**

Match the rate of progression to endometrial cancer from the hyperplasia type.

   (A) 1%
   (B) 4%
   (C) 10–19%
   (D) 20–29%
   (E) 30–49%

58. Complex hyperplasia

59. A complex atypical hyperplasia

60. Simple hyperplasia without atypia

**Questions 61 through 63**

   (A) serous tumor
   (B) mucinous tumor
   (C) endometrioid tumor
   (D) clear cell tumor
   (E) Brenner tumor

61. The ovarian epithelial neoplasm with the lowest malignancy rate

62. The ovarian epithelial neoplasm with the highest rate of bilaterality

63. The ovarian epithelial neoplasm similar in histologic appearance to primary tubal carcinoma

**Questions 64 and 65**

  (A)  radiation therapy
  (B)  chemotherapy
  (C)  both of the above
  (D)  neither of the above

Which of the above therapies for ovarian cancer increases the risk of the following?

**64.**  Bone marrow suppression

**65.**  Bowel obstruction

**Questions 66 through 71**

  (A)  dysgerminoma
  (B)  endodermal sinus tumor
  (C)  choriocarcinoma
  (D)  mature teratoma
  (E)  struma ovarii
  (F)  carcinoid
  (G)  granulose
  (H)  gonadoblastoma

Which of the above germ cell tumors is most likely to produce large amounts of the following?

**66.**  Thyroxine

**67.**  Alpha-fetoprotein

**68.**  hCG

**69.**  lactate dehydrogenase (LDH)

**70.**  inhibin

**71.**  androgens

# Answers and Explanations

1. **(B)** D&C has been the traditional method used to diagnose abnormalities of the endometrial lining. Dilation refers to opening of the cervix with a series of dilators to gain access to the intrauterine cavity; curettage refers to scraping of the uterine lining to obtain endometrial tissue. Unfortunately, pain accompanying cervical dilation usually requires that D&C be performed with paracervical or general anesthesia. D&C has been replaced by endometrial biopsy techniques performed as an office procedure. Endometrial biopsy has approximately 90% accuracy in detecting endometrial hyperplasia and cancer. Techniques that obtain endometrial tissue are more accurate than those relying on endometrial cytology. Careful sampling of the intrauterine cavity by some method is mandatory, since some women with the histologic diagnosis of adenomatous hyperplasia have coexisting endometrial carcinoma. When an endometrial biopsy cannot be completed for technical reasons, a fractional D&C must be performed. Hysteroscopy is usually done at the same time as D&C to visualize and remove pathologic findings such as polyps or submucous fibroids. Transvaginal sonography is currently used in the evaluation of abnormal bleeding. When combined with injecting saline into the uterine cavity via the cervix (sonohysterography), abnormalities in the endometrial cavity such as submucous fibroids or polyps can be identified. However, no tissue is obtained for pathologic diagnosis. Also, an endocrinopathy causing anovulation is the most likely reason for the patient's irregular vaginal bleeding. Endometrial biopsy might prove this if prolifera-tive endometrium is seen in the luteal phase of the menstrual cycle.

2. **(B)** The most frequent symptom of endometrial hyperplasia is abnormal vaginal bleeding. Fortunately, this usually occurs early and allows early detection of the dysplastic changes often prior to actual cancer.

3. **(C)** Oral contraceptives used for at least 1 year confer up to a 30% to 50% risk reduction for hyperplasia and carcinoma of the endometrium. In obese women, there is an overproduction of endogenous estrogen and oligoovulation. Without concurrent increases in progesterone, there is estrogenic stimulation of the endometrium. Similarly, unopposed exogenous estrogen is also a risk factor. Hormone replacement therapy should therefore include a progestin for endometrial protection. Tamoxifen, a selective estrogen-receptor modulator is proliferative or estrogenic on the endometrium. Women on tamoxifen have a 2- to 3-fold higher risk of endometrial hyperplasia and cancer. Both early menarche and late menopause increase lifelong exposure to endogenous estrogens.

4. **(C)** Endometrial hyperplasia causes the endometrium to thicken and acquire a velvety, lobulated texture with a yellowish appearance. Dilation of endometrial glands often occurs in a hyperplastic endometrium and is referred to as cystic hyperplasia or simple hyperplasia. It is considered weakly premalignant because it progresses to endometrial carcinoma in approximately 1% of women. This may regress in some

women but this patient has abnormal uterine bleeding as well. Therefore, progestin therapy is indicated and will usually correct the hyperplasia and the irregular vaginal bleeding. Treatment with estrogen is contraindicated. Hysterectomy is always an option but should be considered after medication with progestins.

**TABLE 22–1.  Classifications of Endometrial Hyperplasias**

| Traditional | International Society of Gynecologic Pathologists |
|---|---|
| Cystic hyperplasia | Simple hyperplasia |
| Adenomatous hyperplasia | Complex hyperplasia (adenomatous hyperplasia without cytologic atypia) |
| Atypical adenomatous hyperplasia | Atypical hyperplasia adenomatous hyperplasia with cytologic atypia) |
| Architectural atypia (mild, moderate, severe) | |
| Cytologic atypia (mild, moderate, severe) | |

5.  **(C)** Endometrial polyps arise as fingerlike endometrial projections and commonly occur under conditions of unopposed estrogen stimulation. They may be small in size (1 to 2 mm) or large enough to protrude through the cervix. Although frequently asymptomatic, abnormal bleeding is the most common symptom of an endometrial polyp. Pelvic pain may also occur if extrusion of the polyp through the cervix causes cervical dilation. Their histologic pattern consists of glandular and stromal elements and a central vascular channel surrounded on three sides by epithelium. Two-thirds of endometrial polyps contain immature endometrium unresponsive to progesterone, occasionally associated with cystic hyperplasia. Endometrial polyps originate from functional endometrium undergoing cyclic histologic changes. Less than 1% of endometrial polyps are malignant. Malignant transformation develops in 1% to 2% of polyps. Several endometrial polyps can occur together and may not be removed entirely by using forceps at the time of D&C. Endometrial polyps frequently coexist with other endometrial pathology. It is important to separately examine polyps and endometrial lining to determine the source of irregular vaginal bleeding.

6.  **(A)** An endometrial stripe of less than 5 mm in a postmenopausal woman confers minimal risk of cancer. It is reasonable not to proceed with other evaluation (supported by ACOG and Society of Radiologists in Ultrasound). A stripe of more than 10 mm correlates with a 10% to 20% risk of hyperplasia or cancer. The data on endometrial stripe thickness for premenopausal women are more difficult to interpret, but it appears that less than 12 mm confers little risk of cancer. A hysterectomy is not appropriate until a tissue diagnosis is obtained.

7.  **(B)** The mass the internist describes is likely to be a polyp. It could be endocervical or endometrial in origin, and the latter type can prolapse through the cervix. Adenomatous polyps may antedate endometrial hyperplasia, and abnormalities range from benign polyps to frank adenocarcinoma. The appropriate therapy is to remove the mass for pathologic evaluation. This can be done simply without performing a cone biopsy. Even with a negative Pap smear, the mass should be removed.

8.  **(B)** Progestins oppose estrogen action in endometrial tissue by decreasing the number of estrogen receptors and changing the lining to a secretory endometrium. Progesterone receptors are high in late proliferative and early secretory phases but even higher in endometrial hyperplastic states. The regression of endometrial hyperplasia often occurs within 3 months. There are some reports of the disease being successfully controlled for more than 3 years, even after only 6 weeks of therapy. However, if an endocrinopathy (such as polycystic ovarian disease), obesity, estrogen-producing tumor, or other factor contributing to chronic endometrial exposure to estrogen still exists, the disease is likely to recur. Therapy with progestins can be continued for a long term.

9.  **(E)** A neoplasm is defined as an abnormal tissue growth that persists and grows independently of its surrounding structures. The most common uterine neoplasms are benign leiomyomas. Myomas are clinically apparent in approximately 25% of reproductive-age women. This number may be up to 80% when using ultrasound or other imaging and histologic data from hysterectomies. Adenomyosis is diagnosed on the basis of histologic findings after hysterectomy and

the reported incidence ranges from 20% to 60%. One in approximately 40 women will develop endometrial adenocarcinoma during her lifetime. In the United States in 2009, the American Cancer Society (ACS) estimated that there would be 42,160 new cases of uterus cancer, most arising from the endometrial lining. Sarcomas account for less than 5% of uterine cancers. Choriocarcinoma in association with a pregnancy is rare.

10. **(D)** Breast cancer is the leading gynecologic cause of cancer death. It is also the primary cause of all deaths in women 40 to 44 years old. Approximately one in eight (12%) American women develops breast carcinoma during her lifetime. For 2010, the ACS estimated that 207,090 women would be diagnosed with breast and that 39,840 women would die from that condition in the same year. Endometrial carcinoma is the next most common gynecologic cancer, with 43,470 new cases estimated for 2010 and 7,950 deaths. Ovarian cancer would affect 21,880 women in 2010 with 13,850 deaths. Cervical cancer was estimated to affect 12,200 women, with 4,210 deaths. Vulvar cancer was estimated to affect 3,900 women and 920 women would die from this disease in 2010. So although endometrial cancer is more common, only 2% of women die from it. Breast cancer is very common with approximately 20% of patients dying. Although 65% or more of women with ovarian cancer die from their disease, it is fortunately less common.

11. **(A)** A chest radiograph (CXR) should be performed because the lung is the main site of extrauterine spread from endometrial carcinoma (36% of cases). CXR is the only required preoperative imaging study. Additional imaging is not necessary, however; MRI or CT may aid in surgical planning. Endometrial cancer is surgically staged.

12. **(C)** Adenocarcinoma of the endometrium with extension to the cervix is a stage II lesion (Table 22–2).

13. **(A)** Seventy to seventy-five percent of endometrial cancers are diagnosed as stage I disease. Ten to fifteen percent of endometrial cancers are stage II at the time of diagnosis, while the re-

**TABLE 22–2. Corpus Cancer Staging**

| Stage | Characteristic |
| --- | --- |
| IA | Tumor limited to endometrium |
| IB | Invasion to <1/2 myometrium |
| IC | Invasion to ≥1/2 myometrium |
| IIA | Endocervical glandular involvement only |
| IIB | Cervical stromal invasion |
| IIIA | Tumor invades serosa and/or adnexae, and/or positive peritoneal cytology |
| IIIB | Vaginal metastases |
| IIIC | Metastases to pelvic and/or para-aortic lymph nodes |
| IVA | Tumor invasion of bladder and/or bowel mucosa |
| IVB | Distant metastases including intra-abdominal and/or inguinal lymph node |

Source: Adopted from International Federation of Gynecology and Obstetrics (FIGO), 1987.

maining 10% to 15% are stages III and IV. The ability of women to seek medical advice at the onset of abnormal vaginal bleeding probably accounts for the early detection of disease.

14. **(E)** In women with stage I and II disease, exploratory laparotomy with total (not radical) abdominal hysterectomy, bilateral salpingo-oophorectomy, and pelvic and para-aortic lymphadenectomy treats early disease and determines extent of disease spread for planning of postoperative therapy. Peritoneal washings for malignant cells are obtained on entering the abdomen. The uterus is opened in the operating room and examined for evidence of tumor invasion into the myometrium. Bilateral salpingo-oophorectomy should be performed as 6% to 10% of patients with clinical stage I disease will have metastasis to the adnexa.

15. **(B)** Treatment of early endometrial cancer depends on prognostic factors, pattern of disease spread, and probability of metastatic disease. The presence of extrauterine disease (nodal and/or adnexal metastases, malignant cells in peritoneal cytology) is associated with a high rate of disease recurrence. Generally, women with stage IA, grade 1 or 2 lesions are adequately treated with surgery alone since the risk of metastatic disease is low (4%). However, patients with stage I disease and poor prognostic factors (e.g., poorly differentiated tumor, tumor invasion beyond the inner half of the myometrium, nodal and/or adnexal metastases, and malignant peritoneal cytology) and women

with stage II disease involving the cervical stroma benefit from postoperative radiation therapy. This patient has stage IC disease. Radiotherapy may be:

- External irradiation (external beam pelvic radiation): Reduces the risk of recurrent disease at the vaginal vault and pelvic wall. The radiation field may be extended to the para-aortic region in patients with nodal metastasis in this area.
- Brachytherapy (a form of radiation therapy in which the radioactive source is placed in proximity to tumor): Reduces the risk of recurrent disease at the vaginal vault but not the pelvic wall. A common form of brachytherapy used in the treatment of endometrial cancer is intravaginal irradiation (radium, cesium, or cobalt).

16. **(B)** Early and late complications from radiation therapy occur. Acute reactions, including cessation of mitotic activity and tissue edema with or without necrosis, may be associated with cystitis (hematuria, urgency, frequency), proctosigmoiditis (tenesmus, diarrhea, hematochezia), enteritis (nausea, vomiting, diarrhea, abdominal pain), and bone marrow suppression. Chronic reactions to radiation, occurring 6 to 24 months after completion of radiation, include obliteration of small blood vessels, fibrosis, and reduced number of epithelial and parenchymal cells. Chronic reactions may be associated with enteropathy (proctosigmoiditis, ulceration, fistula, stenosis), vaginal vault necrosis and/or stenosis, and urologic injuries (cystitis, vesicovaginal fistula, uterovaginal fistula, ureteric stenosis).

17. **(E)** Ninety percent of recurrences of endometrial adenocarcinoma occur within 5 years of the initial diagnosis. Half of the recurrences occur in the pelvis and vagina, while the most frequent sites of nonpelvic metastases are lung (17%), upper abdomen (10%), and bone (6%). One-third of recurrent endometrial cancers have sex steroid receptors. High-dose oral progestin therapy (i.e., medroxyprogesterone acetate and megestrol acetate) with or without chemotherapy is often effective in controlling advanced or recurrent disease-containing progesterone receptors (15% to 30% response rate for progestins alone). The use of progestin combined with tamoxifen, an antiestrogen, in these women is controversial but attractive since tamoxifen increases the progesterone receptor content of some tumors. Tumors without sex steroid receptors are usually treated with cytotoxic agents since their response to hormone therapy is poor. Some chemotherapeutic agents used singly and in combination for treatment of endometrial cancer include doxorubicin and cisplatin. These are the most active agents. Other agents that might be used include paclitaxel and ifosfamide.

18. **(D)** Uterine sarcomas consist of malignant mesenchymal (sarcomatous) components arising from endometrial stroma, myometrium, or uterine connective tissue. They comprise fewer than 5% of uterine cancers and are classified according to whether the sarcomatous element resembles tissue indigenous (homologous) or foreign (heterologous) to the uterus and exists alone (pure) or admixed with malignant epithelial (carcinomatous) tissue (Table 22–3). The most common sarcoma is the malignant mixed Müllerian tumor (up to 43%), followed by leiomyosarcoma (up to 33%).

**TABLE 22–3. Classification of Uterine Sarcoma**

 I. Pure sarcoma
   A. Homologous
      1. Leiomyosarcoma
      2. Endometrial stromal sarcoma
         a. Low-grade: endolymphatic stromal myosis
         b. High-grade: endometrial stromal sarcoma
   B. Heterologous
      1. Rhabdomyosarcoma
      2. Chondrosarcoma
      3. Osteosarcoma
      4. Liposarcoma
 II. Malignant mixed müllerian tumors
   A. Homologous (carcinosarcoma): carcinoma + homologous sarcoma
   B. Heterologous: carcinoma + heterologous sarcoma
 III. Other sarcomas

19. **(D)** Radical hysterectomy and lymphadenectomy are not indicated. Although the presence of involved lymph nodes may be of prognostic significance, lymphadenectomy is not therapeutic, since outcomes are similar for similarly

staged patients who did and did not undergo lymphadenectomy. Lymphadenectomy should be reserved for only patients with clinically suspicious nodes. Adjuvant radiation therapy probably improves local control, but its impact on survival is unclear; there is no role for intraoperative radiation. Leiomyosarcoma does tend to spread locally and hematogenously and chemotherapy offers fair results. In leiomyosarcoma, doxorubicin has significant activity with a response rate of approximately 25%.

20. **(A)** The incidence of sarcomatous degeneration in a uterine leiomyoma is less than 1%. The tumors usually originate from uterine myometrium but occasionally develop from preexisting leiomyomas. An important microscopic criterion for distinguishing leiomyosarcoma from leiomyoma is the number of mitoses present in tumor tissue (mitotic index):

    - Greater than 10 mitoses per 10 high-power fields (hpf) is associated with frank malignancy (leiomyosarcoma).
    - Between 5 and 10 mitoses per 10 hpf may be associated with malignant behavior, especially if atypia is seen.
    - Less than 5 mitoses per 10 hpf and no atypia is associated with benign behavior (leiomyoma).

21. **(D)** Malignant mixed müllerian tumors develop from menopause (median age of patients, 62 years) as large, soft, polypoid masses filling the uterine cavity. One-third of women with this disease have a history of pelvic irradiation for benign disease or cervical cancer. These tumors are derived from totipotential endometrial stromal cells that have the capacity for epithelial and stromal differentiation. They contain carcinomatous epithelial (glandular) elements and sarcomatous tissue resembling normal uterine mesenchyme (homologous or carcinosarcoma) or tissue foreign to the uterus (heterologous), such as cartilage bone or striated muscle. Malignant mixed müllerian tumors have a poor prognosis, since up to 50% of patients have metastatic disease at the time of diagnosis.

22. **(B)** Her risk with two first-degree relatives having ovarian cancer is 7%. For a single affected first-degree relative, the risk is 4% to

5%. Given the poor prognosis with treatment of advanced ovarian cancer and no workable screening for early detection of disease, it is not unreasonable to consider bilateral salpingo-oophorectomy. This can usually be accomplished via laparoscopy. However, if she desires childbearing, she may wish to delay surgical therapy until her family is complete. The use of OCPs or other combined hormonal contraceptive that prevents ovulation may provider some protection.

23. **(C)** Lynch type II hereditary cancer syndrome includes nonpolyposis colorectal cancer and endometrial, ovarian, and other gastrointestinal and genitourinary malignancies. Genetic abnormalities account for apprivimately 10% of ovarian cancers. If she had known mutations of *BRCA1* or *BRCA2*, her risk would be even greater. The lifetime risk for developing ovarian cancer with *BRCA1* is 20% to 45% and for *BRCA2* is 10% to 20%, as compared to the general population lifetime risk of 1.3%.

24. **(E)** Unlike previously thought, ovarian cancer may indeed produce symptoms. Goff et al. (2004) demonstrated in a prospective case–control study that women with both early and advanced ovarian cancers often have multiple and recurring symptoms prior to the diagnosis. These symptoms include pain (abdominal, pelvic, back), bloating, constipation, difficulty eating, fatigue, urinary urgency, increasing abdominal girth. No longer is this cancer considered as a "silent killer." Symptoms generally occur often in the several months, not years, before a diagnosis is made. Unfortunately these are often vague enough to be dismissed by the patient and the provider as indigestion, dietary indiscretions, menopausal complaints, or depression.

25. **(C)** Most women with ovarian carcinoma have a palpable abdominal or pelvic mass. The pelvic examination remains the cornerstone for detection of ovarian neoplasia. The presence of a fixed, irregular, adnexal mass with cul-de-sac nodularity should be considered an ovarian carcinoma until proven otherwise. Unfortunately, no good screening test exists. The US Preventive Services Task Force has graded the routine

screening of ovarian cancer with a "D" ranking, which is defined as fair evidence to recommend its exclusion in a periodic health examination. Screening ultrasound and CA-125 should be reserved for women in clinical trials or those with *BRCA1* or *BRCA2* abnormalities. CA-125 is not a specific marker for ovarian cancer.

26. **(A)** The percentage of ovarian neoplasms (benign and malignant) derived from epithelial cells, germ cells, and all other cell types is 65, 25, and 5 to 10, respectively.

27. **(E)** Ovulation appears to play a role in the pathogenesis of epithelial ovarian carcinoma. These tumors rarely develop in other mammals ovulating infrequently but occur commonly in fowl that ovulate regularly. Nulliparous women who are ovulatory and experience late menopause are at increased risk for developing ovarian cancer. OC use, pregnancy, and breast-feeding inhibit ovulation and protect against this disease. There are conflicting reports on other risk factors for developing ovarian cancer. Perineal use of talc powder (allowing an irritant to enter the peritoneal cavity via the reproductive tract), fat intake, and a history of mumps infection before menarche may be risk factors. Obesity and alcohol have also been weakly linked to ovarian cancer. The incidence of ovarian cancer is increased in affluent, industrialized countries such as the United States. Women's Health Initiative (WHI) showed a nonsignificant increase in the risk of ovarian cancer in women who had taken combined hormone replacement therapy. Prior data also support a possible increased risk in women who took estrogen-only therapy. WHI data on that specific issue are still unavailable.

28. **(A)** The incidence of ovarian carcinoma increases with age until the seventh decade of life. The malignancy rate of ovarian tumors in women between the ages of 20 and 40 and older than 50 is 10% and 50%, respectively. Recent data show that patients actually do experience a variety of symptoms, even with early stage ovarian cancer. Symptoms include pelvic or abdominal pain, fatigue, bloating, constipation, and urinary frequency. Elderly women are more likely to have their disease diagnosed at an advanced stage, contributing to a poorer prognosis compared to women with disease who are younger than 65 years.

29. **(E)** Approximately 10% of ovarian epithelial cancers are tumors of low malignant potential. However, they account for up to 20% of all ovarian epithelial tumors. The cells of these tumors do not invade ovarian stroma. Ovarian tumors of low malignant potential tend to occur in reproductive-age women and have an excellent prognosis regardless of stage (5-year survival rate more than 90%), although late recurrences are possible. A conservative surgical approach is advisable for early-stage disease in women desiring fertility. The most common types of "borderline" tumors are serous and mucinous, although other epithelial types also occur. Its external capsule is smoother and has a bluish-gray appearance; its interior is divided by septa into lobules. Each lobule contains clear viscid fluid produced by a single layer of columnar epithelium rich in mucin. The rate of bilaterality varies based on histologic type but ranges from 10% to 50%. Pseudomyxoma peritonei may also result from mucinous tumors of low malignant potential. Careful microscopic examination of these tumors is crucial to assure that invasive elements are not present.

30. **(E)** Gynecologic surgeons recognize that intraoperative analysis of a large borderline tumor may fail to recognize small areas of invasive elements. It is important to conduct a thorough surgical staging to guard against the possibility that a borderline ovarian tumor harbors a malignant component. The standard operation for ovarian epithelial cancer (without gross disease beyond the ovary) is total abdominal hysterectomy, bilateral salpingo-oophorectomy, omentectomy, and complete surgical staging. Patients wishing to preserve fertility may undergo conservative surgery (e.g., unilateral salpingo-oophorectomy) under the following conditions:

- Tumor is confined to the ovary.
- Tumor is well differentiated without invasion of ovarian capsule, lymphatics, or mesovarium.
- Peritoneal washings are negative for tumor cells.

- Close surveillance is possible.
- Patient will consider excision of the contralateral ovary after childbearing is completed.

Biopsy of a normal-appearing contralateral ovary is not done because it is unlikely to uncover tumor and increases the risk of pelvic adhesions leading to infertility.

31. **(C)** The ovaries of reproductive-age women are usually palpable, measuring approximately 1.5 × 2.5 × 4.0 cm in diameter. The postmenopausal ovary is usually nonpalpable because it decreases in size to 2.0 × 1.5 × 0.5 cm. Therefore, a palpable ovary in a woman beyond menopause always warrants diagnostic studies to rule out the possibility of malignancy. Prior to the advent of diagnostic studies (e.g., tumor markers and vaginal ultrasonography), most postmenopausal women with a palpable ovary underwent exploratory laparotomy. It now appears that in postmenopausal women unilocular cysts less than 5 cm in diameter are usually benign. Ovarian masses that are solid, multiloculated, more than 5 cm in diameter, or associated with elevated serum CA-125 levels should be removed. The decision to proceed with surgery depends on the patient's age, operative risk, serum CA-125 levels, and sonographic characteristics of the ovarian mass.

32. **(C)** CA-125 is produced by normal tissue derived from coelomic epithelium, including the epithelial component of the müllerian system, and the mesothelial cells of the pleura, pericardium, and peritoneum. It is not found in normal fetal or adult ovaries. Although it is a circulating antigenic marker for epithelial ovarian carcinoma, serum CA-125 measurement for detection of pelvic malignancy is controversial. An elevated serum CA-125 level (>35 U/mL) occurs in more than 80% of patients with nonmucinous epithelial ovarian carcinomas and also accompanies other malignancies and benign diseases, including pregnancy, endometriosis, fibroids, PID, hepatocellular disease, chronic peritonitis, and carcinomas of the endometrium, fallopian tube, endocervix, pancreas, colon, breast, and lung. Evaluation of a pelvic mass should not be based solely on a serum CA-125 but should also depend on history, pelvic examination, and

ultrasound. A serum CA-125 level greater than 200 U/mL in any individual suggests the presence of an ovarian malignancy. An elevated CA-125 at the time of surgery is useful to monitor tumor progression and to follow the clinical response of the patient to therapy.

33. **(D)** A 65-year-old woman with ascites and a fixed pelvic mass is most likely to have ovarian epithelial cancer. Preoperative studies are used to exclude other etiologies for a pelvic mass. Mammography is used to detect primary mammary cancer with metastases to the ovary. Stool guaiac examination, sigmoidoscopy, and intestinal tract imaging are useful for detecting gastrointestinal cancers in patients with appropriate symptoms. A chest X-ray will detect pulmonary disease and/or pleural effusions. Cervical Pap smear and endometrial biopsy (if necessary) eliminate cervical and endometrial disease. An IVP is useful if the patient is symptomatic for genitourinary disease. It will detect ureteral obstruction and will also show pelvic calcifications suggestive of benign or malignant disease. Laboratory tests including a complete blood count, blood chemistries, and urinalysis are also helpful. Ultrasonography and/or a CT scan of the abdomen and pelvis will also be of assistance.

34. **(A)** Although further studies are required to improve long-term survival, several statements can be made about the current treatment of ovarian epithelial cancer. The most important principle in ovarian cancer therapy is removal of all gross disease if the risk of fatal complications is minimal. A midline incision should be used and bowel may be removed if necessary. Most gynecologic oncologists will recommend a bowel preparation to minimize bowel injury and its inherent challenges in repair.

First-line multiagent chemotherapy with paclitaxel plus a platinum compound (carboplatin or cisplatin) is used for patients with stage IA to IB, grade 3 (some oncologists treat grade 2), stage II to IV, or with residual disease after initial tumor removal.

35. **(D)** The stage of ovarian cancer is determined by physical examination, roentgenologic studies,

surgical findings, histologic analysis of tumor, pelvic organs, omentum, and biopsies of suspicious areas, and cytology examination of peritoneal fluid. At surgery, careful inspection of the pelvic viscera, peritoneal serosa, gastrointestinal tract, omentum, liver, diaphragm, retroperitoneal nodes, pancreas, and biliary structures is mandatory. Peritoneal fluid should be collected for cytologic examination. Omentectomy is performed because the omentum is a common site for metastases. Lymph node sampling is recommended, and palpable nodes should be excised in all but obviously advanced cases. The staging system for ovarian carcinoma, as defined by the FIGO, is based on the following:

- *Stage I*: Growth limited to the ovaries but can include malignant cells in the peritoneal cavity, ovarian surface excrescences, capsule rupture, or involvement of both ovaries.
- *Stage II*: Growth involving one or both ovaries with pelvic extension to the uterus, tubes, or other pelvic structures.
- *Stage III*: Abdominal metastases and their size, positive retroperitoneal lymph nodes, or extension to small bowel or omentum.
- *Stage IV*: Distant metastases, including liver metastases or malignant pleural effusion (see Figure 22–3).

36. **(B)** Despite the benefit of cytoreductive surgery, the 3-year survival rate of patients with stage III ovarian cancer without residual disease after cytoreduction is only 30%. Therefore, combination chemotherapy (e.g., *cis*-platinum and paclitaxel) is commonly given after cytoreductive surgery. The use of combination chemotherapy for the treatment of high-stage disease appears to provide superior survival rates compared to single-agent chemotherapy. The response to chemotherapy is related to the amount of residual disease after surgery. Younger patients achieve results from postoperative therapy superior to those of older patients. The response to chemotherapy usually occurs within 6 months. If the patient with a stage III cancer appears to have a complete response to chemotherapy (by physical examination and diagnostic testing), a second-look operation is sometimes performed. Under this condition, about one-half

of women thought to be free of cancer have disease present at second-look operation.

37. **(D)** Pediatric ovarian malignancies are rare (1.7 per 100,000 per year) so only 36% to 64% of cases are identified before surgery. The most common incorrect diagnosis is acute appendicitis since the most common presenting symptom is abdominal pain. Germ cell tumors represent 70% of ovarian neoplasms in children. Germ cell tumors are believed to originate from primitive germ cells that differentiate toward developmental tissues of either embryonic (e.g., ectoderm, mesoderm, and endoderm) or extraembryonic (e.g., yolk sac and trophoblast) origin. They are the most common neoplasms in women younger than 30 years (representing 70% of ovarian neoplasms in infants and children). Germ cell tumors are the main cause of ovarian malignancy in young women but account for only 3% of all ovarian malignancies. However, when reviewing any ovarian enlargement, 67% of masses are benign and are frequently nonneoplastic follicles or theca lutein cysts.

38. **(E)** Bowel perforation is a well-recognized although uncommon complication of laparoscopy and injuries are not always recognized at the time of surgery. Most patients present with postoperative symptoms within 10 days. The diagnosis is not always clear. While ileus and severe obstipation from narcotics give similar symptoms, the marked fever and elevated WBC count argue for bowel perforation. Similarly, although chemical peritonitis has been reported with dermoids, bowel perforation is more likely, given the clinical scenario.

39. **(A)** The likely diagnosis is endodermal sinus tumor given the elevated alpha-fetoprotein. The majority of cases are stage I, and bilaterality is rare so unilateral adnexectomy is appropriate. However, simple surgical therapy results in frequent recurrences so chemotherapy is also indicated. These tumors are very sensitive to chemotherapeutic agents and the majority of women are cured with surgery plus adjuvant chemotherapy. This tumor accounts for about

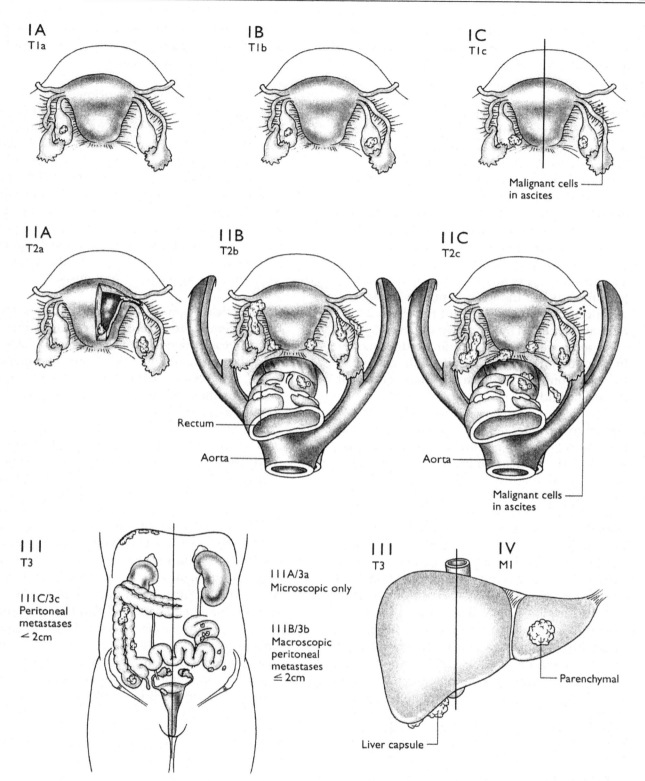

**IA**
T1a

**IB**
T1b

**IC**
T1c

Malignant cells
in ascites

**IIA**
T2a

**IIB**
T2b

Rectum

Aorta

**IIC**
T2c

Aorta

Malignant cells
in ascites

**III**
T3

**IIIC/3c**
Peritoneal
metastases
≤ 2cm

**IIIA/3a**
Microscopic only

**IIIB/3b**
Macroscopic
peritoneal
metastases
≤ 2cm

**III**
T3

**IV**
M1

Parenchymal

Liver capsule

Figure 22–3.

one-fifth of all germ cell tumors. Almost all cases have elevated alpha-fetoprotein levels, and it is a useful marker for following these tumors clinically.

40. **(E)** Germ cell tumors represent one quarter of all ovarian tumors and occur anatomically anywhere along the migration route of primordial germ cells from the yolk sac to the genital ridge. Germ cell tumors are commonly unilateral and are usually seen during the second and third decades of life. Most germ cell tumors are benign. The mature teratoma, or dermoid cyst, is the most common germ cell tumor, accounting for 95% of all germ cell tumors. In addition, it accounts for 25% of all ovarian neoplasms. Dysgerminomas are the most common malignant germ cell tumors and account for 1% to 2% of ovarian cancers. Three percent of germ cell tumors are malignant and occur predominantly in prepubertal girls. Abdominal enlargement is the most common sign of a malignant germ cell tumor in children.

41. **(D)** Immature teratomas contain embryonal (immature) tissue, resembling that normally found in the human embryo. Tumor grade is based on the maturity of the ectodermal neural tissue. Hair is present in 40% of tumors, and calcified bone is usually grossly evident. Immature teratomas are the second most common malignant germ cell tumor (the first being dysgerminoma). Seventy-five percent of these tumors are discovered during the first two decades of life. Survival varies from 81% to 30% for grades 1 to 3. Bilaterality is rare, although 5% of immature teratomas are associated with a mature teratoma in the contralateral ovary. Stage I, grade 1 disease may be treated by unilateral salpingo-oophorectomy, but adjuvant chemotherapy is required for higher grades or more advanced stages. Pure immature teratomas do not produce alpha-fetoprotein or hCG.

42. **(A)** Dysgerminoma is the most common malignant germ cell tumor of the ovary. Histologically, dysgerminoma is composed of primordial germ cells and intervening connective tissue infiltrated by lymphocytes. The tumors are usually smooth, rounded, and thinly encapsulated. Rupture of the capsule may lead to intra-abdominal hemorrhage.

43. **(D)** Dysgerminoma occurs primarily in women younger than 30 years. It has the highest rate of bilaterality (10% to 15%) of all malignant germ cell tumors. The 5-year survival rate following unilateral salpingo-oophorectomy for tumor confined to one ovary is more than 90%. Survival rates drop to approximately 60% when disease extends beyond the ovary. Dysgerminoma is sensitive to chemotherapy and radiotherapy. Other germ cell tumors (e.g., teratoma and gonadoblastoma) may coexist with dysgerminomas and may worsen the prognosis.

44. **(B)** Physical examination strongly suggests testicular feminization, a disorder in men due to defective androgen action. The uterus is absent and the vagina ends blindly, causing amenorrhea. The testes are located in the pelvis or within an inguinal hernia and contain immature seminiferous tubules.

45. **(D)** Gonadoblastoma is the most common neoplasm associated with dysgenetic gonads. Eighty percent of patients with this tumor are phenotypic women, most of whom are virilized and have a Y chromosome. Adolescent patients with gonadoblastoma may experience delayed puberty due to primary gonadal failure. Many of these tumors are small and contain calcifications. Bilaterality occurs in at least half of the patients. Fifty percent of gonadoblastomas contain malignant germ cell elements, predominantly dysgerminoma, which reduce the chance for survival. Bilateral salpingo-oophorectomy is usually performed in patients with dysgenetic gonads containing a gonadoblastoma because malignant germ cell elements may be present and bilaterality is common. Gonadectomy is usually delayed until after puberty in patients with testicular feminization to allow hormone-dependent pubertal changes.

46. **(B)** The presence of a Y chromosome in an individual with dysgenetic gonads carries a 25% chance of developing a germ cell tumor (e.g., gonadoblastoma, dysgerminoma, endodermal

sinus tumor, and choriocarcinoma). Most of these malignant changes occur after puberty and before the age of 30.

47. **(E)** Metastatic tumors to the ovary usually originate in the breast, gastrointestinal tract, or uterus. They account for 4% to 8% of ovarian carcinomas. Lymphatic channels are probably the most important route of ovarian metastasis. Other means of cancer spread to the ovaries include direct extension, intraperitoneal dissemination, metastasis via the lumen of the fallopian tube, and hematogenous metastasis.

48. **(E)** Tumor grade is a major determinant of prognosis when survival is examined for each stage of disease. Tumor cell type also affects prognosis (e.g., serous tumors have a worse prognosis than mucinous, endometrioid, and clear cell tumors). Serous tumors tend to be more poorly differentiated and identified at a higher stage than other tumors. Other factors adversely affecting survival from stage I ovarian epithelial carcinoma include pelvic adhesions and ascitic fluid (250 mL). Women with well-differentiated tumors confined to the ovary do not require further treatment after surgery. Individuals with poorly differentiated stage I and stage II disease usually receive postoperative adjuvant therapy (e.g., radiotherapy or chemotherapy). Psammoma bodies have no prognostic significance in gynecologic cancer.

49. **(D)** Fibromas and the comas are benign tumors derived from stromal mesenchyme. They can occur at any age but are most common in peri- and postmenopausal women. The tumors are solid, irregular, and mobile, ranging in size from small to several thousand grams. The fibroma is the most common benign solid ovarian tumor. It does not produce hormones but can be associated with Meigs' syndrome. The thecoma is almost always unilateral and is composed of endocrinologically active stromal cells bearing a resemblance to lipid-laden thecal cells. Its yellow appearance on cross section is due to the presence of steroid-producing cells. Granulosa cell tumors produce estrogen; hilar cell and Sertoli–Leydig tumors produce androgens.

50. **(D)** GTD occurs in approximately 1 in 600 therapeutic abortions and 1 in 1,500 pregnancies. Twenty percent of patients will develop malignant sequelae, requiring chemotherapy after primary evacuation with D&C. Primary treatment with D&C usually by suction is curative in most patients. The most common symptom is abnormal bleeding in the first trimester and abnormally high serum hCG level. Fetal tissue is often present in partial moles but absent in complete moles.

51. **(C)** Choriocarcinoma used to be almost universally fatal. It can now be cured in nearly 100% of cases when it is not metastatic and in 90% of all cases. Surgery to evacuate the uterus is still used, but it is not the most effective mainstay of treatment. The incidence of this condition is 1 per 20,000 to 40,000 pregnancies.

52. **(D)** Tumors grow exponentially because of disruption in the regulation of programmed cell death (apoptosis), not because of rapid proliferation. Gompertzian growth is the concept that as the tumor grows larger, the rate of growth slows.

53. **(D)** The stem cell theory states that only certain undifferentiated cells (stem cells) are able to divide to reproduce a tissue. The remainder of the cells are well differentiated (specialized) and cannot undergo this change. Tumors are thought to arise from an individual stem cell. Malignant cells are thought to escape the normal regulation of cells in some as yet undetermined manner.

54. **(A)** In multiagent chemotherapy, each drug should be effective against the tumor. If each is not, effect is less. Toxicity at comparable dosage is no different than in single-agent therapy, and each drug must be monitored for its own side effects. Multiagent chemotherapy is used in the same general doses as if the agents were used alone. Generally, the faster growing a tumor is, the more susceptible it is to chemotherapeutic agents. Agents from different classes are often combined for an effective multidrug treatment.

55. **(D)** Chemotherapy commonly induces neutropenia, which puts patients at risk for serious

infections including bacteremia. Often, fever is the only complaint of patients with neutropenia and bacteremia. These infections can progress rapidly. The diagnosis is made by blood culture, chest X-ray, and urine culture. Any febrile, neutropenic patient should be admitted and placed on two antibiotics, although some investigators recommend single-antibiotic therapy with agents like imipenem. Giving the sixth course of chemotherapy is contraindicated with the current neutropenia and should be delayed. Granulocyte colony-stimulating factors (GCSFs) may decrease the duration of neutropenia.

56. **(B)** Only a few cases (approximately 2%) of simple hyperplasia without atypia will progress to carcinoma and progression is slow. The D&C alone often removes the hyperplasia. Progestin is a standard treatment. Appropriate follow-up includes repeat endometrial sampling in 6 months to assure resolution of the process. A hysterectomy is not indicated unless bleeding problems persist despite hormonal treatment or the disease progresses to hyperplasia with atypia.

57. **(D)** Severe atypical hyperplasia may progress to endometrial carcinoma so hysterectomy is warranted. In severe atypia, approximately 25% develop carcinoma, 25% regress, and 50% persist. She is likely to have polycystic ovarian syndrome (PCOS), causing anovulation and prolonged estrogen exposure.

58. **(B)** Three to five percent of patients with complex hyperplasia will ultimately develop endometrial cancer. The precise mechanism of progression to carcinoma is unknown.

59. **(D)** Probably 21% to 29% of women with atypia in the hyperplasia will progress to a malignant cancer. This is why hysterectomy is offered when childbearing is completed.

60. **(A)** Simple hyperplasia without atypia rarely progresses to endometrial cancer.

61. **(E)** Less than 5% of Brenner tumors are malignant. The malignancy rates for mucinous and serous tumors are 15% and 30%, respectively.

Almost all endometrioid and clear cell tumors are malignant.

62. **(A)** The risk of bilaterality is an important issue in the treatment of ovarian tumors. Malignant tumors have a higher rate of bilaterality than benign tumors. The bilaterality rates of ovarian epithelial neoplasms are in decreasing order of frequency: serous cystadenocarcinoma (33% to 66%), mucinous cystadenocarcinoma (10% to 20%), endometrioid carcinoma (13% to 30%), and Brenner tumor (6%).

63. **(A)** Serous ovarian tumors have an appearance similar to that of tubal epithelium. Ovarian and tubal tumors also may contain papillae or papillary structures. Ovarian disease metastatic to the fallopian tube is diagnosed when the tubal mucosa is intact and malignant cells are present in the subepithelial lymphatics. Some patients have small ovaries (<4 cm in diameter) and widespread serous carcinoma in the abdomen, referred to as papillary serous carcinoma of the peritoneum. Occasionally the primary site of papillary serous carcinoma is difficult to determine.

64. **(C)** Bone marrow suppression may accompany chemotherapy or radiation therapy. It is common when abdominopelvic radiation follows chemotherapy.

65. **(A)** Radiation-induced bowel obstruction can lead to a surgical emergency. In addition, intestinal injuries commonly occur when surgery is performed after abdominopelvic radiation. Adhesions resulting from intestinal injury may cause symptoms of bowel obstruction (e.g., postprandial crampy abdominal pain, vomiting, and anorexia), which are similar to those of recurrent disease.

66. **(E)** Struma ovarii refers to a teratoma in which thyroid tissue represents more than half of the tumor. One-quarter of these tumors are associated with clinical hyperthyroidism.

67. **(B)** Alpha-fetoprotein is produced by endodermal sinus tumors. It can be detected in the serum of patients with primary and recurrent disease.

The prognosis for patients with endodermal sinus tumor has improved markedly with the recent use of multidrug chemotherapy (stage I, 80%; stage II, 60%; stage III, 30% survival).

68. **(C)** Choriocarcinoma may develop from a germ cell (nongestational) or a pregnancy (gestational) arising in the ovary or elsewhere in the genital tract. All of these tumors produce hCG and contain sheets of cytotrophoblastic and syncytiotrophoblastic tissues. Nongestational choriocarcinoma is less responsive than gestational choriocarcinoma to chemotherapy. The prognosis of patients with nongestational choriocarcinoma is poor.

69. **(A)** Pure dysgerminomas occasionally produce large amounts of LDH. They do not secrete significant amounts of alpha-fetoprotein or hCG.

70. **(G)** Inhibin is produced by granulosa cell tumor and may be used as a serum marker for this tumor.

71. (H) Gonadal tumors may produce androgens directly (gonadoblastoma) or indirectly through the secretion of chorionic gonadotropin (e.g., nongestational choriocarcinoma, embryonal carcinoma, and mixed germ cell tumor).

# CHAPTER 23

# Breast Cancer

## Questions

**DIRECTIONS (Questions 1 through 31): For each of the multiple choice questions in this section, select the lettered answer that is the one *best* response in each case.**

1. A 55-year-old patient who had her first child at age 38 is overweight and smokes. She had a grandmother who was diagnosed with breast cancer at age 63 years. The patient's breast biopsy reveals atypical epithelial hyperplasia. Which of the following is her greatest risk factor for the development of breast cancer?

   (A) delayed childbearing
   (B) a family history of breast cancer
   (C) increased dietary fat intake
   (D) smoking
   (E) atypical epithelial hyperplasia

2. You have to give a talk about breast cancer to a women's group. You can correctly tell them which of the following is most likely to detect early breast cancer?

   (A) bloody discharge from the nipple
   (B) a palpable mass on self-examination
   (C) a palpable mass on annual examination at the caregiver's office
   (D) mammographic abnormalities
   (E) a mobile tender cyst

3. A 60-year-old woman has the following findings on an examination of her breast. Which one is the most likely to be a late finding of breast cancer?

   (A) greenish-gray discharge
   (B) drooping of the breasts
   (C) darkening of the areola
   (D) asymmetry of the breast size
   (E) skin or nipple retraction

4. A 20-year-old nulligravid woman with a history of breast cancer in a paternal grandmother presents with increasing bilateral breast pain. The breast pain is worse before her menses. On physical examination a tender 2-cm mass is palpable in the upper outer quadrant of her right breast. There is no adenopathy. What is the best next step in her evaluation?

   (A) magnetic resonance imaging (MRI)
   (B) ultrasound
   (C) mammogram
   (D) core needle biopsy of the mass
   (E) excisional biopsy of the mass

5. A patient has found a mobile discrete lump in the lower outer quadrant of her breast. What is the most common site for breast cancer to occur?

   (A) upper outer quadrant
   (B) upper inner quadrant
   (C) lower outer quadrant
   (D) lower inner quadrant
   (E) under the nipple

6. A 44-year-old patient has a clear discharge from the left nipple. What is the diagnostic accuracy for cancer from cytology of nipple discharge or fluid from breast cyst aspiration?

   (A) It has generally been shown to be of little benefit.
   (B) It has an extremely high false-positive rate.
   (C) It is diagnostically correct approximately 75% of the time.
   (D) It is accurate approximately 100% of the time in diagnosing breast cancer.
   (E) It has a low false-negative rate.

7. A 48-year-old patient is deciding whether she will have a mammogram given the latest conflicting recommendation between national organizations on when to start mammogram screening in a low-risk population. She asks you about the advantages and disadvantages of the procedure. Which of the following should you advise her?

   (A) Mammography can be performed with a radiation exposure of 1 rad.
   (B) Mammography can be used to evaluate suspicious breast masses and save women from biopsy in many cases.
   (C) Mammography and physical examination are equally effective in the diagnosis of all types of breast cancer.
   (D) Mammographic screening of new populations for breast cancer will identify about 1 cancer for every 1,000 women screened.
   (E) Mammography is a much more effective technique for diagnosing breast cancer than is breast ultrasound.

8. A patient has been given a BI-RADS (American College of Radiology Breast Imaging, Reporting and Data System) terminology designation of zero. What does this designation mean?

   (A) normal mammogram
   (B) benign lesion
   (C) probably benign lesion

   (D) suspicious for malignancy
   (E) needs additional evaluation

9. A 38-year-old patient has been asked to get an ultrasound of the breast after a mammogram revealed a mass. What is ultrasound most useful to diagnose?

   (A) fibroid adenomas
   (B) invasive cancer
   (C) in situ carcinoma
   (D) interductal papillomas
   (E) benign cysts

10. A breast cancer is usually not detected by palpation until it has grown to 1 cm or more. How many years of growth does the average perimenopausal/menopausal breast cancer require to reach a diameter of 1 cm?

   (A) 1.5
   (B) 2
   (C) 4
   (D) 6
   (E) 10

11. Approximately what percentage of breast cancers that are not seen on mammography can be found by clinical breast examination?

   (A) <1%
   (B) 5–8%
   (C) 15–20%
   (D) 25–28%
   (E) >33%

12. Which of the following is the most appropriate response to a reproductive-aged woman who asks, "When should I perform breast self-examination to have the best results?"

   (A) at the onset of menses
   (B) just after menses
   (C) at midcycle
   (D) just before the onset of menses
   (E) monthly at any time during the cycle

13. A 25-year-old G2P2 healthy woman's mother developed breast cancer at age 52. The patient's sister was diagnosed with breast cancer at age 30. Both her mother and sister are living. She wants to know if there are any tests she should get to help her evaluate the risks of her getting breast cancer. In her case, which of the following tests would most likely help evaluate her risk?

    (A) Decreased T- and B-cell levels cause a decline in immunity.
    (B) Human epidermal growth factor receptor 2 (*HER-2*)/*neu* gene levels are associated with later development of breast cancer.
    (C) *BRCA1* and *BRCA2* mutations may predict increased risk of breast cancer.
    (D) Serum androgen levels are associated with a decreased risk of breast cancer.
    (E) CA-125 is a good prognostic marker for breast cancer.

14. What is the most common pathologic type of breast malignancy?

    (A) lobular in situ
    (B) ductal in situ
    (C) Paget's disease
    (D) infiltrating lobular carcinoma
    (E) infiltrating ductal carcinoma

15. A woman has a stage II, estrogen receptor-positive (ER+) and progesterone receptor-positive (PR+) breast cancer. What is the major importance of knowing the ER status in breast cancers?

    (A) If a tumor lacks ERs, it is generally more amenable to treatment.
    (B) Tumors with ERs and/or PRs generally do not require adjuvant chemotherapy.
    (C) Antiestrogen therapy (such as tamoxifen) may improve survival in patients with a positive ER status.
    (D) Diethylstilbestrol (DES) may be given as a curative agent in many of these patients.
    (E) The long-term prognosis is better in patients with ER– and PR– tumors.

16. A 59-year-old woman presents with a 3-cm, irregular, mobile mass in the upper outer quadrant of her breast. Her right axilla has two palpable, very small, rubbery, mobile lymph nodes. If the primary mass is malignant, what is the most likely stage of her disease?

    (A) 0
    (B) I
    (C) II
    (D) III
    (E) IV

17. A woman is operated on for stage II breast cancer with a lumpectomy and axillary node dissection on the involved side. Two lymph nodes are positive for breast cancer. Which of the following statements best describes her prognosis?

    (A) Her chance of 5-year survival should be approximately 85%.
    (B) Her chance of 10-year survival is nearly the same as her 5-year survival rate.
    (C) Breast cancer with one to three positive axillary nodes gives approximately 60% chance of survival at 5 years.
    (D) She has greater than a 70% chance of dying from her breast cancer.
    (E) She should be cured of her cancer.

18. A patient with what is thought to be stage I breast cancer prior to surgery asks about the chances of finding cancer in her axillary lymph nodes during the surgery. There are no clinically palpable nodes present on her preoperative examination. Which of the following is most likely?

    (A) The chance should be close to 0%.
    (B) The chance is approximately 10%.
    (C) The chance is approximately 30%.
    (D) The chance is greater than 50%.
    (E) Most women have lymph node involvement in any breast cancer.

19. What procedure is designed to prevent many of the surgical complications of axillary lymph node dissection, and has very good positive and negative predictive values for detecting lymph node metastasis?

    (A) MRI
    (B) fine-needle biopsy
    (C) sentinel node mapping
    (D) HER-2/neu detection
    (E) clinical breast examination

20. A 46-year-old woman has an irregular, firm, 2-cm mass on breast examination. Her axillary examination is normal. On clinical grounds, you are very suspicious of a cancer. She asks you, "What are the chances that this will be benign?" How should you advise her?

    (A) nearly 0%
    (B) approximately 15%
    (C) approximately 30%
    (D) approximately 50%
    (E) 70%

21. You are counseling a patient about doing a biopsy on a mass found in her breast. Which of the following should you advise her?

    (A) A needle biopsy has been proven to be as good as open biopsy in nearly all cases.
    (B) Needle biopsy has little or no role in the evaluation of breast masses.
    (C) Needle biopsy can be falsely negative in 15–20% of cases.
    (D) Open breast biopsy should remove an entire breast lobule surrounding the mass.
    (E) General anesthesia is necessary to do an adequate breast biopsy in most cases.

22. A 61-year-old woman has a clinically suspicious, relatively superficial breast mass. Her ipsilateral axilla is normal. A biopsy is recommended. She asks how the biopsy should be done. Which of the following is the best option?

    (A) to do her biopsy in the office today
    (B) a lumpectomy and axillary dissection or mastectomy in your ambulatory surgery center as indicated after gross inspection of the specimen
    (C) an outpatient biopsy in the ambulatory surgery center and await the final pathology reports before proceeding with any further evaluation or treatment
    (D) doing the biopsy in the hospital and proceeding with axillary dissection or mastectomy depending on the pathologist's frozen section report
    (E) a fine-needle aspiration

23. Excluding recurrence of the cancer, what is the most common complication following the treatment of breast cancer?

    (A) edema of the ipsilateral arm
    (B) complications from breast reconstruction
    (C) development of leukemia from adjuvant chemotherapy
    (D) permanent alopecia
    (E) agranulocytosis

24. A 22-year-old patient has a family history of breast cancer and *BRCA1* mutation. She also has the *BRCA1* mutation. Which of the following is the most effective method to prevent breast cancer in this patient?

    (A) bilateral oophorectomy
    (B) tamoxifen
    (C) bilateral mastectomy
    (D) avoid weight gain
    (E) have first term birth before age 22

25. A 32-year-old woman at 15 weeks' gestation with a wanted pregnancy has a 2.5-cm breast lump and no palpable axillary or clavicular nodes. A core needle biopsy reveals a ductal carcinoma that is ER– and PR–. Chest X-ray and bone and liver MRIs are negative. Which of the following is the best management for this woman who wants to keep her pregnancy?

    (A) delay treatment until after delivery
    (B) lumpectomy and radiation

(C) antiestrogens

(D) definitive surgical excision with chemotherapy after delivery

(E) definitive surgical excision with chemotherapy now

26. Which of the following will improve the detection of malignant cells in axillary nodes significantly more than routine cytology in patients with breast cancer?

(A) *BRCA1* testing

(B) palpation

(C) HER-2/neu detection

(D) sentinel node mapping

(E) serial sectioning

27. A 24-year-old G2P2 has a 2-cm firm mobile mass in her left breast, lower inner quadrant. Her examinations are consistent with fibrocystic change. There is no adenopathy in either breast. Breast ultrasound notes a solid mass. What is the best next step?

(A) mammogram

(B) MRI

(C) needle biopsy

(D) excisional biopsy

(E) conservative management

28. A 48-year-old G4P2 sab2 presents with a bloody discharge in her right breast. The discharge is scant and intermittent. Physical examination is unremarkable; no masses are palpable in either breast. The discharge is serosanguinous and seems to be coming from a small area at the edge of the areola. The next best step for diagnosis is which of the following?

(A) cytology of the discharge

(B) ultrasound with ductography

(C) fine-needle biopsy

(D) MRI

(E) CT

29. A 32-year-old African American woman G3P2 had a core needle biopsy of a suspicious breast mass. The results show moderately differentiated ductal carcinoma. Lumpectomy showed good margins of a 2-cm tumor with small areas of ductal carcinoma in situ with disease-free margins. Sentinel node was positive for a 0.8 mm (micrometastases) area of a tumor. Other nodes were negative. The tumor is triple negative in addition to breast radiation. This woman should be considered for which of the following?

(A) tamoxifen

(B) trastuzumab (Herceptin)

(C) aromatase inhibitor

(D) chemotherapy with alkylating agents

(E) no further therapy

30. A 38-year-old woman presents for her annual examination. As her history is updated, she states that her first cousin on her mother's side was diagnosed with breast cancer the past year. Her cousin was 54. Her self-breast examination and clinical breast examinations are unremarkable. She asks about her risk of breast cancer. Your next step in assessing her breast cancer risks should be which of the following?

(A) recommend *BRCA* and *BRCA2* testing

(B) referral to a genetic counselor

(C) obtain a screening mammogram

(D) use the Gail BRCA model

(E) explain that the risks are no greater than the background risks

31. A 48-year-old woman 2 years after TAH/BSO for benign uterine disease is found by the Gail model to be at threefold increased risk for breast cancer. She should be offered which of the following?

(A) tamoxifen

(B) danazol

(C) aromatase inhibitors

(D) trastuzumab (Herceptin)

(E) annual MRI of the breast

# Answers and Explanations

1. **(E)** Increasing age, delayed childbearing, non–breast-feeding, high-fat diet, a positive family history, late menopause, early menarche, and mammary dysplasia are all risk factors in the development of breast cancer. Of the options listed, atypical epithelial hyperplasia is the greatest risk factor. Smoking is not proven to increase the risk of breast cancer.

2. **(D)** While most cases of breast cancer are found by the patient during self-examination, the earliest detectable lesions are most likely to be discovered using screening mammography in an asymptomatic, postmenopausal population.

3. **(E)** Late findings in breast cancer include skin or nipple retraction, axillary adenopathy, sudden breast enlargement, redness, edema, chest wall pain, and fixation of a mass to the chest wall. Greenish gray discharge is most often ductal epithelial breakdown. Drooping of the breasts is a phenomenon of aging. Darkening of the areola is a progesterone effect most often seen in pregnancy. Most women have slightly asymmetric breast development, but this should be a life-long condition. Skin or nipple retraction suggests interference with normal breast architecture, which occurs with malignancy.

4. **(B)** This patient has findings consistent with fibrocystic change. Bilateral pain that is menstrually related is considered a classic finding. The tender 2-cm mass is most likely a cyst. However, it should be imaged before being aspirated. Ultrasound is the best modality for imaging at this time. Mammography and MRI are second and third steps, respectively. Biopsy of any type is not indicated until imaging is complete. As this is most likely a cyst that will resolve after aspiration, no further biopsy will be needed. If the mass is not cystic then fine-needle biopsy is acceptable in this situation.

5. **(A)** The presenting complaint of approximately 70% of women with breast cancer is a painless lump. Approximately 90% of these masses will be discovered by the patient herself. Breast cancer is usually slow growing. By the time a mass is palpable (1 to 2 cm), it may have been present 8 years! Nearly one-half of breast cancers will occur in the upper outer quadrant and another 25% under the nipple and areola. A discrete lump in any position must be evaluated.

6. **(A)** Cytology of nipple discharge and breast cyst aspirate is seldom diagnostic. It also has a high false-negative rate. Most experienced evaluators do not send the fluid for cytologic examination routinely unless the fluid is bloody. The fluid can be checked for blood by microscopy or guaiac. If it is bloody, further evaluation may be indicated. Negative results of such evaluation, however, cannot be considered reassuring.

7. **(E)** Mammography is an excellent screening procedure in appropriate patients (postmenopausal and premenopausal patients with risk factors). The radiation is very low (approximately 0.1 rad with new equipment) and can be considered noncarcinogenic. It can detect nonpalpable breast cancer very accurately. When combined with physical examination in screening programs for new populations, a diagnosis rate for breast cancer as high as 6 per 1,000 is

attained. Approximately 80% of affected women diagnosed by mammogram have negative axillary lymph nodes, compared to 45% of those diagnosed by physical examination alone. However, mammography is not as good in diagnosing medullary carcinoma of the breast, and it has been reported that as high as 40% of some types of cancer can be diagnosed by palpation but do not show on mammography. While mammography is certainly indicated to aid in the diagnosis of a suspicious breast mass, the mass itself needs to be removed. Mammography is not a substitute for biopsy. Mammography is a much more effective technique than ultrasonography in detecting cancer, but ultrasound is useful to distinguish cystic from solid masses in the breast.

8. **(E)** BI-RAD was devised to make mammographic terminology more standardized and to reduce confusion. Zero means more evaluation is needed, such as repeat mammogram film or ultrasound. One is a normal mammogram. Second is a benign lesion. For both of these, yearly screening is recommended. Third is probably a benign lesion, which demands a shorter follow-up. There is a low (<2%) chance of malignancy. Four and five are suspicious or highly suspicious of malignancy, usually demanding biopsy.

9. **(E)** Ultrasound helps most in distinguishing whether a mass detected on mammogram is cystic or solid. If the mass is cystic with a thin lining and no excretions, it can be safely aspirated, as it is almost always benign.

10. **(D)** Although a few breast carcinomas grow very rapidly, most grow slowly and give time for screening to pick them up early enough for treatment to be highly efficacious. Women who do routine breast self-examination find lesions that are approximately 2 cm in size.

11. **(C)** Clinical breast examinations can discover between 15% and 20% of breast cancers that are not detected by mammography. The examination will detect more masses if it is done systematically by both inspecting and palpating the breasts and taking 3 to 5 minutes to accomplish the examination.

12. **(B)** Examination is best performed just after menses when the breasts are usually in the most quiescent state. Breast self-examination is generally recommended for all women older than 20 years. Beginning at this age helps women get used to doing a normal examination and establish a routine, and provides them with a valuable cost-free disease prevention technique. Examining during the luteal phase of the cycle increases the probability of finding breast cysts and other changes in the parenchyma that are hormonally influenced. These changes can make the examination confusing in the menstrual-age patient.

13. **(C)** The *BRCA1* gene is located on chromosome 17. It is a suppressor gene, and if a patient has a mutation, the risk of breast cancer in her lifetime is quite high, with small subsets of patients having an 80% to 85% risk during their lifetime. *BRCA2*, which is located on chromosome 13, also results in a similar increased breast cancer risk. As both members of this patient's family with breast cancer are alive, they can be checked for a *BRCA1* or *BRCA2* gene mutation. If one is found, the patient can be evaluated for a similar mutation. Women with either *BRCA1* or *BRCA2* mutations are at increased risk for ovarian cancer as well. These women should use recognized screening procedures to help detect cancer at an early stage. *HER-2/neu* is associated with a poorer prognosis of known breast cancer but has not been of use as a screening diagnostic test. Neither T- nor B-cell levels are breast cancer screening tests. T cells are associated with cell-mediated immunity and B cells with antibody production. CA-125 has been found helpful to follow ovarian cancer but has not been helpful for screening. It is not helpful for screening for breast cancer. Androgen levels in 25-year-olds are unhelpful as well.

14. **(E)** Infiltrating ductal carcinoma comprises 65% of breast cancer. Ductal carcinoma in situ comprises approximately 10%. Lobular carcinoma in situ comprises approximately 2% of breast cancer, while 8% of breast cancer is invasive lobular. Other types are less common.

15. **(C)** Generally, patients with positive hormone receptor status are more amenable to hormonal therapy (80% responders when metastatic disease is present). Tamoxifen is effective as an adjuvant to surgery or radiation, especially in receptor-positive patients. Chemotherapy is a benefit in both ER+/PR+ and ER–/PR– tumors. DES was once given to induce receptors, but it is no longer administered.

16. **(C)** A stage I tumor is less than 2 cm in diameter. Stage II tumors are less than 5 cm in diameter and without any suspicious nodes. In this case, the nodes found are small and rubbery, and not suspicious for metastatic disease. Stage III disease demonstrates tumor greater than 5 cm in diameter or tumor of any size with invasion of skin or attached to the chest wall. Supraclavicular nodes must be negative, and there should be no sign of distant metastases. Stage IV disease shows evidence of distant metastases (Table 23–1).

**TABLE 23–1.   Clinical and Histologic Staging of Breast Carcinoma and Relation to Survival**

| Clinical Staging (American Joint Committee) | Crude 5-Year Survival (%) |
|---|---|
| Stage I | 85 |
| Tumor <2 cm in diameter | |
| Nodes, if present, not felt to contain metastases | |
| Without distant metastases | |
| Stage II | 66 |
| Tumor <5 cm in diameter | |
| Nodes, if palpable, not fixed | |
| Without distant metastases | |
| Stage III | 41 |
| Tumor >5 cm or— | |
| Tumor any size with invasion of skin or attached to chest wall | |
| Nodes in supraclavicular area | |
| Without distant metastases | |
| Stage IV | 10 |
| With distant metastases | |

17. **(C)** The histologic findings of lymph node dissection are extremely important in prognosis of early stage breast cancers. Stage II breast cancer should have approximately a 66% survival rate at 5 years (stage I, 85%; stage III, 41%; stage IV, 10%), but lymph node involvement can greatly alter prognosis. Unlike most other cancers, breast cancer survival at 5-year survival does not equate with cure. A patient with one positive lymph node has a 5-year chance of survival of approximately 60% and a 10-year chance of approximately 40%. A patient with more than four axillary lymph nodes positive for cancer has a 32% chance of survival at 5 years but only a 13% chance at 10 years (see Table 23–2). The survival rate appears to be increasing.

**TABLE 23–2.   Clinical and Histologic Staging of Breast Carcinoma and Relation to Survival**

| Histologic Staging | Crude Survival (%) | |
|---|---|---|
| | 5 Years | 10 Years |
| All patients | 63 | 46 |
| Negative axillary lymph nodes | 78 | 65 |
| Positive axillary lymph nodes | 46 | 25 |
| 1–3 positive axillary lymph nodes | 62 | 38 |
| >4 positive axillary lymph nodes | 32 | 13 |

18. **(C)** Studies show that approximately 30% of patients who have clinically negative axillary nodes actually have spread their breast cancer to these nodes. When the experienced clinician thinks nodes are involved at the time of surgery, cancer is found approximately 85% of the time.

19. **(C)** The routine removal of all lymph nodes in the axilla creates a high incidence of chronic lymphedema. A method of injecting radioactive tracers and dye in the area of the tumor allows the lymph nodes that drain that tumor to be identified and removed without doing a complete axillary dissection unless those nodes are positive.

20. **(C)** Approximately 30% of lesions thought to be cancerous prior to biopsy are benign, and approximately 15% (roughly one in seven) thought to be benign are cancerous. This emphasizes the need for biopsy for an accurate diagnosis.

21. **(C)** Needle biopsies are excellent at making a diagnosis in most cases but have been reported to have false-negative rates as high as 20%. A negative biopsy, therefore, may have to be followed with an open biopsy in some patients. Open breast biopsies can usually be done as outpatient procedures with local anesthetic. In most cases, there is no need to remove more than the

lump with a small margin of normal tissue surrounding it.

22. **(C)** The first two options are unacceptable. Many patients will not have cancer on their biopsy, even when an experienced surgeon predicts it will be. These patients should be well informed about their problem, its diagnostic course, and possible outcomes, but they do not need to be unnecessarily frightened or subjected to uncertainties, such as "What will I find when I wake up?" For these reasons, the National Cancer Institute recommends a two-step approach. First, the patient is educated about the need for biopsy and the procedure of biopsy. After the biopsy, final reports are obtained and discussed so that she has time to consider treatment options, including reconstructive surgery. She should make a decision based on all the facts. Different patients have different needs, and evaluation regimens might have to be modified in some cases. The delay of the two-step regimen has not been shown to adversely effect prognosis for breast cancer. In this case fine-needle aspiration will only unnecessarily delay the workup; if it is negative a biopsy will need to be done, and if it is positive it will not give enough information to make definite plans.

23. **(A)** Following either local excision of tumor plus radiotherapy or radical surgery, there is a 10% to 30% incidence of chronic edema of the ipsilateral arm. Breast reconstruction or implants seldom cause problems for the patient, despite what our media would have us believe. Still, many women choose not to have reconstructive surgery. Alopecia and leukocytopenia are almost always transient. Leukemia is a rare complication of combination chemotherapy, occurring most often with alkylating agents.

24. **(C)** Bilateral mastectomy is the most effective means of preventing breast cancer in high-risk patients with up to 91% prevention. Bilateral oophorectomy may prevent up to 70% but makes future pregnancies with her own eggs unlikely. However, it will also protect her against ovarian cancer. First term birth before age 20 provides some prevention, as will tamoxifen.

Avoiding weight gain is the best lifestyle modification, which also includes the avoidance of smoking and drinking alcohol.

25. **(D)** Treatment should begin as soon as the diagnosis is known and the workup is done. Modified radical mastectomy with adjunctive chemotherapy would be the best management especially if the nodes were positive, although chemotherapy increases survival even if the nodes are negative and can be given during pregnancy, especially after the first trimester. Radiation could be done after delivery. Antiestrogens are not indicated in ER– cancers or during pregnancy. Lumpectomy and radiation are good treatments in nonpregnant women with negative nodes but would not be wise in this case because of radiation scatter to the nearby pregnant uterus. The diagnosis of breast cancer is often delayed during pregnancy because of changes in breast architecture and a lowered index of suspicion, but stage-for-stage prognosis is the same in pregnant and nonpregnant women. Treatment can be carried out at any stage of pregnancy and by any technique in most cases. While not common, the incidence of breast cancer is approximately 10 to 30 per 100,000 pregnancies. By the time breast cancer is diagnosed and treated, about two-thirds of pregnant patients have axillary metastases.

26. **(E)** Many women will have negative nodes at initial surgery, but 30% to 40% who do not appear to have grossly positive nodes have metastasis discovered during histologic examination. By adding immunohistochemical staining for cytokeratin and serially sectioning the axillary nodes, 10% to 30% of women who were initially thought to have negative nodes by routine histologic evaluation will be found to have positive nodes. Serial sectioning decreases the sampling error. *BRCA1* and HER-2/neu are good markers but do not increase detection of malignant cells.

27. **(C)** In a 24-year-old the most likely diagnosis in this setting is a cyst or fibroadenoma. The ultrasound has noted the mass to be solid. Although fibroadenoma is most likely a tissue diagnosis should be made. Mammography is rarely

indicated in young women and MRI as a secondary imaging technique is also not necessary. Needle biopsy is the next step to obtain the tissue diagnosis. After that excisional biopsy may be desired by the patient. Conservative management is also acceptable

28. **(B)** The most likely diagnosis is intraductal papilloma. However, cancer may also produce a bloody discharge. Cytology is rarely helpful being fairly sensitive. Ductography with ultrasound provides the best diagnosis. It also can help direct the excisional biopsy for both definitive diagnosis and treatment.

29. **(D)** This woman is at the edge of stage I and with a micrometastases in her lymph node is almost a stage II. However, because her tumor is the most aggressive type of breast tumor—"Triple Negative"—most oncologists would offer adjuvant systemic therapy. The fact that she is 32-year-old is another factor for offering adjuvant therapy. Triple negative tumors are found more commonly in younger women. African American and Latino women and women with *BRCA* mutations. They have a greater likelihood for earlier metastases within 2 to 5 years and brain and lung than other types of ductal carcinoma. Thus, chemotherapy would be offered even though this is stage I. Because this woman is ER negative, hormones would not be helpful nor would Herceptin, which is an agent directed against the (HER-2/neu) receptor.

30. **(D)** To assess a woman's risks of breast cancer, the Gail model (and the Claus model) was developed and then modified by the National Cancer Institute to form the BCRAT (Breast Cancer Risk Assessment Tool), which evaluates factors such as age, menstrual history, breast, and family history. The patient may not be a good candidate for genetic testing, which accounts for approximately 10% of breast cancer. Without a better history BRCA testing is inappropriate. If the history is complete then referral to a genetic counselor is appropriate. A mammogram may be indicated in the next year of the patients wont assess further risk.

31. **(A)** Tamoxifen has been approved for the prevention (prophylactic therapy) of breast cancer. A main side effect is uterine cancer, but she has had a hysterectomy. Herceptin is for treatment. MRI is not a prophylaxis, only a screening tool, and only indicated for a 20 times increased risk. Danazol and aromatase inhibitors are not indicated in primary prophylaxis.

# CHAPTER 24

# Infectious Diseases in Obstetrics and Gynecology

## Questions

**DIRECTIONS (Questions 1 through 25): For each of the multiple choice questions in this section, select the lettered answer that is the one *best* response in each case.**

1. A 23-year-old woman at 29 weeks' gestation ruptures her amniotic membrane. She is admitted to the hospital, and 3 days later, she is found to have a temperature of 101.1°F, a white blood cell (WBC) count of 15,000, fetal tachycardia, and mild tenderness over her lower abdomen. Which of the following is the most likely diagnosis for this patient?

   (A) intra-amniotic infection
   (B) lower urinary tract infection (UTI)
   (C) pyelonephritis
   (D) genital herpes
   (E) cytomegalovirus (CMV)

2. Three weeks after delivery, a 29-year-old primipara, who is breast-feeding twin girls, presents to the clinic, complaining of a tender right breast mass. On physical examination, you find a 5-cm fluctuant, swollen, reddened mass in her right breast that is exquisitely tender to the touch. Axillary lymph nodes on the ipsilateral side are enlarged and tender. What is the most appropriate next step in the management of this patient?

   (A) excisional biopsy of the mass
   (B) needle aspiration of the mass

   (C) intravenous antibiotic therapy for the mother and infants
   (D) have the patient continue to breast-feed on the other side
   (E) incision and drainage of the mass plus oral antibiotics for the mother

3. Two weeks after the birth of her infant, a new mother brings the child in to see you. The child's eyes are edematous, with conjunctival erythema and a mucopurulent discharge. Your evaluation and treatment should include which of the following?

   (A) a pelvic examination (using a small scope) of the infant
   (B) culture maternal genital tract for GC and chlamydia
   (C) anaerobic cultures of the infant's and mother's eyes
   (D) immunoglobulin M (IgM) titers of the infant
   (E) penicillin VK for both the mother and the infant

4. Three days after an elective termination of pregnancy, a 29-year-old woman presents to the emergency department with a history of mild abdominal pain and fever, a physical examination showing pelvic tenderness, and a purulent cervical discharge. A Gram's stain of the cervical discharge shows gram-negative intracellular diplococci. What is the most likely causative agent in this patient's case?

(A) *Neisseria gonorrhoeae*
(B) *Chlamydia trachomatis*
(C) *Escherichia coli*
(D) *Treponema pallidum*
(E) *Staphylococcus aureus*

5. A 31-year-old woman in her first trimester presents for her initial visit. She complains of a painless raised lesion in her vulva. Examination reveals a chancre. Rapid plasma reagin (RPR) test with elevated titer is positive along with fluorescent treponemal antibody absorption (FTA-ABS), confirming the diagnosis of primary syphilis. The patient should be offered which of the following counseling or treatment options?

(A) Offer the woman termination, as the fetus will be infected and develop congenital syphilis.
(B) Immediately treat her with parenteral penicillin G.
(C) The causative agent for syphilis, *T. pallidum*, does not cross the placenta; therefore, there is no risk for congenital syphilis.
(D) Penicillin-allergic women should be treated with erythromycin.
(E) If a fetus is affected, the anatomic ultrasound will always be abnormal.

6. A woman has a stillborn infant covered with a petechial rash. Which of the following infections would be most likely?

(A) herpes zoster
(B) herpes simplex
(C) *Listeria monocytogenes*
(D) human papillomavirus (HPV)
(E) chronic active hepatitis

7. Regarding immunization during pregnancy, which of the following vaccines would be the safest to receive during pregnancy?

(A) mumps
(B) polio
(C) rabies
(D) rubella
(E) rubeola (measles)

8. A patient presents to labor and delivery in active labor and has a precipitous delivery within 15 minutes of arrival. Her prenatal care has been erratic. During the repair of a second-degree laceration, you note ulcerations on the labia consistent with herpes simplex virus (HSV). On further questioning of the patient, her history is consistent with a primary outbreak of herpes. You send cultures but recommend immediate treatment of the newborn for HSV while waiting for the results. When the patient inquiries why, you tell her that HSV infection in pregnancy is associated with a neonatal mortality rate for untreated infected infants. What is this mortality rate?

(A) 10%
(B) 25%
(C) 50%
(D) 75%
(E) 95%

9. An infant, seemingly well when born, demonstrates microcephaly, chorioretinitis, deafness, and delayed development later in life. Which of the following is the most likely cause?

(A) type 2 herpes hominis virus acquired at the time of delivery
(B) CMV infection during pregnancy
(C) vitamin K deficiency in the newborn
(D) late-onset group B streptococcal infection
(E) parvovirus infection

10. A 19-year-old woman who has never had chickenpox has just been exposed to the disease (approximately 36 hours ago) at 16 weeks' gestation. What is the most appropriate next step in the management of this patient?

(A) reassurance only

(B) a measurement of maternal varicella titer 3 weeks after exposure

(C) a measurement of maternal varicella titer 6 weeks after exposure

(D) the patient should be advised to consider termination

(E) the administration of varicella zoster immune globulin (VZIG)

11. A 27-year-old gravida you have been following throughout her pregnancy presents at 22 weeks' gestation not feeling well. She complains of fever, cough, a runny nose, conjunctivitis, and on examination has white spots surrounded by a halo of erythema on her buccal mucosa and an erythematous maculopapular rash on her abdomen. What is the most likely cause of this patient's condition?

(A) varicella zoster

(B) rubella

(C) rubeola (measles)

(D) syphilis

(E) herpes

12. A 25-year-old G1 is newly pregnant. She is found to be rubella nonimmune. She asks you about the implication of this. You should inform her about which of the following?

(A) A significant percentage of fetuses of women who develop rubella infection during pregnancy will develop congenital rubella syndrome.

(B) Rubella infection increases maternal mortality.

(C) Treatment with antiviral medications is effective.

(D) She should receive rubella immunization during this pregnancy.

(E) If she is infected, she will likely develop significant fever and rash.

13. Of the following individuals, who would theoretically be at highest demographic risk for toxoplasmosis infection during pregnancy?

(A) country western singer

(B) medical technologist

(C) plumber

(D) cat breeder

(E) kitchen worker in Los Angeles

14. A 25-year-old sexually active woman complains of a "fishy" smelling gray-white vaginal discharge. You examine this on wet mount and see epithelial cells with clusters of bacteria obscuring their borders. The vaginal pH is 5.5. This infection has been most closely implicated in which of the following complications of pregnancy?

(A) intrauterine growth restriction

(B) preterm birth

(C) congenital cataracts

(D) learning disabilities during childhood

(E) preeclampsia

15. A 45-year-old Laotian woman is visiting her daughter. She comes to your office complaining of frequent intermenstrual bleeding for years. You examine her and feel that her pelvis is "firmly fixed," with little mobility of the organs. You perform an endometrial biopsy. The pathology report returns stating that "frequent giant cells, caseous necrosis, and granuloma formation" are seen. Which of the following is the most likely cause of this woman's condition?

(A) syphilis

(B) *C. trachomatis*

(C) tuberculosis

(D) *N. gonorrhoeae*

(E) *L. monocytogenes*

16. A 43-year-old woman has had a history of frequency, urgency, and dysuria for the past 8 years. She has had five negative urine cultures and urinalyses in the last year. Cystoscopy 1 month ago showed a normal bladder and reddened urethra. An intravenous pyelogram (IVP) is normal. What is the most likely diagnosis?

    (A) surreptitious use of antibiotics by the patient to mask her laboratory results
    (B) tuberculous urethritis
    (C) vulvar vestibulitis syndrome
    (D) urethral syndrome
    (E) urethral gonorrhea

17. A 51-year-old woman presents complaining of dysuria, dyspareunia, frequency of urination, dribbling of urine from the urethra when she stands after voiding, and a painful swelling under her urethra. Which of the following is the most likely diagnosis?

    (A) simple cystitis
    (B) urethral syndrome
    (C) infection of the Skene's glands
    (D) infected urethral diverticulum
    (E) urethral carcinoma

**Questions 18 and 19 apply to the following patient:**

On the evening after a vaginal hysterectomy, a patient develops a temperature of 100.4°C. You are called to evaluate her.

18. Which of the following do you consider most likely prior to examining the patient?

    (A) She probably has a UTI.
    (B) Ureteral obstruction is likely.
    (C) Her fever may be factitious.
    (D) She may be having an allergic reaction to her medications.
    (E) The temperature elevation is most likely unrelated to a surgical infection.

19. The same patient continues to have fever in the 102°F to 104°F range over the next few days. A pelvic examination is repeated and a midline, tender mass approximately 8 cm in diameter is noted over the vaginal cuff. What is the most appropriate next step in this patient's management?

    (A) obtain an ESR and WBC, and start or change antibiotics
    (B) get an infectious disease consult
    (C) send a vaginal culture to assess the coverage of your antibiotics
    (D) open the vaginal cuff in the midline
    (E) aspirate the vaginal cuff for culture

20. The hospital is reviewing its protocols to decrease the iatrogenic infection rate within the hospital. For which of the following procedures would prophylactic antibiotics be appropriate?

    (A) amniocentesis
    (B) laparoscopy
    (C) tubal sterilization
    (D) vaginal hysterectomy
    (E) episiotomy repair

21. A 35-year-old woman undergoes a cesarean section after a failed induction for postmaturity. Three days after surgery, she develops a high spiking fever. Ampicillin and gentamicin are administered. Complete physical examination shows no abnormality except a tender uterus. Blood, urine, and sputum cultures are negative. On the fifth day after surgery, a hectic (spiking) fever is still present. The antibiotics are changed to ampicillin, gentamicin, and clindamycin in high dosage. Forty-eight hours later, the fever persists, and examination shows a tender uterus. A chest X-ray is normal. Pelvic CT is consistent with parametrial thrombosed vessels but no abscess. Which of the following is the next best step in managing this patient?

    (A) reoperate to find the source of the fever
    (B) anticoagulate the patient with heparin
    (C) get an infectious disease consult
    (D) discontinue all antibiotic medication and reculture the patient
    (E) change antibiotics again

22. A 34-year-old woman (gravida 2, para 1) is at 13 weeks' gestation by last menstrual period (LMP) with a desired pregnancy. She presents to the emergency department very anxious with a 10-hour history of low abdominal cramping and vaginal bleeding. Her temperature is 102.2°F, and her uterus is markedly tender on bimanual examination. Ultrasound shows an intrauterine pregnancy with a crown–rump length consistent with her LMP and fetal cardiac activity present. Her cervix is dilated by 1 cm. Her WBC count is 26,000. What is the best management for this patient?

   (A) place a cervical cerclage immediately after administering antibiotics
   (B) administer antibiotics and expectantly manage her
   (C) evacuate her uterus after administering antibiotics
   (D) administer antibiotics, and if she does not spontaneously abort after 24 hours of observation, place a cervical cerclage
   (E) place her on bed rest and administer both a tocolytic and antibiotics

**Questions 23 through 25 apply to the following patient:**

An asymptomatic 24-year-old African-American woman with sickle cell trait is found on routine prenatal screening at 14 weeks' gestation to have symptomatic bacteriuria ($10^5$ colonies/mL).

23. What is her risk of developing pyelonephritis if untreated?

   (A) 5–10%
   (B) 20–30%
   (C) 40–50%
   (D) 60–70%
   (E) 90–100%

24. What is the most likely organism to be cultured?

   (A) group B streptococcus
   (B) *Klebsiella pneumoniae*
   (C) *C. trachomatis*
   (D) *Proteus* species
   (E) *E. coli*

25. What is an appropriate choice of antibiotic therapy for this patient pending culture results?

   (A) ampicillin
   (B) tetracycline
   (C) ciprofloxacin
   (D) nitrofurantoin
   (E) metronidazole

**DIRECTIONS (Questions 26 through 43): The following groups of questions are preceded by a list of lettered options. For each question, select the one lettered option that is most closely associated with it. Each lettered option may be used once, multiple times, or not at all.**

**Questions 26 through 32**

   (A) candidal vaginal infections
   (B) *Trichomonas*
   (C) bacterial vaginosis
   (D) atrophic vaginitis
   (E) mucopurulent cervicitis
   (F) foreign body

26. Most common type of vaginitis with a high pH in the sexually active patient.

27. In cases of treatment failure, combined oral and intravenous therapy with metronidazole may be indicated.

28. The patient complains of a white, curdy discharge, and vaginal burning and itching; on examination, the copious discharge is confirmed. The vaginal pH is 3.0.

29. Associated most commonly with chlamydia or gonorrhea.

30. Diagnosis may require vaginoscopy.

31. The treatment should include intravaginal estrogen therapy.

32. The most likely causative organism also has a highly associated incidence of upper genital tract infection.

**Questions 33 through 43**

   (A)  uncomplicated anogenital gonorrhea

   (B)  disseminated gonococcal infection

   (C)  syphilis

   (D)  chancroid

   (E)  lymphogranuloma venereum

   (F)  donovanosis

   (G)  pediculosis pubis

   (H)  scabies

   (I)  molluscum contagiosum

   (J)  genital herpes infection

   (K)  HPV infection

   (L)  genital mycoplasma

**33.** Diagnosis can be made from culture on Thayer–Martin or Transgrow media.

**34.** An asymptomatic disease on the vulvar skin, spread by close contact; it can be found as a disseminated disease in children that is not necessarily spread by sexual contact.

**35.** The causative organism for genital condyloma, an etiologic agent, cofactor, or enhancer for the development of most intraepithelial neoplasias of the genital tract.

**36.** A 44-year-old schoolteacher returns from a vacation in Haiti, where she had unprotected intercourse with a native Haitian approximately 3 weeks previously; she now has a painless vulvar ulcer.

**37.** A 48-year-old Nigerian woman presents with vesicular and pustular lesions with ulceration of the vulvar areas. She also has painful elevated inguinal nodes.

**38.** One of the most infectious of all sexually transmitted diseases (STDs); characteristic lesions are found at the base of hair follicles.

**39.** One week after her first intercourse, an 18-year-old college student presents to your office with intense, constant itching in the area of her pubic hair; on examination, you think you see red "moles" that are moving.

**40.** A patient reports having had intercourse with a new sexual partner approximately 8 days ago and now complains of general malaise and fever, vulvar pain, pruritus, and vaginal discharge; genital examination shows tender inguinal lymphadenopathy and vesicles and ulcers on the labia majora bilaterally.

**41.** A 41-year-old woman returns from a job on a Caribbean cruise ship. She had several new sexual partners during the 3-week cruise. A few days before coming to see you, she noticed the growth of an asymptomatic vulvar nodule. The skin ulcerated over the nodule, and she now has a beefy-red ulcer. She thinks additional nodules may be developing. The ulcer is painless, and there are no associated groin lesions or enlarged lymph nodes.

**42.** Caused by *Hemophilus ducreyi*, the disease is characterized by a painful ulcer, most commonly of the vaginal vestibule.

**43.** Frequently isolated from the cervix and vagina, its role as a cervical pathogen is unclear.

# Answers and Explanations

1. **(A)** The diagnosis of intra-amniotic infection (also called chorioamnionitis) is often one of the exclusions. The most common physical findings are fever, maternal/fetal tachycardia, uterine tenderness, foul-smelling vaginal discharge, and preterm labor. The most common causative organisms are bacteria and probably most often are polymicrobial. Organisms include group B streptococcus, *Gardnerella vaginalis*, and *Mycoplasma hominis*. The primary treatment is delivery and secondarily initiation of broad-spectrum antibiotic therapy. The most common neonatal sequela is pneumonia.

2. **(E)** This is a classic presentation of puerperal mastitis with a localized breast abscess. The most common causative organism is *S. aureus* from the infants' normal mouth flora. Approximately 10% of women with mastitis will develop an abscess. The abscess needs to be drained and an appropriate antibiotic, such as dicloxacillin or erythromycin, should be given to the mother. Women with mastitis or abscess should continue to evacuate the breast frequently by nursing or pumping, if possible.

3. **(B)** The infant is very likely to have a *C. trachomatis* conjunctivitis from passage through the birth canal of the infected mother. It causes conjunctivitis 1 to 2 weeks after delivery in the infant and may be an indolent organism that causes pelvic infection in the mother. The diagnosis is made from immunologic enzyme assay in most cases. The mother can be treated with a tetracycline or preferably with erythromycin if she is breast-feeding. The infant should be treated with oral erythromycin and/or sulfa ointment to the eyes. Tetracycline can stain the infant's permanent teeth.

4. **(A)** While not pathognomonic, the finding of gram-negative intracellular diplococci combined with the history of intrauterine instrumentation makes the likelihood of gonorrhea approximately 100%. A syphilitic lesion should be sought on all patients with venereal disease, but it is not a high-prevalence STD in most settings. Given the likelihood of gonorrhea as the causative organism, the patient and all recent partners should be treated.

5. **(A)** The incidence of syphilis has been increasing in recent years in the United States. It is due to spirochete *T. pallidum*. Because of fetal immunocompetence, these organisms seldom clinically affect the fetus before 18 weeks' gestation. The fetus can acquire syphilis via placental passage or via contact with vaginal or vulvar lesions at the time of delivery. Women diagnosed and treated early may avoid any negative effect on their fetus. Maternal treatment would consist of immediate parenteral penicillin G. There are no proven alternatives to penicillin during pregnancy and women with penicillin allergy should undergo skin testing to confirm risk of anaphylaxis and then undergo desensitization. Fetal ultrasound may be suggestive of infection with hydrops, ascites, and hepatomegaly; however, some infected fetuses will be sonographically normal.

6. **(C)** Listeriosis is characterized by abortion, stillbirth, septicemia, and encephalitis. It has a characteristic rash in infants that is often

described as petechial or granulomatous in appearance and is a good candidate for the stillbirth. It causes overwhelming sepsis in infants much like group B streptococcus. Maternal septicemia is also common. It is unusual for listeriosis to cause repetitive pregnancy loss.

7. **(B)** Polio vaccine is generally a vaccine made from an inactive virus and, therefore, safe to receive during pregnancy. Mumps, rabies, rubella, and rubeola are live virus vaccines and, therefore, not generally felt to be as safe in pregnancy. Other inactive virus vaccines include hepatitis B and influenza vaccines. Killed bacterial vaccines include pertussis, typhoid, typhus, cholera, meningococcus, and rickettsia. Toxoids include diphtheria and tetanus. Killed bacteria vaccines and toxoids are also thought to be safe during pregnancy.

8. **(C)** Genital herpes is usually symptomatic in mothers when infants are overtly infected. Genital lesions can usually be found. Transmission rates to infants are probably approximately 30% in mothers who have primary outbreak late in pregnancy and only 3% when maternal infections are recurrent. Infant infection is associated with high neonatal mortality rates, nearly 50% among nontreated infants. Preexisting antibody to HSV-2 but not to HSV-1 reduces the risk of vertical transmission of HSV-2. Acyclovir has been demonstrated to be effective in diminishing the rate of recurrent genital herpes outbreaks.

9. **(B)** CMV is an asymptomatic maternal infection passed to the infant during gestation. Virus can be isolated from any body fluid. Nearly all of the infected infants will be asymptomatic at birth, but 5% to 15% will develop the central nervous system manifestations during early childhood. Vitamin K deficiency causes neonatal coagulopathy. Late-onset group B streptococcal infection is typically manifested by bacteremia, meningitis, and pneumonia. In utero infection with parvovirus is a cause of fetal hydrops. Infection in young children is generally associated with fever, malaise, adenopathy, and a characteristic rash.

10. **(E)** Varicella zoster is a highly contagious virus that causes chickenpox. It is a more severe disease in adults than in children and has been reported to cause pneumonia in 10% of infected pregnant women. Approximately 10% of fetuses can become infected in utero when the gravida is exposed in early pregnancy. Severe congenital malformation of the limbs, chorioretinitis, and cerebral cortical atrophy are possible as a result of exposure. The administration of VZIG within 96 hours of exposure will attenuate most infections. Before administering VZIG, maternal serum can be tested to see if the patient is immune.

11. **(C)** This is a classic presentation of measles (rubeola), especially the pathognomonic (Koplik) spots. It seldom has an effect in midgestation. Vaccination is not indicated during pregnancy, and if you already have the infection, vaccination is of no value. Some authorities would recommend passive immunity.

12. **(A)** Congenital rubella is teratogenic and often fatal to the fetus or neonate. Eighty percent of fetuses will be affected if the mother was infected during the first trimester and manifested a rash. By the end of the trimester, the fetal infection rate drops to 25%. Maternal symptoms are usually quite mild with low-grade fever and maculopapular rash; however, 50% are subclinical. It is seldom dangerous to the gravida but has been increasing in frequency in recent years. Vaccination is the key to prevention and should be performed shortly after pregnancy or when adequate contraception is being used. Vaccination during pregnancy is not recommended.

13. **(D)** Those who eat raw meat and those who handle cat feces (litter box cleaners) are at greatest risk for toxoplasmosis infection during pregnancy. The cat breeder is at greatest risk. The rate of primary infection in pregnancy is low (approximately 1 per 1,000) and only 10% of those infected will have serious neonatal sequelae. Women who desire to be tested for this disease will show appropriate immunoglobulin (IgG) titers that can be measured before pregnancy. During pregnancy, the most appropriate test is to follow titers to see if a dramatic rise can

be demonstrated. A patient with a household pet is highly unlikely to be exposed to toxoplasmosis and so screening is not typically offered. These women may opt not to be responsible for cleaning the litter box if they are concerned.

14. **(B)** The infection described is bacterial vaginosis, which results from an overgrowth of many anaerobic bacteria. It has been associated with preterm birth, and oral, rather than topical, therapy is preferred in pregnancy. The treatment of choice is metronidazole; clindamycin and amoxicillin/clavulanic acid are also effective. Douching is not a recommended practice because it can disturb the natural flora (i.e., lower the concentration of lactobacillus), which can make women more prone to vaginal infections. The male partner is not symptomatic and does not generally require treatment.

15. **(C)** Tuberculosis of the female genital tract is found in Asia, Latin America, and the Middle East as a cause of infertility and pelvic inflammatory disease (PID). The diagnosis can be established by biopsy in the secretory phase of the cycle. Treatment consists of 24 months of combination antituberculous drugs. Surgery is reserved for those who fail medical therapy.

16. **(D)** Urethral syndrome has same symptoms as cystitis. Its etiology is unknown, and the only physical findings may be tenderness and redness of the urethra on urethroscopic examination. While tuberculosis and gonorrhea may give you sterile cultures (because a special medium is needed) with urethral infection, both do produce pyuria, which is not present in this patient. Antibiotics should make the symptoms better and not mask a diagnosis of simple cystitis.

17. **(D)** This patient has the classic triad of symptoms for urethral diverticulum: dysuria, dyspareunia, and dribbling of urine after voiding. The tender suburethral mass is the most common physical finding. The mass needs to be excised as it is a source of chronic infection.

18. **(E)** Seventy-five percent of women may show some elevation of temperature during the evening after having had surgery, more so after vaginal than abdominal hysterectomy. Only one-fifth of postoperative fevers is related to infection. UTI is the most common cause of true infection in any patient who has been catheterized at the time of surgery. It is not the most common cause of an isolated temperature elevation. Ureteral obstruction, factitious fevers, and febrile allergic reactions are uncommon. Postsurgical atelectasis is by far the most common cause.

19. **(D)** This history, combined with the finding of a tender mass, gives you the diagnosis of pelvic abscess. Abscesses need to be opened and drained. Opening the vaginal cuff is easy, and material for culture usually comes flowing out. This alone will lead to cure in 12 to 36 hours in most cases.

20. **(D)** There has been no benefit shown from antibiotic prophylaxis for minor procedures unless the patient is immunocompromised or is at high risk for infecting an abnormal heart valve. Prophylactic use of antibiotics has been shown to be of benefit in both abdominal and vaginal hysterectomies. The typical antibiotic of choice is a cephalosporin given 30 to 60 minutes prior to the incision.

21. **(B)** In this case, the patient has all the classic findings of septic pelvic thrombophlebitis, especially a spiking (hectic) fever. She has had an adequate trial of a broad-spectrum antibiotic followed by combination broad-spectrum antibiotics without success. It is thought that tiny, inflamed clots need to be anticoagulated while waiting for resolution.

22. **(C)** This woman is undergoing a septic abortion, a potentially fatal condition if not treated promptly and appropriately. The fetus is not salvageable. After adequate blood levels of broad-spectrum antibiotics are achieved, her uterus must be promptly evacuated.

23. **(B)** The prevalence of asymptomatic bacteriuria in pregnancy is 5% to 10%, and all pregnant women should have urine cultures at their first prenatal visit to detect this. Treatment

reduces the risk of acute cystitis and pyelonephritis. Approximately 20% to 30% of women with untreated lower UTI will develop pyelonephritis. Pyelonephritis in pregnancy can result in preterm labor, septic shock, and adult respiratory distress syndrome.

24. **(E)** *E. coli* is the most frequent organism identified on urine culture, responsible for 80% to 90% of initial infections. Other common organisms include *Staphylococcus, Saprophyticus, K. pneumoniae, Proteus* sp., and *Enterococci.*

25. **(D)** In recent years, 20% to 30% of *E. coli* strains have developed resistance to ampicillin, so this is not a good choice unless sensitivity tests are known. Tetracycline and ciprofloxacin are contraindicated in pregnancy because of their teratogenic effects. Metronidazole is effective against anaerobes that are a cause of pelvic infection but are not common uropathogens. Nitrofurantoin is the best choice. It has activity against most gram-negative aerobic bacilli and its cost is relatively low.

26–32. **(26-C, 27-B, 28-A, 29-E, 30-F, 31-D, 32-E)** Vulvovaginitis and mucopurulent cervicitis are the two most common symptoms of infections in the lower genital tract. Vaginitis is more common, affecting nearly every woman at some time in her life. Bacterial vaginosis (previously called *Gardnerella* vaginitis) is the most common cause of vaginitis with a pH > 4.7. Laboratory evaluation of vaginitis includes taking a pH of the vaginal secretions and looking at wet mounts of the secretions diluted, respectively, with normal saline and potassium hydroxide (KOH). *Candida* does not change the normal pH of the vagina (3 to 4.5). *Trichomonas* and bacterial vaginosis are treated with metronidazole, but *Trichomonas* may be resistant to standard doses and require both oral and intravenous therapies in some cases. Children also are susceptible to the same types of vaginal infections but foreign bodies (the most common one being toilet paper) must also be considered as a common cause. Because of the small vagina in children, a small diameter scope might have to be used to make the diagnosis and perhaps used for removal of the foreign body (vaginoscopy). Elderly women may also have vaginitis symptoms because of the vaginal atrophy induced by lack of estrogen. Replacement therapy with estrogen will generally alleviate this problem. Finally, it must be remembered that not all discharge from the vagina is from vaginal infection. Cervicitis from gonorrhea, *Chlamydia*, herpes simplex, and flat condyloma can cause excessive discharge. Whenever discharge from the cervix is seen, STDs must be strongly suspected, and the caregiver must realize that the patient is at great risk of infection in the upper genital tract (Figure 24–1).

33. **(A)** Uncomplicated anogenital gonorrhea is most often asymptomatic in women. The most common symptom when present would be vaginal discharge followed by dysuria and/or anogenital itching. Diagnosis is made by culture onto a selective media such as Thayer–Martin or Transgrow media, or more currently by nucleic acid amplification tests for DNA. Patients with gonorrhea may have a 20% to 40% chance of also being infected with *Chlamydia*.

34. **(I)** Molluscum contagiosum is a viral disease. Women are generally asymptomatic other than for the unpleasant appearance of the lesions on the vulvar skin. The disease is spread by close contact but is not very contagious, despite what the name implies. It may be a disseminated disease in children that is not necessarily spread by sexual contact. The incubation period is weeks to months. Characteristic small nodules or firm vesicles with a waxy appearance and some with umbilicated centers are present. Either the gross appearance or biopsy is diagnostic. They are treated by simple debridement.

35. **(K)** HPV is the causative organism for genital condyloma acuminata (not condyloma latum, which is associated with syphilis). HPV is also the etiologic agent for the development of most intraepithelial neoplasias of the genital tract.

36. **(C)** Primary syphilis is associated with painless genital ulcers (chancre) on the labia, vulva, vagina, cervix, anus, lips, or nipples. The lesion appears 10 to 90 days after the initial infection. The chancre lasts 1 to 5 weeks and will resolve without treatment; however, the infective

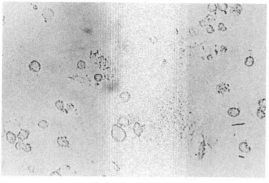

A. Trichomonads

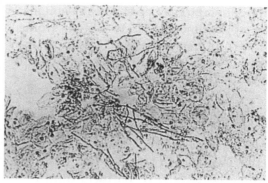

C. *Candida albicans* on normal saline prep

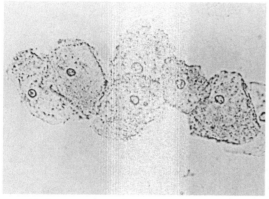

B. Clue cells of BV on normal saline prep

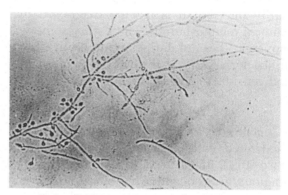

D. *Candida* showing budding on KOH prep

**Figure 24–1.** Vaginitis.
(Reproduced, with permission, from DeCherney AH, Nathan L. *Current Obstetric and Gynecologic Diagnosis & Treatment*, 9th ed. New York: McGraw-Hill, 2003.)

organism remains. The disease is treated with penicillin, erythromycin, or tetracycline. Haiti is endemic for syphilis.

37. **(E)** In lymphogranuloma venereum, the causative organism is *C. trachomatis*. Transmission is venereal with men affected six times more frequently than women. It presents as vesicular and pustular lesions with ulceration of the inguinal and vulvar areas. The characteristic exquisitely painful inguinal lesion is called a bubo. Late complications include rectal strictures. The disease is treated with doxycycline, tetracycline, erythromycin, or sulfa drugs.

38. **(G)** Pediculosis pubis is an infestation by the crab louse, *Phthirus pubis*, and is generally confined to the hairy areas of the vulva but occasionally may be found in the eyelashes. It may

be the most infectious of all STDs. Characteristic lesions are found at the base of hair follicles; colposcopy is an excellent way to see these lesions.

39. **(H)** Scabies is caused by *Sarcoptes scabiei*, a parasite with a red appearance resulting from blood consumption. They may be found anywhere on the body. Both pediculosis pubis and scabies are treatable with 5% permethrin (Nix) or lindane (Kwell) shampoo or cream.

40. **(J)** Genital herpes can produce systemic symptoms, including general malaise and fever, in women during the primary infection. Symptoms of vulvar pain, pruritus, and discharge peak between days 7 and 11 of the primary infection. The patient has severe symptoms for 14 days in these cases. However, the primary infection may be relatively asymptomatic and they are unrecognized in half of the early cases.

Severity of symptoms necessitates hospitalization for approximately 5% to 10% of women with known primary infection. Notorious as a recurring disease, genital herpes may be prophylactically treated with acyclovir.

41. **(F)** This is a classic presentation of donovanosis (granuloma inguinale), caused by *Calymmatobacterium granulomatis*. It is an STD (in most cases) that incubates in 1 to 12 weeks. It is transmitted to 10% to 50% of partners during intercourse. It presents as coalescing, ulcerating nodules that may not be painful unless secondarily infected. It is usually diagnosed by its clinical manifestations. The pathognomonic Donovan bodies are dark-staining (with silver stain) bacteria found in the cytoplasm of the infected cells. It is generally treated with tetracycline.

42. **(D)** Chancroid is an STD that is very uncommon in the United States. It is predominantly a male disease (10:1). It is caused by *H. ducreyi*, a very contagious, gram-negative rod-shaped bacteria. The disease cannot penetrate normal skin, so there must be an area of trauma where it enters. Lesions may be solitary or multiple and begin as a papule that later ulcerates. Lymph nodes are involved about half of the time. The diagnosis is made from a combination of Gram's stain, culture, and biopsy. Tetracycline, cephalosporins, penicillins, and sulfa drugs have all been used successfully for treatment.

43. **(L)** Genital mycoplasmas include *M. hominis* and *Ureaplasma urealyticum*. It is doubtful whether these organisms can cause mucopurulent cervicitis, and it is also doubtful that they cause any genital tract damage. They are often cultured and treated in infertility patients. Little useful information about their pathogenicity exists.

# CHAPTER 25

# Special Topics in Gynecology: Pediatric and Adolescent Gynecology, Sexual Abuse, Medical Ethics, and Medical–Legal Considerations

## Questions

**DIRECTIONS (Questions 1 through 18): For each of the multiple choice questions in this section, select the lettered answer that is the one *best* response in each case.**

1. A mother brings her 4-year-old daughter in for complaints of itching "down there" and staining on the underwear. Which of the following conditions is the most likely cause of vulvovaginal symptoms in children?

   (A) foreign body
   (B) lichen sclerosis
   (C) nonspecific
   (D) physiologic leukorrhea
   (E) trauma

2. A 6-year-old girl is referred by her pediatrician for a friable mass in the genital region. You suspect a urethral prolapse. Which of the following is the most common symptom of urethral prolapse in the prepubertal, unestrogenized girl?

   (A) dysuria
   (B) hematuria
   (C) painless genital bleeding
   (D) urinary frequency
   (E) urinary retention

3. A mother has brought in her 8-year-old daughter because of the development of breasts over the past year. They are now to the size that she is requiring a bra and is being teased by the other children. Premature thelarche differs from true precocious puberty in that premature thelarche is associated with which of the following?

   (A) axillary hair development
   (B) isolated breast development
   (C) pubic hair development
   (D) spontaneous ovulations
   (E) voice changes

4. A 14-year-old girl is brought into the office by her mother because of a concern of a lack of menarche. Her mother is worried that something is wrong since she has not started menstruating. Based on a complete history and limited physical and thorough application of a knowledge of normal pubarche changes, you may be able to calm the mother. Which of the following occurs earliest in preadolescent girls entering puberty?

   (A) axillary hair growth
   (B) breast development
   (C) menarche
   (D) peak growth velocity
   (E) pubic hair growth

5. A 16-year-old girl is seen in the emergency department for evaluation of nausea and vomiting. Her vital signs are blood pressure, 80/40 mm kg; pulse, 130 bpm; and temperature, 102.2°F. Physical examination shows conjunctivitis, oropharyngeal hyperemia, and a sunburn-like macular rash over the face, proximal extremities, and trunk. Palpation of the extremities elicits muscle tenderness. Pelvic examination is normal, and a bloody tampon is present in the vagina. Which of the following is the most likely diagnosis?

   (A) erysipelas
   (B) human immunodeficiency virus (HIV)
   (C) Kawasaki disease
   (D) syphilis
   (E) toxic shock syndrome (TSS)

6. A 14-year-old girl has a chronic cough with copious expectoration. A biopsy of the respiratory mucosa shows ciliated epithelium devoid of dynein arms. Which of the following conditions is most likely to occur in later life?

   (A) abnormal vaginal bleeding
   (B) chronic diarrhea
   (C) infertility
   (D) pelvic pain
   (E) urinary incontinence

**Questions 7 and 8 apply to the following patient:**

An 8-year-old girl is brought in by the mother after finding her crying and having bloody underwear. She will not tell her mother what happened. On examination, there are injuries consistent with vaginal penetration. You advise the mother that it is very important to allow the authorities to speak with the daughter about what happened.

7. What is the percentage of sexually abused children who know their assailant?

   (A) 15
   (B) 35
   (C) 55
   (D) 75
   (E) 95

8. Which of the following is the most commonly reported form of incest?

   (A) brother–sister
   (B) father–daughter
   (C) father–son
   (D) mother–son
   (E) stepfather–daughter

**Questions 9 and 10 apply to the following patient:**

A father brings his 9-year-old daughter to the office after he picked her up for his joint custody visit. He and his ex-wife have been in a long drawn-out custody battle. His daughter told him that her mom's new boyfriend was touching and poking her "down there" last night while mom was shopping.

9. When childhood sexual assault is suspected within the past 72 hours, which of the following should be the next action of the physician?

   (A) bring family members together for an interview
   (B) contact mental health workers
   (C) notify the police
   (D) perform a complete physical examination
   (E) report the incident to Child Protective Services

10. Which of the following is a legal but not a medical responsibility of the physician caring for an alleged sexual assault victim?

   (A) collecting samples of hair and vaginal secretions, and microscopic evaluation of motile sperm
   (B) obtaining a complete gynecologic history
   (C) obtaining informed consent from patient
   (D) offering postcoital hormonal prophylaxis to prevent pregnancy if reproductive age
   (E) providing counseling and emotional support

11. Which of the following legal theories describes the failure of a physician to disclose the risks of a procedure?

   (A) abandonment
   (B) breach of duty
   (C) informed consent
   (D) intentional tort
   (E) lack of diligence

12. Professional liability insurance that protects against claims made during the policy period, regardless of when the suit is filed, is which of the following?

   (A) claims-made policy
   (B) occurrence policy
   (C) tail policy
   (D) nose policy
   (E) time-limited policy

13. An 8-year-old girl is brought to your office soon after suffering a fall on her brother's bicycle. Her mother reports that the girl's foot slipped off the bicycle pedal, which resulted in the girl falling on the center bar of the bicycle. The girl complains of sharp pain between her legs. There has been no obvious bleeding and no other injuries are apparent. The girl is in moderate distress with a pulse of 110 bpm, blood pressure of 118/68 mm Hg, and respirations of 28/min. Physical examination is normal with the exception of inspection of the vulva where a 6-cm tender bluish mass is present in the area of the right labia majora. No further examination is possible because of the girl's discomfort. Which management is most directly related to an uncomplicated outcome?

   (A) topical application of ice
   (B) use of prophylactic antibiotics
   (C) bed rest for the next 24 hours
   (D) examination under anesthesia
   (E) surgical evacuation of the hematoma

14. Which legal document sets out a patient's wishes regarding her future health status, including end-of-life issues?

   (A) living will
   (B) proxy directive
   (C) advanced directive
   (D) informed consent
   (E) durable power of attorney

15. What is a common emotional sequella of rape?

   (A) mania
   (B) depression
   (C) rage
   (D) bipolar disorders
   (E) panic attacks

16. A 6-year-old girl is seen for a 10-day history of intense vulvar itching leading to excoriation. The vulva are noted to be diffusely inflamed. What is the most likely cause for these symptoms?

   (A) *Candida albicans* infection
   (B) foreign body
   (C) sexual assault
   (D) *Enterobius vermicularis*
   (E) atrophic vulvitis

17. Which of the following sales activities would be considered unethical in medical practice?

   (A) sale of a pessary fitted in the office
   (B) sale of prescription medications to be taken at home
   (C) sale of cookies for a local charity
   (D) sale of annual flu vaccine given in the office
   (E) brokered sale of a vacation home to patient

**18.** A patient presents for her new obstetrical visit. During her history, she reports that she is a Jehovah's Witness and will not accept any blood products. You counsel her regarding risks and benefits of receiving blood in case she experiences a massive hemorrhage. She listens to you politely, asks some appropriate questions, and then states she will not accept any blood products and would prefer to die than receive a transfusion. You must either refer the patient or honor this request as an example of which of the following ethical principles?

(A) justice
(B) beneficence
(C) autonomy
(D) nonmalfeasance
(E) religious independence

# Answers and Explanations

1. **(C)** Nonspecific vulvovaginitis (NSV) accounts for 25% to 75% of vulvovaginal symptoms in children. The predominant vaginal organism cultured in NSV is *E. coli*. Although vaginal colonization with *E. coli* occurs in asymptomatic girls, half of 3- to 10-year-old girls with NSV have this organism present in the vagina. Foreign bodies can cause a profuse, foul odor discharge but this is a less likely cause. Physiologic discharge is very uncommon a few months after delivery (due to maternal estrogen) and prior to onset of puberty. Trauma such as straddle injuries or sexual abuse is uncommon but needs to be included in the differential.

2. **(C)** Girls with urethral prolapse typically experience painless genital bleeding. This symptom can be precipitated by straining or constipation. Urinary frequency and retention can also be seen occasionally. Dysuria and hematuria occur only with significant irritation and inflammation. Conservative management with estrogen cream and sitz baths is appropriate with surgical intervention only in extreme cases.

3. **(B)** Premature thelarche is the spontaneous development of breast tissue as an isolated event without other pubertal changes. It is caused by presence of estrogen only and not the normal cascade of pubertal events and may represent estrogen-secreting tumor such as a granulosa cell tumor. Premature onset of puberty involves activation of the full pubertal cascade that includes androgenic as well as estrogenic effects such as pubic hair along with breast development.

4. **(B)** Pubertal changes are marked by various stages of sexual and somatic development. A growth spurt, but not peak growth velocity, generally precedes the more readily identifiable sexual changes of puberty. Breast development or thelarche is the first sexual sign of puberty in the female, usually occurring between 9 and 11 years of age. Breast development is complete within 3.5 years after onset. Adrenarche is the onset of sexual hair growth. Pubic hair growth occurs between 11 and 12 years of age, while axillary hair growth occurs later. Menarche is the final stage of puberty and occurs after 12 years of age. Thus if the patient has breast and pubic hair but only recently, she is likely having a slightly delayed but normal timing of her puberty. If none of these changes are occurring then she may be experiencing a delayed puberty or some difficulty.

5. **(E)** TSS has an incidence of only about 1–2 per 100,000 menstruating women annually. It was originally associated with one brand of superabsorbent tampon (Rely) but the incidence has been dramatically reduced since the removal of that tampon from the market in 1980. (The last active surveillance for TSS was in 1987.) TSS still occurs occasionally with the use of diaphragms, vaginal sponges, cervical caps, and postoperative wound infections. Symptoms of TSS occur during menstruation and include sudden high fever, flulike symptoms (sore throat, headache, diarrhea), erythroderma, signs of multisystemic failure, and hypotension. TSS is usually associated with vaginal strains of *S. aureus* producing an exfoliative exotoxin (toxic shock syndrome

toxin [TSST-1]). Adolescent females are at greatest risk for TSS because they have not yet developed immunity against TSST-1. Treatment of TSS includes aggressive supportive therapy (e.g., hydration, transfusion, replacement of coagulation factors, and use of vasoactive agents) and antistaphylococcal antibiotic therapy. Mechanical ventilation and hemodialysis may be required to treat adult respiratory distress syndrome and renal failure. Risk for recurrence of TSS is 30% and may be reduced by intermittent use of tampons during menses or by not using tampons.

6. **(C)** Immobile cilia syndrome, or Kartagener syndrome, refers to the congenital absence of dynein arms in ciliated epithelium. Abnormalities of microtubular structure may coexist. Patients with Kartagener syndrome have chronic cough, sinusitis, bronchiectasis, and airway obstruction. The diagnosis is usually made by microscopic examination of the respiratory mucosa. Immobile cilia may coexist in the fallopian tube epithelium and may increase the risk of infertility in some individuals.

7. **(D)** About 75% of sexually abused children know their assailant. At least one-half of these cases involve another family member.

8. **(B)** Incest refers to a sexual relationship between people who are related and cannot legally marry. The most commonly reported form of incest involves the father and his own daughter (75% of reported cases). Brother–sister incest may actually be the most common form of incest but is not reported often. A sexual relationship between a stepfather and child or between a mother's boyfriend and child is called "functional parent incest" because the individuals are not related.

9. **(D)** Any child in whom sexual assault is suspected within the past 72 hours should be examined immediately to document physical findings corroborating the assault. Since the child of an incestuous relationship may not disclose the full history in the presence of the involved family member, the parents and child should be interviewed separately. When sexual assault is suspected weeks to months earlier, the child can be examined after the interviewing process is completed. In many locations, suspected sexual assault at any age requires police notification and when a minor is involved, child protective service must also be contacted, although these notifications should be secondary to the immediate evaluation and care of the patient.

10. **(A)** It is important to distinguish legal from medical responsibilities in the care of an alleged sexual assault victim. The collection of hair and vaginal secretions for the microscopic evaluation of motile sperm and semen is a legal responsibility to provide evidence to the authorities for the sake of documentation. All of the other answers provided represent medical responsibilities to the patient.

11. **(B)** The doctrine of informed consent states that a patient having an unfavorable result from a procedure may seek recovery for failure of the physician to properly disclose the risks of the procedure. This disclosure as a part of the informed consent process is his legal duties to the patient. Recovery is not sought for medical negligence or fault. To avoid lawsuits claiming lack of informed consent, the physician should provide complete, understandable information regarding treatment, document informed discussions about the treatment, and personally obtain written consent from the patient after answering any questions and the likely benefit of the treatment. If the risk of a treatment has a realistic incidence of occurrence, it must be disclosed along with alternative treatments and their pros/cons.

12. **(B)** An occurrence policy protects against claims made during the policy period, regardless of when the suit is filed. This form of insurance is expensive for obstetric coverage. A claims-made policy protects against claims made during the life of the policy. It does not provide coverage if the policy is discontinued and the physician is subsequently sued for an event occurring when the policy was in effect. (For such coverage, an additional tail policy can be purchased when the claims-made policy is discontinued.)

13. **(A)** The first and most effective therapy for this type of vulvar injury is the application of ice. This reduces the pain and produces local vasospasm that reduces further growth of the hematoma. Unless there is evidence of continued growth of the hematoma or a suggestion of other associated trauma, examination under anesthesia or surgical exploration is both unnecessary and potentially harmful. Based on the history provided, there is little to suggest internal injuries that would warrant an examination under anesthesia. Surgical exploration is associated with an increased risk of infection and is associated with technical difficulties of finding the source of bleeding and securing hemostasis in the loose areolar tissues of the vulva. Unless the skin has been broken, there is no indication for antibiotic use. While vulvar hematomas are painful, ice and analgesics are generally sufficient to allow relatively normal activity. Normal activity neither exacerbates a stable hematoma nor hastens its resolution. Most patients can be allowed to increase their activity as tolerated, and bed rest is not indicated.

14. **(C)** An advance directive is the formal mechanism by which a patient may express here values regarding her future health status, including end-of-life issues. This directive may take the form of a living will, a proxy directive, or a durable power of attorney that designates someone else to be able to act in her stead if she were unable to do so by her self. Informed consent refers to process involving all the elements of information and ability that go into the patient's decisions regarding a proposed treatment, rather than a physical document.

15. **(B)** A well-defined rape trauma syndrome including isolation, depression, anxiety, somatic symptoms, suicide attempts, and posttraumatic stress disorder has been well described. There are three sequences in reaction to rape: a short-term, an intermediate, and a long-term reaction. A range of traumatic symptoms, such as somatic complaints, characterizes the short-term reaction; sleep disturbance and nightmares, fear, suspiciousness, anxiety, major depression, and impairment in social functioning are also common. Symptoms generally remain relatively stable for 2 or 3 months. Three months to 12 months after assault (intermediate phase) the diffuse anxiety usually becomes rape specific. Women then experience depression and social and sexual dysfunction. The long-term reaction, 1 year following the assault, involves anger, hypervigilance to danger, sexual dysfunction, and diminished capacity to enjoy life. Some of these symptoms may last for years or a lifetime. More than half of rape victims show some level of rape trauma.

16. **(A)** While the lower estrogen levels of childhood result in a relative atrophy of the vulva and vagina, infections with monilial species are still common and present in the same way as in reproductive women. Intravaginal foreign bodies in children more commonly present with a yellow, malodorous discharge or painless bleeding. Pin worms (*Enterobius vermicularis*) cause perineal itching predominately at night and will be easily differentiated from a monilial infection by inspection and microscopic examination of a vaginal specimen. Suspicion of sexual assault should also be a part of any presenting complaint when there is a discrepancy between the presenting complaint and the physical findings.

17. **(B)** Under most circumstances, the sale of products by physicians violates several generally accepted principles of medical ethics. First, and most important, the practice of physician sales to patients creates a potential conflict of interest with the physician's fiduciary responsibility to put the interests of patients above their own. When a product or device is only available by prescription and must be used or administered in the physician's office, it is acceptable to sell the item at cost, plus any associated overhead cost associated with having it available. This can also apply to devices, such as pessaries, that may not be readily available in the patient's community. Inexpensive items for the benefit of community organizations (such as Girl Scout cookies) are acceptable as long as the products are sold without pressure, and the physician does not derive a profit from such sales. Sale of products that clearly are external to the patient–physician relationship, would be considered appropriate, especially if brokered by a third party.

**18.** The principle of autonomy includes the ability of the patient, after being given the pros and cons of a procedure (or lack of it), to make a decision that she feels is best for her. In the case of Jehovah's Witnesses, this can pose a problem for some providers but they must acknowledge the patient's autonomy and ability to make an informed decision that we may not agree with. Beneficence means to do good. Although some may feel that to give blood is consistent with this principle, the patient's autonomy trumps it. Nonmaleficence is to do no harm, but a JW feels that to receive blood is having a harm done to her. Justice is complex and one might try to argue that allowing her to die if a major hemorrhage occurs thus leaving the newborn without a mother. Again autonomy trumps. There is no unique ethical principle of religious freedom.

# Primary Health Care for Women

## Questions

1. A 46-year-old patient has her serum cholesterol tested in your laboratory, and it is 280 mg/dL. Which of the following statements regarding this finding would be accurate to tell her?

   (A) Elevated serum cholesterol is the most significant risk factor in the development of ischemic cardiac disease.
   (B) Further evaluation will be needed.
   (C) She needs to see an internist immediately.
   (D) The pizza she had for lunch the previous day probably is responsible for the elevation.
   (E) Unless there is a family history of cardiac disease, she is less likely to develop heart problems than the rest of the population.

2. A 70-year-old woman who is in good health comes to your office for the first time. Her only disease prevention issue is that she smokes. While discussing this with her, which of the following should you tell her?

   (A) Assure her that 70 years of age is too old to be worrying about quitting smoking.
   (B) At 70 years of age, smoking is up to her, and she is certainly mature enough to make her own decisions.

   (C) If she got to be 70-year-old and smokes, it is probably good for her.
   (D) Inform her that her life expectancy may be 15 to 20 more years or longer, and that if she would like to try to quit smoking, you will assist her.
   (E) Thirty-five percent of people will die of cancer, and the greatest risk factor we know of for developing cancer is smoking.

3. There is a great deal of debate about what is the best screening strategy regarding the use of mammography. Which of the following is true about the most important feature of mammography?

   (A) It allays fears in women.
   (B) It can detect lesions as small as 1 mm.
   (C) It essentially misses no cancer.
   (D) It leads to a reduction in mortality in breast cancer in women aged 50 to 64 years.
   (E) It provides the caregiver with a medical–legal safety screen.

4. Many common illnesses are related to life choices that increase risks for developing medical complications. Such life choices include smoking, overeating, and use of illegal substances. The clinician needs to determine where the patient is regarding approaching change in behavior to direct management. A pregnant patient who is smoking 10 cigarettes a day has already arranged with family not to smoke around her, has established a quit date, and is enquiring about nicotine replacement. Which of the following best describes the mindset of this patient?

(A) action
(B) contemplative
(C) maintenance
(D) precontemplative
(E) relapse

**Questions 5 and 6 apply to the following patient:**

A 43-year-old woman, 5 ft 4 in. tall (163 cm) and weighing 176 lb (80 kg), presents for her annual examination and assistance on losing weight.

5. She asks "How many calories would I have to cut out each day to lose 1 pound per week?" Which of the following choices is the best response?

(A) 100
(B) 500
(C) 900
(D) 1,300
(E) 1,800

6. You also encourage her to exercise. Given her current status, which of the following is the best initial form of exercise for her to maximize the calories burned per week?

(A) bicycling
(B) jogging/running
(C) swimming
(D) tennis
(E) walking

7. A 27-year-old woman presents for her annual examination and renewal of her oral contracep-

tive (OC) pills. Her history and physical examination were unremarkable except for a nontender 4 × 4 cm enlargement of the left lobe of her thyroid. Which of the following is key in the evaluation of this finding?

(A) TSH level
(B) free T4 and free T3 levels
(C) radioactive iodine scan
(D) ultrasound with fine-needle aspirate
(E) MRI of neck

8. As part of a premarital examination, a 24-year-old teacher would like a measles vaccination because she is nonimmune. She asks, "Do I need to avoid pregnancy after getting this vaccination?" Which of the following is the most appropriate response?

(A) no, it is a killed vaccine and unnecessary
(B) no, it is a form of passive immunization and therefore noninfective
(C) yes, for 6 weeks
(D) yes, for 12 weeks because it is a live, attenuated vaccine
(E) yes, and if pregnancy is attained before 6 months, abortion is recommended

9. A 28-year-old woman who has been splenectomized as a result of a car accident wonders if there is any special immunization she should have as a result. Of the following choices, how should you answer her?

(A) measles
(B) mumps
(C) meningococcus
(D) pertussis
(E) pneumococcus

10. A patient presents to you with excruciating pain, and you confirm the diagnosis of a kidney stone. You would like to provide the greatest amount of pain relief possible until the stone can be treated or passes. Which of the following narcotics has the greatest analgesic potency (administered parenterally) when compared to morphine?

(A) codeine
(B) hydromorphone
(C) meperidine
(D) methadone
(E) oxycodone

11. A 77-year-old woman comes to see you with her daughter. The mother has recently moved in with the daughter because it is difficult for her to care for herself completely. At night, the mother seems to become confused, does not know where she is, and cannot recognize her daughter. Which of the following is this?

(A) a normal variant of aging and should be accepted
(B) an indication that the mother needs to be restrained at night for fear of hurting herself
(C) an indication of possible early dementia or organic brain syndrome, needing further evaluation
(D) controllable by administration of sleep medication early in the evening
(E) expected to resolve completely as the mother becomes more aware of her new surroundings

12. A 19-year-old patient comes in for an annual re-fill of her birth control pills. For the past 6 years her family physician has treated her for nodular cystic acne with what the patient feels are poor results. Which of the following should you recommend?

(A) isotretinoin
(B) stopping her OCs
(C) oral tetracycline
(D) topical benzoyl peroxide
(E) topical clindamycin

13. A woman and her husband are planning a trip to Mexico for their 25th anniversary. She has heard about "traveler's diarrhea" and wonders what advice you can give her. You should tell her to do which of the following?

(A) not to worry about it; very few people ever get it
(B) she will get it no matter what she does, and it will subside quickly on its own
(C) to be sure to drink plenty of water, not to eat uncooked meat or vegetables, and she will likely be fine
(D) to take oral clindamycin before they get to Mexico and all during their stay
(E) to take trimethoprim–sulfa tablets along and begin them at the first signs of diarrhea

14. A 39-year-old woman comes in complaining that every night just after going to bed she awakens with a severe, substernal burning that is relieved when she drinks a glass of milk. She is allergic to codeine and has a known gallstone. Physical examination shows she is 5 ft 4 in. tall and weighs 209 lb. Her general examination is normal. There is no abdominal tenderness. Her stool is guaiac negative. She would like to know what to do for long-term relief. Of the following choices, how should you advise her?

(A) antacids before bedtime
(B) an upper gastrointestinal X-ray series
(C) cholecystectomy
(D) histamine blockers
(E) weight loss and no eating within 3 hours of bedtime

15. A 34-year-old multigravid patient comes to your office with two complaints. She has difficulty having bowel movements. They occur about twice weekly and are associated with significant straining. She has also noticed a painful mass at the anus and some bright red blood on her toilet paper. On examination you see a bluish lump about 2 cm across the anus, a mild rectocele, and a normal digital rectal examination. A stool specimen is guaiac negative. Of the following choices, how should you advise her?

(A) that a biopsy of the mass is necessary
(B) to have a colonoscopy
(C) to drink 8 to 10 glasses of water each day, increase the amount of fiber in her diet, and soak the area in a tub of warm water twice daily
(D) to see a colorectal surgeon
(E) to use hydrocortisone suppositories for the discomfort

16. A 27-year-old woman has just begun a new job as an administrative assistant after working for years as an account representative at another bank. Over the last few weeks, she has developed a chronic, bilateral, nonpulsatile headache that begins every afternoon. Her 79-year-old aunt has recently died of a cerebral aneurysm, and she had a cousin who she believes died of a "brain tumor." Her neurologic examination is within normal limits. What do you tell her about the origin of her headaches?

(A) Given her family history, an angiogram is indicated.
(B) It is a common migraine headache, and she will need further evaluation.
(C) She needs to see a neurologist.
(D) She needs to see a psychiatrist.
(E) The headaches are most likely stress-related and can be managed without further testing.

17. A 48-year-old patient (gravida 2, para 2) presents for an annual examination. She has had a tubal ligation for contraception. She reports her menses occur every 25 to 28 days and are "normal." Her history and examination, including stool guaiac and skin, are unremarkable other than she appears somewhat pale on examination. Which of the following laboratory results should prompt an evaluation for a cause other than simply iron deficiency from menstrual loss?

(A) hemoglobin <11.5 g/dL
(B) increased total iron-binding capacity (TIBC)
(C) microcytic hypochromic cells on peripheral smear
(D) normal indices on an automatic analysis of peripheral smear
(E) normal to high reticulocyte count once corrected for the anemia

18. A 19-year-old woman (gravida 0, para 0) presents for her annual sports physical. She is 5 ft 10 in. tall and weighs 110 lb. She states that she has been having this weight for "a while" and attributes it to being the star forward for her nationally ranked college soccer team. She does note her last menses was more than 3 months ago. Her urine human chorionic gonadotropin (hCG) is negative. Which of the following findings would be inconsistent that her presentation is due to athletic involvement and instead raise the concern of an anorexic disorder?

(A) increased exercise tolerance
(B) increased physical activity
(C) lanugo hair
(D) low body weight
(E) resting bradycardia and hypotension

19. A 14-year-old patient presents complaining of knee pain that has been increasing over the past few months. Since she is the goalie for the high school soccer team, you suspect patellofemoral dysfunction. Which of the following would decrease a postpubertal girl's risk for this problem?

(A) hyperelastic joints
(B) increased angle from knee to pelvic girdle
(C) shallow trochlear groove configuration

(D) tight vastus lateralis musculature

(E) tight vastus medialis obliquus musculature

20. A 38-year-old woman presents with the complaints of symmetric polyarthritis, especially in the hands and wrists, marked morning stiffness that lasts for up to an hour, and nodules over her elbows. These complaints have been present and increasing over the past 3 to 4 months. Of the following differential list, which is the most likely diagnosis?

(A) ankylosing spondylitis

(B) gout

(C) osteoarthritis

(D) Reiter syndrome

(E) rheumatoid arthritis

21. A patient asks what she can do to minimize her risks of developing skin cancer. You inform her of which of the following?

(A) application of sunscreen is best just before sun exposure

(B) high altitudes are less dangerous for sun exposure dermal injury

(C) one will get sun damage on overcast days

(D) she should use a sunblocker with a sun protection factor (SPF) rating of 8 or less

(E) tanning booths use a form of ultraviolet (UV) radiation that is safer than sun exposure

22. During her annual examination, a patient states that she is very concerned about developing skin cancer due to a strong family history. You instruct her in the components of a skin examination that involves evaluating a lesion for danger signs for melanoma, which would include which of the following?

(A) asymmetry of appearance

(B) consistent dark black pigmentation

(C) diameter of 4 mm

(D) nonraised surface

(E) smooth border

**DIRECTIONS (Questions 23 through 36):** The following groups of questions are preceded by a list of lettered options. For each question, select the one lettered option that is most closely associated with it. Each lettered option may be used once, multiple times, or not at all.

**Questions 23 through 26 apply to the following patient:**

Match the diagnosis to each of the following patients.

(A) alopecia areata

(B) androgenic alopecia

(C) syphilitic alopecia

(D) systemic lupus–related alopecia

(E) telogen effluvium

(F) traumatic alopecia

23. A patient presents with acute hair loss in patches. Inspection of the patches shows complete hair loss without signs of inflammation and scarring. Hair can be easily plucked at the edge of these patches.

24. A patient complains of thinning of her hair on her crown over the past months. She reports her mother had a similar problem.

25. A patient presents 3 months' postpartum complaining that she is going bald. She describes large amounts of hair in her brush each morning and her hairdresser says her hair is thinner.

26. A patient presents complaining of temporal balding. She is African American and has worn her hair in plaited braids for years.

## Questions 27 through 30

The development of a rash in a pregnant woman can represent a simple uncomplicated infectious or allergic response or it can represent a disease process that can place the mother or the fetus at significant risk.

Choose the best diagnosis for each patient presentation.

(A) drug rash

(B) erythema multiforme

(C) Lyme disease

(D) measles

(E) pityriasis rosea

(F) rubella

(G) varicella

27. A 24-year-old woman presents with a generalized eruption of small oval lesions that are aligned along skin lines. She denies any constitutional symptoms. She did note a single large lesion a few days prior to the generalized rash.

28. A 22-year-old schoolteacher presents complaining of a rash that started as a bull's-eye pattern that rapidly enlarged. She had a flulike illness prior to the rash. Although she often hikes, she denies any tick bites.

29. A 19-year-old woman presents with vesicular pustular pruritic lesions on an erythematous base. The rash followed a high temperature. The rash started in the hairline and has rapidly spread to the entire body.

30. An 18-year-old college student from Vietnam presents with the complaint of a maculopapular rash that started on her face and spread rapidly. The rash followed a day of malaise, fever, headache, and conjunctivitis. Lymphadenopathy is evident in the postauricular and suboccipital nodes.

## Questions 31 through 33

Of the following which is the primary cause of mortality for each of the age groups?

(A) accidents

(B) cancer

(C) cerebral vascular disease

(D) chronic obstructive lung disease

(E) heart disease

(F) human immunodeficiency virus (HIV) infection

(G) homicide

(H) suicide

31. Women aged 15 to 34

32. Women aged 35 to 54

33. Women aged 55 to 64

## Questions 34 through 36

Back pain is a common complaint for women much of which is attributed to pregnancy, obesity, activity related, or osteoporosis. The ability to differentiate by history and physical examination those that require further imaging and treatment is necessary for providers who provide care for women. What is the diagnosis for the following patients?

(A) degenerative disease

(B) disk disease

(C) nerve root pain

(D) ankylosing spondylitis

(E) referred pain from pelvic viscera

34. A 65-year-old patient presents with complaints of back pain that is worse after exercise or at the end of the day.

35. A 30-year-old patient complains of back pain that is worse in the morning. Her examination reveals decreased range of motion of the spine and tenderness over the sacroiliac joints. There is a loss of lordosis.

36. A 45-year-old woman presents complaining of back pain that radiates down her legs and is accompanied by numbness, paresthesia, and some weakness. The pain is increased with normal activities and improved with rest.

# Answers and Explanations

1. **(B)** A serum cholesterol of 280 mg/dL is well outside the normal range. Cholesterol as a risk factor may be greatly overemphasized, but further evaluation is needed. You will need to fractionate it to determine her levels of low-density lipoprotein (LDL) and high-density lipoprotein (HDL). You will need to assess any other cardiac risk factors, such as a positive family history, 30% or more over ideal weight, smoking, exercise level, blood pressure, dietary intake, and other medical conditions (diabetes, hypothyroidism, hyperuricemia, and so forth).

2. **(D)** Smoking is associated with heart disease, chronic respiratory disease, and multiple cancers (head, neck, lung, and cervix). While no one lives forever, a 70-year-old woman could easily live to be 90. Would not you help a 20-year-old live to age 40? Offer this woman smoking cessation therapy; she may be more interested than one might think. About 23% of all deaths in the United States are due to cancer.

3. **(D)** Mammography is the most common method of detecting asymptomatic malignant disease in the breast, the second most prevalent of cancers deaths in women. It can be wrong and seldom finds cancer of less than 0.5 cm. It may create as much anxiety as it solves. Given the prevalence of breast cancer, its age-related incidence, the cost of mammography and the ability of mammogram to correctly identify women at significant risk for cancer, there has been a great deal of controversy as to which population of women benefits the greatest from this screening and when it is most cost-effective. Although there is general agreement of screening between ages 50 and 65, there is a great deal of disagreement as to when testing should start (ages 40 or 50) and frequency (every 1 or 2 years in low-risk women). This debate is representative of many of the debates that will be occurring over the next decade as screening strategies are critically reviewed for cost-effectiveness.

4. **(A)** Behavioral change requires a great deal of motivation and investment by the patient. A model commonly used to determine if a patient is ready to try and change is the "stages of change." This allows the provider to determine where the patient is in his or her approach to the problem and the physician can direct the intervention accordingly. Directing intervention inappropriately can create barriers between the physician and the patient. The stages are (1) precontemplative (they really are not considering change at this time—physician input at this stage is to provide information as to why they may want to consider change); (2) contemplative (the patient is considering change but has not developed a plan or time line for initiating change—the provider can provide information to reinforce the benefits of change and help to develop a plan; (3) action (the patient has already initiated steps for change such as setting a date or has initiated behavioral change; (4) maintenance (the patient has successfully achieved change but is at risk for relapse and needs support and monitoring for relapse); and (5) relapse (patients need to be supported that a relapse is not a failure but an opportunity to learn more about why they have the behavior that needs

changing. It is important to help them return to action stage with a more focused plan for change).

5. **(B)** This is a very simple calculation. A negative calorie balance of 3,500 kcal is required to lose 1 lb. So 3,500 kcal/lb divided by 7 means 500 kcal less per day loses about 1 lb per week. She would need to maintain the same level of exercise.

6. **(E)** Although bicycling or swimming will use up to 200 cal/h and tennis and jogging even more, it is difficult for an overweight person who has not been exercising to do these activities for more than a few minutes. However, walking (at 150 cal/h) is more consistent with their abilities. Thus, the patient will typically be more successful at walking for 30 or more minutes per session and do it three or four times per week. As their conditioning improves, they can change to more demanding activities if they prefer.

7. **(D)** An asymmetric enlargement of a lobe of the thyroid is a nodule till proven otherwise. A patient with a hyperthyroidism from Graves or hypothyroidism goiter will have a diffusely enlarged thyroid. Given that the patient is asymptomatic makes it unlikely that this is a case of multinodular thyroiditis. It is essential that a thyroid ultrasound is done and if a discrete nodule is found that a fine-needle aspiration is done to evaluate for cancer. If cancer is found and lymph nodes are appreciated, an MRI might be indicated. Radioactive iodine scans are rarely used since the FNA under ultrasound guidance provides a more accurate diagnosis compared to the classification of a hot or cold nodule. Thyroid cancer rates seem to be increasing and is one of the cancers found in younger women. Given the low cost of a thyroid examination at the well woman examination, the low rate of false-positive examinations, the increasing incidence of thyroid cancer and effectiveness of surgery to cure the cancer, it is probably reasonable to continue to do thyroid examinations for screening at annual well women examinations.

8. **(D)** Measles is a live, attenuated vaccine. It is given as a single subcutaneous (SQ) dose.

It is recommended for all persons born after 1956 who are nonimmune. Pregnancy is recommended to be avoided for 3 months. If a pregnancy does occur, there is no need for a termination solely due to the vaccine exposure since there is no documented congenital anomalies due to congenital rubella from a vaccine.

9. **(E)** Pneumococcus vaccine is given as a single dose of purified capsular polysaccharide to people more than 2 years of age who are at increased risk of infection with pneumococcus. Splenectomy, chronic cardiovascular disease or pulmonary disease (excluding asthma), metabolic or hepatic disease, or immunocompromised state (e.g., HIV) increases that risk. Meningococcus vaccine is typically offered to college students, especially those students living in dormitories or other residential living facilities on college campuses. The others are part of a routine immunization program.

10. **(B)** The relative potency of a parenteral dose of the listed medications would be (most potent to least potent): hydromorphone > oxycodone = methadone > meperidine > codeine. For pain as intense as a kidney stone and a sure diagnosis, maximum pain relief is indicated.

11. **(C)** This is referred to as "sundowning." Confusion in the late afternoon or early evening is the key symptom. It can be associated with dementia, organic brain syndrome, unfamiliar environments, and aging. In this case, the fact that the mother does not recognize her daughter is most worrisome and would lead you to pursue a more detailed cause than simply aging. It may improve over time, but it may well need to be treated. Restraints (physical or chemical) are not the answer. More specific therapy can be recommended.

12. **(A)** Isotretinoin is a vitamin A derivative that is indicated for just this problem. You should be certain that other therapies (especially C, D, and E) have been tried and failed, failing because of ineffectiveness rather than noncompliance. The patient should also be informed of the need to continue effective contraception when using this medication because of its known

teratogenicity. Also, OCs will often help in the improvement of the acne.

13. **(E)** Traveler's diarrhea results from the ingestion of contaminated water or food, so advising large water consumption or consumption of uncooked but washed raw foods is poor advice. The disease is common, and most physicians will recommend either prophylaxis or treatment immediately with the onset of symptoms. Trimethoprim–sulfa or ciprofloxacin is the best choice. The diarrhea without treatment can last for a long time. Clindamycin is a poor choice because it not only provides poor coverage, but also in its oral form may be associated with colitis.

14. **(E)** Most likely, she has simple reflux esophagitis. An upper gastrointestinal series would lend little to the resolution of this problem. Milk calms it, but in the long run probably exacerbates the problem. Antacids at the bedside or chronic administration of histamine blockers could treat the discomfort. However, the real problem is increased intra-abdominal pressure, probably related to her weight and to overeating, especially before bedtime. A gallstone would be associated with a different type of pain and would be unlikely to resolve as a result of the ingestion of milk. The surgical removal of asymptomatic gallstones is debatable.

15. **(C)** This is a simple case of hemorrhoids brought on or exacerbated by constipation. Adding fluids and bulk-forming agents, and providing relief with sitz baths, astringents, or topical anti-inflammatory creams should help. Referral is unnecessary at this point, and biopsy is one of the biggest mistakes you will ever make in the office setting. Bright red blood per rectum on the toilet paper at age 34 is unlikely to be a malignancy, and colonoscopy should be reserved for persistent or changing symptoms.

16. **(E)** The history given is classic for stress-related headache. Her family history is unlikely to contribute in this instance. There is little that is hereditary in either case. Reducing her stress, small doses of analgesic, and patient education about stress-related headaches are most appro-

priate. The only other suggestion may be to have an eye examination to determine if corrective lens are indicated. Otherwise, referral would be inappropriate at this time.

17. **(E)** The most common cause of anemia in a premenopausal–perimenopausal patient is iron deficiency related to menstrual loss or pregnancy. The other choices are all consistent with iron deficiency and support the conservative approach of iron supplementation unless the history would imply a source other than menses for the loss. An elevated reticulocyte count would imply that there are adequate iron stores, and there is another source such as hemolysis for the anemia.

18. **(C)** The diagnosis of anorexia is very important since this can become life threatening. A patient may be embarrassed by her problem or not see it as a problem and provide the physician with a number of "explanations" for her body mass. Conversely, as more women become involved in sports, the lean build may reflect this athletic involvement and not an eating disorder. Athletes tend to have increased exercise tolerance with purposeful training and muscle development. They have a more accurate body image with body fat levels within a defined normal range. This contrasts with anorectics who have more aimless physical activity with poor exercise performance and muscle development. They have a flawed body image with body fat below normal. They may have cold intolerance and dry skin. Both groups tend to share dietary faddism, controlled caloric consumptions, low body weight, increased physical activity, resting bradycardia and relative hypotension, and menstrual cycle abnormalities typically amenorrhea. Although increased exercise tolerance is mainly associated with the athletic individual, the findings other than the lanugo hair are common in both groups.

19. **(E)** As more women become involved in sports at a competitive level, physicians are seeing more knee injuries. The exact reason for this is unclear but is partially due to the wider pelvic girdle, which causes more lateral placement of the proximal attachments of the anterior thigh muscles. This, along with a common finding of

an asymmetry in the strength of the knee muscles with more strength evident laterally, encourages the patella to track abnormally with resultant patellofemoral irritation and pain. Activities that involve repetitive hyperextension (such as punting a soccer ball) will often precipitate this problem. Muscle strengthening exercises (to improve muscle strength medially to overcome the lateral pressures), appropriate bracing or taping, and modification of activity are all part of the therapy.

20. **(E)** This is classic for rheumatoid arthritis. It is two to three times more common in women. The etiology is unknown. Occasionally, the arthritis may begin in a more asymmetric manner but will generally become more symmetric as it progresses. Unlike osteoarthritis, this is a systemic disease, hence the nodules. Although osteoarthritis of the hip occurs at the same rate in men as women, women are more likely to have problems with knees and hands. Factors that predispose to osteoarthritis are prior injury or stresses to the affected joint. Ankylosing spondylitis and Reiter syndrome are spondyloarthropathies and tend to be more central in their location (e.g., vertebral and sacroiliac joints). Gout involves isolated joints that are swollen, warm, erythematous, and markedly tender.

21. **(C)** The recommendation is to use SPF 32 sunscreens and apply approximately 2 hours prior to sun exposure to allow skin absorption. The damage is from the UV light waves, which are present on cloudy days and are at high intensity at higher altitudes due to thinner atmosphere. The UV lights in tanning booths are just as bad as natural sunlight and perhaps worse since one does not get hot and hence may increase time of exposure and the amount of skin exposed.

22. **(A)** When evaluating a skin lesion for potential malignant risks, one should look for the ABCD of melanoma: A is for asymmetry of the lesion; a benign lesion is very symmetrical. B is for border, which should be smooth and distinct. C is for color; blackness is not as much of a problem as is a variation of coloring within a malignant

lesion. The diameter should be smaller than the diameter of the eraser on a No. 2 pencil (6 mm). If larger, it is suspicious for melanoma.

23. **(A)** The hairs that are plucked will often show a clubbed hair root. Usually there is spontaneous regrowth of hair in 2 to 6 months. Because of the spontaneous recovery, it is hard to know what the best therapy is. The cause is unknown.

24. **(B)** This is similar to the form of alopecia in men as they get older. This condition is genetic, with onset in reproductive-age women. A biopsy may be helpful in diagnosis, and topical minoxidil will help some patients.

25. **(E)** This is the loss of resting hairs. Pregnancy and other stresses appear to cause a synchronization of hair follicles so a larger portion enter telogen at the same time and then are shed at once. This is usually time limited, and the hair regrows within 6 months.

26. **(F)** The constant tension placed on a hair follicle can cause permanent damage and scarring, resulting in permanent hair loss in the affected areas. Some of the current hairstyles, especially among blacks, are predisposed to this complication.

27. **(E)** This is classic pityriasis rosea with the herald patch. If one looks at the back, the rash will line up with the skin in a diagonal Christmas-tree look. This rash is self-limiting and is probably viral in origin.

28. **(C)** This is likely to be early Lyme disease despite the lack of a history of a tick bite. Laboratory confirmation is difficult as many of the serologic assays are not reliable. Since early Lyme disease is easily treated with 14-day course of tetracycline, it is often wise to treat it if one suspects the diagnosis.

29. **(G)** This is classic varicella. In a healthy adult, treatment is symptomatic, with careful monitoring for the development of varicella pneumonia. Acyclovir has no place in the treatment of an uncomplicated case of varicella.

30. **(F)** This is classic rubella. This is not commonly seen in the United States because of mandatory immunization of schoolchildren but still occurs occasionally. Since this has grave implications for a fetus, it is important to make the diagnosis and then to assure that the patient is not pregnant and that she does not expose other pregnant women.

31. **(A)** More than 25% of deaths in the 15 to 34 age group are related to accidents. The next most frequent cause is cancer, which accounts for about 15%. Homicide and suicide are third and fourth.

32. **(B)** Forty percent of deaths in the 35 to 54 age group are related to cancer. The second most common cause is heart disease, accounting for 15%. Accidents and cerebrovascular accidents follow as third and fourth.

33. **(B)** Cancer is the number one killer in women aged 55 to 64, with heart disease second, and chronic obstructive lung disease third.

34. **(A)** This is typical of degenerative disease. It occurs in older patients and is worse at the end of the day.

35. **(D)** There may also be a decrease in chest expansion. Aortic stenosis and uveitis can be seen in some patients. There is a strong association with human leukocyte antigen (HLA)-B27.

36. **(C)** Anything that stretches the nerve, such as bending, will increase the pain. Sciatica is a form of nerve root pain. If clear muscle weakness is demonstrated, active intervention may be indicated and a referral to an orthopedist may be wise. Otherwise, conservative therapy with anti-inflammatory medications, analgesics, and muscle relaxants is the first-line therapy.

# CHAPTER 27

# Practice Test

## Questions

**DIRECTIONS (Questions 1 through 146): For each of the multiple choice questions in this section, select the lettered answer that is the one *best* response in each case.**

1. A patient wishes you to explain the concept of cervical intraepithelial neoplasia (CIN) III, which has been diagnosed from her cervical biopsy after a low-grade squamous intraepithelial lesion (LGSIL) was found on a Pap smear. What can you correctly tell her about CIN III?

   (A) It is an invasive cancer.
   (B) It includes carcinoma in situ (CIS).
   (C) It requires no further treatment.
   (D) It is due to a bacterial infection.
   (E) It corresponds to the LGSIL shown on her prior Pap smear.

2. Which of the following elements is not necessary for the plaintiff to prove to win a medical professional liability claim?

   (A) duty
   (B) breach of duty
   (C) causation
   (D) intention
   (E) damage

3. A woman wishes to know how she can prevent toxic shock syndrome (TSS). Which of the following would be the most protective?

   (A) use tampons with high absorbency
   (B) change tampons often
   (C) maintain a neutral vaginal pH
   (D) maintain a high vaginal oxygen content
   (E) use pads rather than tampons

4. Universal blood donors have a blood type whose alleles do not produce an antigen. Which of the following alleles has no detectable product?

   (A) A of the ABO blood group
   (B) B of the ABO blood group
   (C) O of the ABO blood group
   (D) D of the Rh group
   (E) K of the Kell blood group

5. A patient needs a kidney transplant. Who among the following is most likely to be the best donor?

   (A) father
   (B) mother
   (C) grandfather
   (D) aunt
   (E) brother

6. A 22-year-old patient is involved in a skiing accident with severe head injuries. Six months after her apparent recovery she has not had a menstrual cycle. She also complains of hot flushes. Her luteinizing hormone (LH), follicle-stimulating hormone (FSH), and estradiol levels are all very low. Which of the following is most likely to have been injured?

   (A) periventricular nucleus
   (B) supraoptic nucleus
   (C) suprachiasmatic nucleus
   (D) arcuate nucleus
   (E) paraventricular nucleus

7. A male infant is born with hypertension and hypokalemia. You suspect an absence of 17-alpha hydroxylase. An elevation in the amount of which of the following hormones will verify this suspicion?

   (A) 17-alpha hydroxyprogesterone
   (B) androstenedione
   (C) testosterone
   (D) deoxycorticosterone
   (E) cortisone

8. Precocious puberty has a number of physical and psychological consequences. However, one of the steroid effects is not reversible or correctable and has major long-term implications. For this reason, which of the following steroid effects would be the prime consideration in management of precocious puberty?

   (A) epiphyseal closure
   (B) hair growth
   (C) genital development
   (D) breast tissue development
   (E) fat redistribution

9. An infant has an absence of 17-alpha hydroxylase. This deficiency is associated with which of the following?

   (A) hypergonadotropic hypogonadism
   (B) hypogonadotropic hypogonadism
   (C) true precocious puberty

   (D) pseudoprecocious puberty
   (E) normal puberty

10. Before and during a menstrual cycle, several follicles begin to grow. What is the ultimate fate of most of these follicles?

   (A) ovulation
   (B) cyst formation
   (C) atresia
   (D) arrest
   (E) regression

11. Which of the following physical findings should prompt an evaluation of a pathologic process in a menopausal woman?

   (A) atrophic vaginal mucosa
   (B) clitoromegaly
   (C) small labia minora
   (D) amenorrhea
   (E) seborrheic cysts of the vulva

12. Prior to making the uterine incision during a cesarean section, the surgeon should examine the uterus to be sure the incision is properly placed. Which of the following situations generally applies to the uterus during pregnancy?

   (A) rotates to the right because of the sacral promontory
   (B) exhibits no rotation
   (C) rotates to the right because of the rectosigmoid
   (D) rotates to the left because of the sacral promontory
   (E) rotates to the left because of the sigmoid colon

13. A patient develops excessive salivation during pregnancy. What is this called?

   (A) deglutition
   (B) pruritus
   (C) emesis
   (D) eructation
   (E) ptyalism

14. During normal pregnancy a lowered hemoglobin is a physiologic finding. What is its major cause?

    (A) low iron stores
    (B) blood lost to the placenta and fetus
    (C) increased plasma volume
    (D) increased cardiac output resulting in greater red-cell destruction
    (E) decreased reticulocytosis

15. The average woman can expect to retain as much as 7 L of water during a normal gestation. What is a major reason for this retention?

    (A) decreased venous pressure in the lower fourth of the body
    (B) increased plasma oncotic pressure
    (C) increased capillary permeability
    (D) marked increase in the maternal serum sodium
    (E) a physiologic cardiac failure resulting in edema, fluid retention, and enlargement of the heart

16. You are examining a 34-year-old woman (gravida 3, para 2) at 38-$^5/_7$ weeks' gestation. She is in labor (5 cm). There is no fetal part in the pelvis. Ultrasound report notes a transverse lie with the fetal back toward the maternal legs. Which of the following is the procedure of choice?

    (A) expectant management anticipating spontaneous vaginal delivery
    (B) tocolysis
    (C) external version
    (D) cesarean delivery
    (E) expectant management expecting forceps rotation after complete dilation

17. Normally, the pregnant woman hyperventilates. Which of the following compensates for this?

    (A) increased tidal volume
    (B) respiratory alkalosis
    (C) decreased $P_{CO_2}$ of the blood

    (D) decreased plasma bicarbonate
    (E) decreased serum pH

18. A 26-year-old G2P1 at 39 weeks' gestation is in active labor. At 5-cm dilatation she experiences spontaneous rupture of membranes. Shortly after she begins to experience bloody amniotic fluid and late decelerations. There is loss of beat-to-beat variability with fetal heart rate in the 190s. Which of the following is the best management at this point?

    (A) set up for amnioinfusion
    (B) begin antibiotics
    (C) terbutaline to slow contractions
    (D) prepare for cesarean section
    (E) ultrasound to verify placental position

19. A 22-year-old presents for prenatal care. This is her first pregnancy. She had had a left lower leg thrombosis 3 years prior, while on oral contraceptives (OCs). A thrombophilia workup identified her as heterozygous for the prothrombin mutation. She is currently without symptoms. What therapy would you recommend for her condition?

    (A) unfractionated heparin
    (B) no therapy antepartum unless she is confined to bed rest
    (C) warfarin until 38 weeks, and then changing to heparin until labor
    (D) aspirin (81 mg daily)
    (E) ibuprofen until 28 weeks, 600 mg, bid, and then low-dose aspirin (81 mg) for the rest of pregnancy

20. A patient presents at 30 weeks' gestation in labor that cannot be stopped. Lung maturity is unlikely. Fetal lung surfactant production may be increased by a number of factors. Which of the following is proven clinically useful?

    (A) estrogen
    (B) prolactin
    (C) thyroxine
    (D) glucocorticosteroids
    (E) alpha-fetoprotein

21. Which of the following is the only class of hormones relevant to the embryogenesis of the external genitalia?

    (A) androgens
    (B) estrogens
    (C) cortisol
    (D) human chorionic gonadotropin (hCG)
    (E) progesterone

22. During an attempted vaginal birth after cesarean at 7 cm, contractions suddenly are not recording by tocometry; the fetal parts are palpated abdominally on examination, and fetal heart tones (FHTs) are heard at 80/min. You can feel fetal feet at –2 station. You should do which of the following?

    (A) perform immediate laparotomy
    (B) perform an immediate ultrasound to evaluate fetal positioning and well-being
    (C) given oxytocin to prevent maternal bleeding
    (D) perform breech extraction as soon as possible
    (E) give terbutaline to stop the contractions

23. When asked about the fetal safety of a category B drug when taken by a pregnant woman, you should respond that a drug in this category has which of the following?

    (A) proven risks that outweigh its benefits
    (B) fetal risk, but the benefits far outweigh the risks
    (C) studies showing adverse effects in animals, but there are no human data
    (D) animal studies showing no fetal risks, or if there are risks, they are not shown in well-controlled human studies
    (E) no fetal risks and the medication is thus considered safe in pregnancy

24. An Rh-negative pregnant woman at 18 weeks' gestation was found to have a titer of 1:32 anti-Lewis antibodies and no other evidence of sensitization to red-cell antigens. What should your next step be?

    (A) perform a repeat blood test at 4 weeks to see if the titer increases
    (B) advise termination of pregnancy
    (C) plan serial amniocentesis, starting at 24–26 weeks
    (D) plan middle cerebral artery velocity measurements at 24 weeks
    (E) plan to give D-immunoglobulin at 28 weeks' gestation

25. When counseling a patient regarding fetal abnormalities during prenatal care, which of the following is the greatest advantage of chorionic villus sampling (CVS) over amniocentesis?

    (A) the ability to provide results early
    (B) the ability to perform enzyme studies
    (C) a decreased fetal risk
    (D) obtaining far superior cellular sample
    (E) a lack of maternal cell contamination

26. When performing clinical pelvimetry in a gynecoid pelvis, the diagonal conjugate should be at least how many centimeters?

    (A) 7.5
    (B) 9.5
    (C) 11.5
    (D) 13.5
    (E) 15.5

27. An infant has an Apgar score of 0 at 1 minute despite clearing the airway and gentle stimulation. Which of the following is the next best step in management?

    (A) immediately intubate and ventilate
    (B) dry and warm the baby
    (C) administer intracardiac epinephrine
    (D) administer a narcotic antagonist
    (E) initiate electrical cardioversion

28. You are called to the bedside of a laboring patient who has just received an injection in her epidural. She has become panicked. She cannot breathe and begins to convulse. Which of the following is your first step in treating a severe systemic reaction to this local anesthetic agent?

(A) oxygen administration
(B) intravenous (IV) fluids
(C) stopping convulsions
(D) supporting blood pressure
(E) clearing the airway

29. A patient has a profuse, thin, acellular cervical mucus with a high degree of stretchability and a palm-leaf crystallization pattern upon drying. Which of the following situations is compatible with this finding?

(A) the secretory phase of the menstrual cycle
(B) preovulatory estrogen surge
(C) on combination birth control pills
(D) being postmenopausal
(E) second trimester of pregnancy

30. What is the implantation of a placenta in which there is a defect in the fibrinoid layer at the implantation site, allowing the placental villi to invade and penetrate into but not through the myometrium called?

(A) placenta accreta
(B) placenta increta
(C) placenta percreta
(D) placental infarct
(E) placenta previa

31. You are checking a term patient in labor. The examination of the fetal presentation feels unusual. Which of the following would be incompatible with a spontaneous delivery?

(A) occiput posterior
(B) mentum posterior
(C) brow asynclitic
(D) occiput transverse
(E) sacrum posterior

32. Ritodrine is a beta-adrenergic receptor stimulator that is used to arrest preterm labor. Which of the following is the most major maternal risk associated with its use?

(A) hypertension
(B) decreased plasma glucose
(C) decreased serum potassium
(D) cardiac arrhythmias
(E) asthma

33. You are taking care of a 29-year-old primigravida with an uncomplicated history, having a postpartum hemorrhage. The placenta delivered spontaneously and intact. Labor was 9 hours and 45 minutes and was unremarkable. There are no obvious lacerations. The infant weighed 9 lb 14 oz. What is your next best step of management?

(A) order coagulation studies
(B) add oxytocin to her IV solution
(C) ultrasound for retained placental parts
(D) observance of a tube of whole blood
(E) uterine curettage with a large "banjo" curette

34. A 21-year-old nulliparous woman presents for preconception counseling. Her history is remarkable only for having been told her vagina is abnormally shaped. On pelvic examination, there is a complete longitudinal vaginal septum. She is concerned as to the implications of this regarding conceiving, continuing the pregnancy and delivery. In the presence of a complete longitudinal vaginal septum, which of the following is true?

(A) delivery is usually difficult
(B) the uterus is less likely to be abnormal
(C) conception is nearly impossible
(D) there is an above-average incidence of urinary tract abnormalities
(E) prophylactic cesarean delivery is indicated

35. The hemostatic mechanism most important in combating postpartum hemorrhage is which of the following?

    (A) increased blood clotting factors in pregnancy
    (B) contraction of interlacing uterine muscle bundles
    (C) markedly decreased blood pressure in the uterine venules
    (D) intramyometrial vascular coagulation due to vasoconstriction
    (E) enhanced platelet aggregation during pregnancy

36. A 32-year-old woman (gravida 4, para 3) at 38 weeks' gestation by good dates presents in your office with painless moderate vaginal bleeding (soaking two pads) after an otherwise uneventful gestation. The bleeding presently has ceased and no uterine contractions are present; the FHTs are 140. What is the best course of action?

    (A) perform a complete pelvic examination
    (B) reassure the patient and send her home to await spontaneous labor
    (C) admit the patient to the hospital the following morning for induction of labor
    (D) perform an ultrasound
    (E) perform an immediate cesarean section

37. A patient has an uncomplicated vaginal delivery of a 3,500-g infant. The placenta delivers spontaneously in 15 minutes. Forty-five minutes after this delivery, you are notified by a nurse that the patient has an unusual amount of bleeding but that vital signs are stable. What is the best course of action?

    (A) examine the patient
    (B) have the nurse call you back in 1 hour if bleeding persists
    (C) order Pitocin IV
    (D) reassure the nurse and wait
    (E) type and crossmatch 2 units of blood

38. A patient wishes to breast-feed. With which of the following active infections in the immediate postpartum period would it still be acceptable for a woman to breast-feed?

    (A) cytomegalovirus (CMV)
    (B) genital herpes
    (C) hepatitis B
    (D) human immunodeficiency virus (HIV)
    (E) varicella

39. Which of the following is normally found in the immediate postpartum period after an uncomplicated spontaneous term vaginal delivery?

    (A) elevated erythrocyte sedimentation rate (ESR)
    (B) large drop in hematocrit (>8%)
    (C) leukopenia
    (D) rapid fall in plasma fibrinogen
    (E) retention of fluid

40. Once respirations are established, which of the following is the most important aspect of immediate care of the newborn?

    (A) doing a brief physical examination
    (B) drying the skin
    (C) measuring the hematocrit
    (D) placing identification bands
    (E) warming the infant

41. Which of the following is the most common cause of newborn jaundice (icterus neonatorum)?

    (A) bottle-feeding
    (B) direct bilirubin
    (C) indirect bilirubin
    (D) lack of carotene production in the newborn liver
    (E) meconium obstruction of the newborn digestive system

**42.** A newborn is noted to have a darkened swelling of the scalp that does not cross the midline. This is most likely which of the following?

(A) caput succedaneum
(B) cephalhematoma
(C) subarachnoid hemorrhage
(D) subdural hemorrhage
(E) tentorial tear

**43.** After delivery, paralysis is noted on one side of the face in a newborn. This is most often associated with which of the following?

(A) abnormalities of the central nervous system (CNS)
(B) facial swelling
(C) forceps-induced nerve injury
(D) neonatal sepsis
(E) pressure on the trigeminal nerve during delivery

**44.** A male infant is born with prominent epicanthal folds, a flattened nose, skin that appears "loose," and large, low-set ears and flexion contractures of the extremities. The baby does not spontaneously breathe, and you intubate the child and find it almost impossible to ventilate. Which of the following is the most likely diagnosis?

(A) diaphragmatic hernia
(B) normal pressure hydrocephalus
(C) postmaturity syndrome
(D) pyloric stenosis
(E) renal agenesis

**45.** A couple returns to your clinic after initial evaluation of their infertility condition. Semen analysis revealed 35 million sperm/mL, 50% motility and 50% normal forms both to 60%. Hysterosalpingogram demonstrated a normal endometrial cavity with unilateral proximal tubal obstruction. The female patient has regular menstrual cycles with appropriate basal body temperature (BBT) rise indicating a 14-day luteal phase. A serum progesterone level was 15.2 ng/mL. A diagnostic laparo-

scopy showed no adhesions or endometriosis, with bilateral free spill of dye from her tubes. What is the most appropriate diagnosis in this case?

(A) luteal-phase deficiency
(B) male factor infertility
(C) oligo-ovulation
(D) tubal factor infertility
(E) unexplained infertility

**46.** Which of the following is the most common chromosomal abnormality found in tissue from first-trimester spontaneous abortions?

(A) autosomal trisomy
(B) sex-chromosome monosomy
(C) sex-chromosome polysomy
(D) triploidy
(E) tetraploidy

**47.** A 31-year-old patient comes to your clinic with irregular menstrual cycles and infertility of 2 years' duration. After evaluation, you determine that clomiphene citrate would be the appropriate mode of therapy. Which of the following statements should be explained to the patient?

(A) Approximately 25% of patients will respond by ovulating with this medication.
(B) Ovulation usually occurs 3 weeks after the last day of clomiphene citrate ingestion.
(C) The risk of multiple pregnancy is 7%.
(D) The risk of severe ovarian hyperstimulation syndrome is 25%.
(E) There is an increased risk of fetal anomalies if pregnancy results.

48. A 23-year-old woman with irregular menses complains of facial hair increasing in amount over several years. She is sexually active but does not wish to conceive. Examination demonstrates hirsutism, obesity, and hyperpigmentation of the neck and axillae. The ovaries are bilaterally enlarged and cystic. A serum testosterone value is 1.2 ng/mL (normal, <0.8 ng/mL). Serum levels of DHEAS, 17-hydroxyprogesterone (17-OHP), and prolactin are normal. Which of the following is the best single therapeutic agent for this patient?

    (A) Oral combination contraceptive
    (B) glucocorticoids
    (C) clomiphene citrate
    (D) antiandrogens
    (E) gonadotropin-releasing hormone (GnRH) analogue

49. A 22-year-old woman experiences amenorrhea of 6 months' duration. Physical examination demonstrates normal breast development and normal pelvic organs. There is no hirsutism or galactorrhea. Serum thyroid-stimulating hormone (TSH) and prolactin levels are normal. A serum pregnancy test is negative. What would be the next course of action?

    (A) administer progesterone
    (B) administer estrogen followed by progesterone
    (C) measure circulating estrogen levels
    (D) measure circulating testosterone levels
    (E) obtain radiologic evaluation of the sella turcica

50. A 33-year-old woman cannot feel the string of her intrauterine contraceptive device (IUCD). Her last menstrual period (LMP) was 1 week ago. A serum pregnancy test is negative. Which of the following is the best immediate action?

    (A) insert another IUCD to replace the lost one
    (B) obtain an abdominal radiogram
    (C) obtain a pelvic ultrasound

    (D) perform a hysterosalpingogram
    (E) probe the cervical canal gently to pull down the string

51. A 45-year-old patient presents with hypermenorrhea with a negative evaluation. Given this is likely ovulatory dysfunction due to approaching menopause and the patient has no contraindications you offer OC pills for cycle control since she desires hormonal and not surgical intervention. She reports having used OCs about 20 years ago prior to her husband having a vasectomy without difficulty except for some mild headaches. Given that she likely was on a 50-$\mu$g estrogen pill, you counsel her that with the lower-dose (25–30 $\mu$g) OCs the most common side effect is which of the following?

    (A) breakthrough bleeding
    (B) chloasma
    (C) dysmenorrhea
    (D) mastalgia
    (E) nausea

52. A 35-year-old woman complains of irregular vaginal bleeding and abdominal pain. Her LMP was 8 weeks ago. A laparoscopic tubal fulguration was performed 2 years ago for permanent sterilization. She wants to know if her symptoms are related to the previous surgical sterilization. The most appropriate response is to advise her that a known complication of female sterilization is which of the following?

    (A) dysmenorrhea
    (B) anovulation
    (C) irregular bleeding
    (D) ovarian cyst formation
    (E) pregnancy

53. A 32-year-old woman has an intrauterine fetal demise at 25 weeks' gestation. Which of the following pregnancy termination methods is associated with the highest rate of complications?

    (A) IV oxytocin
    (B) IV prostaglandin (PG)
    (C) intravaginal PG

(D)  intramuscular (IM) PG

(E)  dilation and evacuation (D&E)

54.  A 58-year-old woman consults you for vulvar pruritus. On pelvic examination, you note thin, atrophic skin with whitish coloration over the entire vulva. Which of the following diagnoses is most likely in this patient?

(A)  vulvar carcinoma

(B)  vulvar intraepithelial neoplasia

(C)  hyperkeratosis

(D)  atrophic vulvitis

(E)  lichen sclerosis

55.  A 53-year-old woman who has not menstruated for 1 year is started on cyclic hormonal replacement therapy. She has scant vaginal bleeding of 2 days' duration as she starts her second cycle of replacement. She is healthy, body mass index (BMI) 21, normal blood pressure, and used OCs until age 42. She refuses an endometrial sampling. Of the following, which is the most appropriate next step in the management of her bleeding?

(A)  begin a menstrual (bleeding) calendar

(B)  take a Pap smear, including endocervical sampling

(C)  insist on an endometrial sample

(D)  perform colposcopy

(E)  perform a transvaginal ultrasonography to measure endometrial thickness

56.  An 18-year-old college student presents with complaints of severe menstrual cramps that are causing her to miss classes. This has been a problem since shortly after her menses started. While in high school, this had not been a major problem but now as a premedical student she is concerned this will have a negative impact on her education and grade. The remainder of her history, physical examination and limited laboratory testing are unremarkable and you diagnose primary dysmenorrhea. She is not sexually active and is not interested in contraception at this time. Currently, the most effective treatment for primary dysmenorrhea in a woman who does not require contraception is which of the following?

(A)  depot-medroxyprogesterone acetate

(B)  birth control pills

(C)  GnRH agonist

(D)  estrogen supplement in the luteal phase

(E)  PG synthetase inhibitors

57.  Endometriosis treated with prolonged estrogen and progesterone combination therapy exhibits which of the following histologic characteristics?

(A)  marked edema

(B)  atrophy

(C)  glandular hypertrophy

(D)  inflammatory infiltrate

(E)  cyclic changes

58.  Luteectomy before 42 days' gestation is most likely to result in which of the following?

(A)  prolonged (postdates) gestation

(B)  spontaneous miscarriage

(C)  reduction of basal body temperature (BBT)

(D)  masculinization of a female fetus

(E)  hypospadias in a male fetus

59.  A 35-year-old complains of increasing dysmenorrhea and pelvic pain. She has not become pregnant despite 3 years of unprotected intercourse. Her pelvic examination demonstrates tenderness and nodularity over her uterosacral ligaments and a 4-cm right ovarian cyst. Which of the following is her most likely diagnosis?

(A)  adenomyosis

(B)  pelvic congestion syndrome

(C)  chronic ectopic pregnancy

(D)  endometriosis

(E)  chronic pelvic inflammatory disease (PID)

**60.** A 65-year-old woman G3P3 is being counseled regarding the risks of having a Burch operation for stress incontinence. She has had a prior hysterectomy. On examination, she has a second-degree cystocele. Urodynamic testing confirmed genuine stress incontinence. Which of the following is the most common early complication of this procedure?

(A) vaginal bleeding
(B) urinary retention
(C) ureteral injury
(D) development of an enterocele
(E) continuous urinary leakage

**61.** A vigorous 79-year-old woman with worsening urinary incontinence over the past year comes to see you. The leakage seems to be without warning. Small volumes leak frequently. It is interfering with her exercise program. She denies neurologic symptoms, stress incontinence symptoms, or voiding problems. She is on insulin for diabetes. Physical examination reveals normal neurologic and pelvic findings. Postvoid residual urine was 240 mL. Urodynamic testing shows uninhibited detrusor contractions with leakage. She generated a low-level detrusor contraction with voiding but has incomplete bladder emptying with residuals around 200 mL. Her bladder capacity is 350 mL. Which of the following is the most appropriate management of this patient?

(A) teach her clean intermittent self-catheterization (CISC)
(B) place a Foley catheter
(C) start her on anticholinergic-type medication
(D) start her on PG inhibitor medication
(E) offer her a urinary diversion

**62.** A 1-year-old girl has an abdominal mass. Rectal examination demonstrates a mass extending into the right pelvis. The cervix is not palpable. Abdominal sonography shows that the uterus and vagina are absent. Both ovaries appear normal. What is the most likely origin of the mass?

(A) gastrointestinal (GI)
(B) renal
(C) musculoskeletal
(D) hepatic
(E) pancreatic

**63.** A 6-cm nontender, mobile, right adnexal mass is present in a 19-year-old woman. One year ago, while using OCs, she was hospitalized for left leg deep vein thrombophlebitis. Transvaginal sonography shows a 4-cm unilocular smooth ovarian cyst without internal excrescences. A serum pregnancy test is negative. Which of the following is the most appropriate next step in this patient's management?

(A) observation
(B) OCs
(C) estrogen therapy
(D) laparoscopy
(E) laparotomy

**64.** A 17-year-old girl experiences sudden right lower abdominal pain. Her LMP was 7 weeks ago. She has severe nausea and breast tenderness. Vital signs are blood pressure, 120/80 mm Hg; pulse, 80 bpm; and afebrile. Abdominal examination is unremarkable. Pelvic examination shows blood in the vagina and a normal-appearing cervix. The uterus is slightly enlarged. A tender 4-cm right adnexal mass is present. Which of the following is the most appropriate initial diagnostic test?

(A) hematocrit
(B) white blood count (WBC)
(C) ESR
(D) serum hCG determination
(E) transvaginal sonogram

**65.** A 28-year-old woman is seen for her first obstetrical visit. Her LMP was 8 weeks ago. Her history is significant for infertility due to chronic salpingitis and she required in vitro fertilization (IVF) with multiple embryo transfer. A serum pregnancy test is positive. A transabdominal ultrasound shows an enlarged uterus containing five viable fetuses. You advise her that the optimal outcome can be achieved only with which of the following?

(A) close supervision
(B) embryo reduction
(C) intramuscular prostaglandin
(D) progestin therapy
(E) termination of the pregnancy

66. A 69-year-old woman presents with a 2-cm firm nodule in the right labium majus without signs of inflammation. Which of the following is the most appropriate course of action?

(A) excisional biopsy
(B) reassurance
(C) hot packs
(D) topical cortisone cream
(E) simple vulvectomy

67. While viewing a cervical biopsy, squamous cell atypia is noted. It extends from the basal layer to a little more than one-half the thickness of the epithelium. Beyond that level, maturation is evident. There is no invasion of stroma. Which of the following is the correct diagnosis based on these biopsy findings?

(A) adenocarcinoma
(B) microglandular hyperplasia
(C) moderate dysplasia (CIN II)
(D) CIS
(E) invasive squamous cell carcinoma

68. The diagnosis of carcinoma of the cervix, International Federation of Gynecology and Obstetrics (FIGO) stage III, is assigned when which of the following occurs?

(A) The carcinoma has infiltrated the bladder base.
(B) The carcinoma involves the distal vaginal mucosa.
(C) The carcinoma has extended into the parametria, but not to the pelvic sidewall.
(D) X-ray reveals tumor.
(E) Adenocarcinoma is present.

69. A patient is referred to you from her primary care provider because of the finding of a large cystic structure in the vagina that prevented visualization of the cervix and the performance of a Pap smear. The patient notes that her boyfriend had mentioned feeling something there but it did not hurt so she had not had it checked until she needed an examination to initial OC pills. On examination, there is a large cyst (5 × 4 cm) on the lateral vaginal wall. You biopsy the wall of the cyst for diagnostic confirmation and to decompress the cyst so a Pap can be done. The pathology returns with the description that the cyst wall is lined with cuboidal, nonciliated epithelium. This type of cyst is most likely to be which of the following?

(A) paramesonephric duct remnants
(B) mesonephric duct remnants
(C) epidermoid inclusion cysts
(D) endometrial implants
(E) adenomatous hyperplasia

70. A 62-year-old obese woman on unopposed estrogen develops abnormal vaginal bleeding. Her cervical Pap smear is normal. She is best evaluated by which of the following procedures?

(A) transvaginal sonography
(B) cervical conization
(C) endometrial biopsy
(D) endometrial cytology
(E) colposcopy and cervical biopsy

71. In which of the following patients is uterine sarcoma most likely to be found?

(A) 10-year-old girl with recent onset vaginal bleeding
(B) 9-year-old girl with a rapidly enlarging pelvic mass
(C) 55-year-old woman with a rapidly enlarging uterus
(D) 40-year-old woman with a slowly enlarging uterus
(E) 25-year-old woman with a rapidly enlarging uterus

72. A patient has ovarian carcinoma. What is the most common site of metastases from this tumor?

(A) contralateral ovary
(B) uterus
(C) peritoneum
(D) liver
(E) lung

73. A patient has a mucinous cystadenoma that ruptures. Which of the following sequelae is most likely to result?

(A) pulmonary metastases
(B) cerebral metastases
(C) liver metastases
(D) pseudomyxoma peritonei
(E) ureteral obstruction

74. A 35-year-old G5P5 patient who is using a tubal ligation as contraception for the past 5 years is noting increasing dysmenorrhea over the past year. Her examination 2 days prior to her menses reveals a large boggy mobile uterus that is tender. This examination is consistent with adenomyosis. Which of the following is the best therapy for secondary dysmenorrhea thought to be due to adenomyosis?

(A) cervical dilation
(B) cyclic OCs
(C) analgesics
(D) hysterectomy
(E) testosterone injections

75. A 19-year-old woman is seen in the emergency room with a history of amenorrhea for 8 weeks, and 1 week of unilateral adnexal pain. On physical examination, she is found to have a diffuse tenderness and fullness in the right adnexa. Laboratory evaluations reveal a hematocrit that is roughly normal, and a positive pregnancy test. Which of the following is the most appropriate imaging modality to establish a diagnosis in this case?

(A) transvaginal ultrasonography
(B) transabdominal ultrasonography

(C) IV pyelography
(D) computed tomography of the pelvis
(E) magnetic resonance imaging

76. A 56-year-old woman has gradual virilization and is found to have a 5-cm left ovarian mass, which contains nests of luteinized thecal cells within the stroma. Which of the following conditions is her most likely diagnosis?

(A) pituitary tumor
(B) polycystic ovarian syndrome (PCOS)
(C) stromal hyperthecosis
(D) Sertoli–Leydig cell tumor
(E) Krukenberg's tumor

77. Currently many screening tests are being evaluated for the most cost-effective population that should receive the test and what interval it should be done. Currently mammograms are being recommended by some to be done only every 2 years in the low-risk woman who is between 50 and 65 years of age with annual clinical examinations. This means that the provider must determine during the clinical examination whether the patient is potentially at more high risk for an early can and should be screened annual. Which of the following findings in a patient would be the most suspicious for an increased risk of a breast carcinoma?

(A) diffuse nodularity in both breasts
(B) a single cyst in the lower inner quadrant of the left breast
(C) a single nodule in the upper outer quadrant of the right breast
(D) multiple cystic masses in both breasts
(E) a lump in the breast that appears just before menses

78. A patient has stage III cancer of the cervix and will be treated with radiation. Which of the following is of greatest concern while delivering this therapy?

(A) harming small bowel
(B) inducing sarcoma of the uterus
(C) destroying the bladder or rectum

(D) causing infection or necrosis

(E) destroying surrounding pelvic muscles

79. You are advising a 27-year-old nurse in good health. What would be the best time of the year for her to get her flu shot?

(A) spring

(B) summer

(C) fall

(D) winter

(E) at age 27, you advise against it

80. A 32-year-old woman (G2P0101) who had a classical C-section with her last pregnancy due to cord prolapse with spontaneous rupture of membranes and a transverse lie at 34 weeks. She presents at 34 weeks EGA with abdominal cramping and pain. What is the best method for determining the extent and severity of uterine damage when uterine rupture is suspected?

(A) transabdominal ultrasonography

(B) transvaginal ultrasonography

(C) computed tomography

(D) magnetic resonance imaging

(E) exploratory surgery

81. A 21-year-old college student presents to the student health clinic with complaints of increasing nervousness, fatigue, weight loss, and palpitations. She is a premedical student with a stressful academic load. She reports normal monthly menses. Her examination is remarkable for a documented 10-lb weight loss since her last clinic visit 6 months ago, warm skin, no goiter, and tachycardia without a murmur or click. What is the next step in her evaluation or therapy?

(A) schedule an echocardiogram to rule out mitral valve prolapse

(B) initiate antianxiety medications

(C) provide psychiatric/psychological referral for stress management

(D) perform thyroid scan

(E) measure TSH levels

82. When making a lower midline abdominal incision, where would you find the lower border of the posterior rectus fascia sheath?

(A) at the insertion of the rectus muscles

(B) at the same position as the lower end of the anterior rectus sheath

(C) at the arcuate line (linea semicircularis)

(D) at the area approximately 2–3 cm above the pubic symphysis

(E) at the symphysis pubis

83. A 21-year-old G1P0 patient has made it to second stage after a slightly prolonged active phase. She has been pushing effectively for 2 hour without descent from 0 station. As you evaluate for reasons that are preventing descent you check for the positioning of the vertex presentation. This is important since there is great variation in the diameter of the vertex depending on the positioning and in turn the fetal ability to negotiate the pelvic axis and descend in second stage. The greatest diameter of the normal fetal head is which of the following?

(A) occipitofrontal

(B) occipitomental

(C) subocciputal bregmatic

(D) bitemporal

(E) biparietal

84. You are going back to do a C-section for a patient with a fetus in a back down transverse lie. To aid in delivery relaxation of the uterus can facilitate an atraumatic delivery from this abnormal lie. Which of the following anesthetic techniques will produce the greatest uterine relaxation?

(A) spinal block

(B) caudal

(C) nitrous oxide

(D) halothane

(E) paracervical

85. You are describing the normal ovaries to a fellow student. Which of the following characteristics of the normal ovary is correct?

    (A) They normally remain constant in size throughout a woman's lifetime.
    (B) They are supported by the round ligaments.
    (C) They secrete hormones and store germ cells.
    (D) They lie in the false pelvis.
    (E) They are immobile.

86. A 25-year-old healthy woman complains of breast tenderness and amenorrhea of 6 weeks' duration. She uses condoms for birth control and does not take any medication. Examination demonstrates a whitish breast discharge with milk-containing fat droplets on microscopic examination. A pregnancy test is negative, and a serum TSH level is normal. A serum prolactin is 80 ng/mL (normal, <20 ng/mL). The next step in the management of this patient should be to obtain radiologic assessment of which structure(s)?

    (A) kidneys
    (B) lumbar spine
    (C) sella turcica
    (D) chest
    (E) pelvic organs

87. The relationship of the long axis of the fetus to the long axis of the mother is called which of the following?

    (A) lie
    (B) presentation
    (C) position
    (D) attitude
    (E) axis of the conjugate

88. An unregistered obstetric patient with no prenatal care presents with active labor and a history consistent with estimated gestational age of 37 weeks and an 8-hour history of spontaneous rupture of the membranes. She delivers precipitously. About 8 hours after delivery, her infant develops septic shock, pneumonia, and a positive Gram's stain is obtained from the infant's blood. The clinical picture in this infant is most consistent with which of the following?

    (A) group A streptococcal infection
    (B) group B streptococcal infection
    (C) infant CMV
    (D) maternal syphilis
    (E) neonatal gonorrhea

89. You are caring for a pregnant woman who is a recent immigrant from Southeast Asia and are concerned about tuberculosis (TB). Which of the following statements is most accurate regarding TB in pregnancy?

    (A) All Southeast Asian immigrants should have a chest X-ray in pregnancy.
    (B) If a patient is treated adequately during pregnancy, TB generally has no deleterious effect on mother or child.
    (C) Skin tests have an unusually high false-positive rate in pregnancy.
    (D) The best single drug for therapy of TB in pregnancy is streptomycin.
    (E) Two-drug antituberculous therapy in pregnancy is contraindicated.

90. A 37-year-old hemodialysis technician is seen at 31 weeks' gestation. She has a temperature of 100.4°F and a blood pressure of 98/64 mm Hg. She complains of general malaise, myalgia, anorexia, nausea, and vomiting. On physical examination, her liver is slightly enlarged and tender. Her urine protein and bilirubin are elevated on the urine dipstick test. Your plan of action should be which of the following?

    (A) admit the patient to the hospital, begin IV antibiotic therapy, and administer high-dose steroids
    (B) have her come back in a week to repeat her blood pressure and urine dipstick test
    (C) order a serum glutamic-oxaloacetic transaminase (SGOT), serum glutamic-pyruvic transaminase (SGPT) (alanine transaminase [ALT]), and alkaline phosphatase

(D) order an ultrasound of the gallbladder

(E) perform a roll-over test to rule out preeclampsia

91. On the seventh day after abdominal hysterectomy, an extremely obese patient (BMI > 43) stands to go to the bathroom and spontaneously passes "a large amount (more than a liter) of serosanguinous fluid" from her abdominal wound. Which of the following is the most appropriate consideration?

(A) Nurse should stay in the room to see if there is more drainage from the wound.

(B) Remove the skin staples from the wound, as they are likely causing an allergic reaction.

(C) She has a wound dehiscence.

(D) There is a urinary tract injury draining spontaneously through the patient's wound.

(E) Wound hematoma has spontaneously drained.

92. A 2-year-old girl is brought in for evaluation of vaginal bleeding. Physical examination shows grape-like lesions protruding from the vaginal introitus. Which of the following is the most likely diagnosis?

(A) condyloma acuminata

(B) hymenal tags

(C) sarcoma botryoides

(D) urethral prolapse

(E) vaginal polyps

93. A 31-year-old woman (gravida 6, para 0-2-3-1) comes to you at 10 weeks' gestation with the history of having had progressively earlier deliveries, all without painful contractions. Her first child was born at 34 weeks and survived, the next delivered at 26 weeks, the next two at 22 weeks, and the last one at 20 weeks. No congenital abnormalities were found. On examination, her uterus is 10–12-week size, FHTs are present with Doppler, and the cervix is soft, three-quarters effaced, and 2-cm dilated. With this information, your first diagnosis is

intrauterine gestation and which of the following?

(A) fibroid uterus

(B) genetic disease

(C) incompetent cervical os

(D) premature labor

(E) progesterone lack

94. During delivery of a 9.5-lb infant, the mother sustained a third-degree perineal laceration with involvement of the rectal mucosa. What is the best course of action?

(A) leave the tear to heal primarily by itself, because of contamination

(B) pack the defect open for secondary closure

(C) repair the anal sphincter and perineal muscles only

(D) repair the defect in layers

(E) repair the defect with through-and-through sutures

95. You are seeing a 21-year-old with G1,P0, abortion 1. Her last pregnancy was terminated at 17 weeks' gestation for anencephaly. She would like to try to get pregnant again. She asks you if there is anything in particular that you would recommend in this pregnancy. Which of the following should you suggest?

(A) begin folic acid 4 mg daily

(B) ultrasounds beginning at 10 weeks with a vaginal scan because anencephaly may be detected at that point

(C) 1 mg folic acid

(D) first-trimester screening for nuchal thickness and blood acolytes—beta-subunit of hCG, inhibin, and Pap A

(E) alpha-fetoprotein screening at 15 weeks' gestation with Level II ultrasound at 18 weeks

96. A patient after a prolonged second stage delivers the vertex with an immediate turtle sign with the head retracting against the perineum. McRobert's maneuver does not affect delivery. Which of the following would be a helpful maneuver in managing this shoulder dystocia?

    (A) fundal pressure
    (B) internal podalic version
    (C) increased maternal pushing effort
    (D) Ritgen maneuver
    (E) Wood's screw maneuver

97. A 30-year-old G3P2 presents at 6 weeks' gestation. She is currently on supplemental T4 secondary to hypothyroid condition brought on after radioactive iodine for Graves' disease. In your counseling, you should say which of the following?

    (A) You will check her thyroid levels each trimester and adjust accordingly.
    (B) She is at risk for hyperemesis, since that is associated with increased thyroid levels.
    (C) She should increase her thyroid dose at this time.
    (D) You will draw TSH levels at this time and every 6–8 weeks to follow her condition.
    (E) You reassure her that since she no longer has Grave's disease the fetus will be unaffected.

98. A patient who is a G2P1001 has been pushing for 3 hours and is exhausted after a long labor. The fetal tracing is now a Category 2 tracing. The vertex is at +3 station. On examination, the infant feels about 7 lb and the pelvis is roomy. You feel that a vacuum-assisted vaginal delivery is an indicated option to expedite delivery. In your counseling of the patient, you tell her that the most severe fetal complications of vacuum extraction for the fetus include which of the following?

    (A) subgaleal hemorrhage
    (B) cephalhematoma
    (C) fetal rib fractures
    (D) facial lacerations
    (E) fetal retinal hemorrhage

99. A patient presents with a complaint that prompted an assessment of the prolactin level. The level returns as elevated by threefold. Which of the following is a normal physiologic reason for an elevated prolactin without associated pathology?

    (A) enlarged sella turcica
    (B) galactorrhea
    (C) oligomenorrhea
    (D) pregnancy
    (E) secondary amenorrhea

100. The three signs of placenta separation after delivery include which of the following?

    (A) a gush of blood, a change in uterine shape from discoid to globular, and lengthening of the umbilical cord
    (B) descent of the fundus, a gush of blood, maternal valsalva
    (C) a darkening of the perineum, a change in uterine shape from discoid to globular, and a blanching in the umbilical cord
    (D) a rise in maternal blood pressure 10 mm Hg, vaginal retraction, and lengthening of the umbilical cord
    (E) descent of the fundus, vaginal retraction, and blanching of the umbilical cord

101. A 26-year-old nulligravida complains of bilateral, spontaneous milky nipple discharge that has been present for the last 3 months. The patient uses a copper-bearing IUCD for contraception. The remainder of her history and physical examination are unremarkable. Which of the following is the most likely cause of this patient's symptoms?

    (A) pituitary adenoma
    (B) hypothyroidism
    (C) renal failure
    (D) exogenous hormone ingestion
    (E) bronchogenic carcinoma

102. During an annual examination, you determine that your patient is depressed. You offer her one of the newer antidepressant medications but warn her that side effects are common. Which of the following is the most common side effect of these agents?

(A) blurred vision
(B) confusion
(C) abdominal cramping
(D) dry mouth
(E) urinary hesitance

103. You are called to evaluate a 42-year-old diabetic, alcoholic patient who has presented to the emergency room with a vulvar lesion present for the last 24 hours. On examination, you find an obese patient with a diffuse swelling of the right labia (majus and minus), a dusky color, and mild crepitation to the tissue. The tissue is not tender over the area of greatest involvement, but is tender on the periphery of the lesion that extends to the anus posteriorly and the lower quarter of the abdominal wall on that side. Vital signs suggest mild hypotension and tachycardia, but the patient has only a low-grade fever. Which of the following is the most likely diagnosis?

(A) Bartholin's gland abscess
(B) necrotizing fasciitis
(C) Crohn's disease involving the vulva
(D) herpes zoster
(E) incarcerated femoral hernia

104. Which of the following screening activities are recommended by the U.S. Preventative Health Services in a low-risk 50-year-old woman?

(A) serum glucose yearly
(B) mammogram every 2 years
(C) Pap smear yearly
(D) serum creatinine yearly
(E) serum cholesterol yearly

105. Formation of the external genitalia in the fetus is influenced by multiple factors. Which of the following factors is the most important?

(A) genetic sex of the embryo
(B) a normal urogenital sinus
(C) the sperm fertilizing the egg (carrying a Y chromosome)
(D) the presence of fetal androgens
(E) maternal hormonal levels

106. A patient presents to the emergency room with abdominal pain and an approximate LMP of 10 weeks prior that would give an Estimated date of confinement (EDC) of November 15. Ultrasound shows a crown-rump length consistent with 8 weeks giving an EDC of November 30. Patient does not return for follow-up until 3 months later. Due to a BMI of 45 fundal height is difficult to determine so an ultrasound is done. Anatomy is normal, singleton fetus and biometry that is consistent with an EDC of November 15. A subsequent ultrasound done 4 weeks later is consistent with EDC of November 8. An additional one gives her a due date of November 1. Which is the most accurate EDC?

(A) November 1
(B) November 8
(C) November 15
(D) November 22
(E) November 30

107. A 25-year-old (G3P0) has had an arrest of labor for 4 hours with no cervical change from 6 cm, −1 station. She has been on oxytocin with adequate contractions for the last 2 hours of that time period. The fetus has a reassuring heart rate tracing. Which of the following is the best management?

(A) continue oxytocin
(B) increase oxytocin
(C) offer vacuum extraction of infant
(D) therapeutic 2-hour pitocin washout period
(E) cesarean section

**108.** A 29-year-old woman (gravida 2, para 1) has a rapid labor. Within minutes of her admission, she is found to be completely dilated, with the vertex at 0 station, and she begins pushing. You are called by her nurse to evaluate her. Contractions are regular, every 2–3 minutes, and palpated to be strong. FHTs are approximately 70 bpm. Cervical examination reveals the vertex to be ROP at 0 station with no caput appreciated. Thick meconium is noted. What should be your first step?

(A) instruct the patient to ambulate

(B) turn the patient on her side and administer oxygen by face mask

(C) begin amnioinfusion and increase IV fluids

(D) await vaginal delivery

(E) give terbutaline to stop contractions

**109.** A 20-year-old primigravida presents at 39 weeks. She has been healthy up to this point. She has a headache and a loss of appetite. Her face and hands are swollen, and she cannot wear her rings. Her BP is 168/90 mm Hg, and she has 1+ protein. The fetus has a reassuring monitoring strip. Which of the following is the best treatment for her preeclampsia?

(A) magnesium sulfate

(B) delivery either by cesarean or by vaginal

(C) an antihypertensive drug that does not affect uterine blood flow

(D) gentle diuresis, with careful monitoring of intake and output

(E) modified bed rest

**110.** The diagnosis of valvular heart disease in pregnancy may be made when there is which of the following?

(A) a history of rheumatic fever

(B) arrhythmia

(C) a diastolic murmur

(D) a soft systolic murmur along the left sternal border (LSB)

(E) an S4

**111.** You are evaluating a pregnant woman for her hemoglobin of 8.3. Her folate levels are reported as deficient. What other results might you expect secondary to the folic acid deficiency?

(A) microcytic anemia

(B) megaloblastic anemia

(C) aplastic anemia

(D) glucose-6-phosphate dehydrogenase (G6PD) deficiency

(E) WBC stippling

**112.** A pregnant patient at 16 weeks' gestation has normal blood pressure, proteinuria (4 g/day), serum albumin (2.0 g/dL), creatinine (0.8 mg/dL), and peripheral edema. Which of the following diagnoses is most appropriate?

(A) glomerulonephritis

(B) pregnancy-induced hypertension

(C) nephrotic syndrome

(D) polycystic kidney disease

(E) chronic renal failure

**113.** The most common reportable sexually transmitted disease (STD) in women that can cause conjunctivitis and neonatal pneumonia is which of the following?

(A) gonorrhea

(B) syphilis

(C) chlamydia

(D) herpes

(E) chancroid

**114.** A 39-year-old woman (G4P4) has had a pregnancy complicated with Graves' disease. She has delivered 4 hours ago. Her thyroid levels and TSH levels have been in the normal range throughout gestation. Among which of the following will her infant most likely be?

(A) hypothyroid infant

(B) mongoloid infant

(C) hyperthyroid infant

(D) infertile infant

(E) infant with ambiguous genitalia

**115.** A 29-year-old G2,P1 is found on ultrasound at 22 weeks to have a 3-cm solid adnexal mass. She states her voice has deepened over pregnancy and she has had increased body hair growth. Her Ca 125 is normal. A pregnancy lutreoma is in your diagnosis. You counsel her that in general luteomas are which of the following?

(A) easily differentiated from a hilus cell tumor

(B) not a part of the corpus luteum of pregnancy

(C) made up of small basophilic cells

(D) cystic

(E) malignant

**116.** Magnesium sulfate is used in the treatment of eclampsia. It has which of the following characteristics?

(A) is metabolized by the liver

(B) has vitamin K as an antidote

(C) can cause convulsions if given in excess

(D) can be given IM or IV

(E) the respiratory arrest reaction is patient-specific idiopathic

**117.** A 24-year-old woman (gravida 3, para 0, abortus 2) comes to you for prenatal care. Her sister had a clot when on the pill and was found to have Factor V Leiden. Her mother and father were tested after her sister's clot, and only her mother is heterozygous for Factor V Leiden. She has never had any problems, even though she took the pill for 4 years. How should you advise her?

(A) She has a 25% chance of having the disease.

(B) She may need low-dose aspirin during this pregnancy.

(C) She needs coumadin starting at 20 weeks and continuing until 36 weeks when she is switched to heparin.

(D) You need to order Factor V levels.

(E) You need to order activated protein C resistance.

**118.** The "stripping" or "sweeping" of the membranes in a term pregnancy is thought to induce labor by the decidual release of a precursor to PGs, which in turn cause labor. Which of the following substances is the precursor to PGs in this setting?

(A) arachidonic acid

(B) isobutyric acid

(C) isoleucine

(D) linoleic acid

(E) phospholipase A

**119.** A 6-year-old girl experiences irregular vaginal bleeding. She is taller than her peers and has early breast development. Serum gonadotropin levels are low and remain unchanged after IV administration of GnRH. What is the most likely diagnosis?

(A) corpus luteum cyst

(B) endometrioma

(C) epoophoron

(D) fibroma

(E) granulosa cell tumor

**120.** During normal pregnancy, which of the following physiologic effects occur?

(A) increased serum beta-globulins (transport proteins) and decreased triglycerides

(B) increased serum corticosteroid-binding globulin and free cortisol

(C) increased levels of immunoglobulins A, G, and M

(D) increased thyroid-binding globulin and iodide levels

(E) decreased serum ionized calcium levels and parathyroid hormone (PTH)

**121.** Which of the following occurs with the increase in red blood cells (RBCs) during pregnancy?

(A) causes the hematocrit to rise

(B) is due to the prolonged life span of the erythrocytes

(C) is due to increased production of erythrocytes

(D) results despite decreased levels of erythropoiesis in maternal plasma

(E) there is no increase in RBCs

**122.** A 18-year-old girl (G1P0) presents to the obstetrical triage unit in the hospital at 34 weeks EGA complaining of shortness of breath. Her pulse ox is 98% on room air, and her lung sounds are clear. You determine that this is a case of physiologic hyperventilation of pregnancy. As she explained the etiology of this, which of the following is noted to probably responsible for physiologic hyperventilation during pregnancy?

(A) decreased functional residual volume (RV)

(B) decreased plasma $P_{O_2}$

(C) increased estrogen production

(D) increased progesterone production

(E) large fluctuations in plasma bicarbonate

**123.** A 29-year-old primigravida at 36 weeks' gestation complains of dizziness and nausea when reclining to read in bed before retiring at night. Suspecting that her symptoms are the result of normal physiologic changes of pregnancy, you recommend which of the following?

(A) elevation of both her feet while lying in bed

(B) improved room lighting

(C) mild exercise before retiring to bed

(D) rolling toward the right or left hip while reading

(E) small late night snack

**124.** A healthy 30-year-old primigravida presents at 34 weeks' gestation. She reports that she has been experiencing abdominal discomfort that increases after eating, especially when in the recumbent position. A series of tests is performed. She has normal vital signs, an unremarkable examination, a fundal height of 33 cm, and a negative urinalysis. Which one of the following represents abnormal test results?

(A) alkaline phosphatase double that of the reference range

(B) hemoglobin of 9.0 g/dL

(C) serum albumin of 3.0 g/dL

(D) serum creatinine level of 0.8 mg/dL

(E) WBC count of 11,000/mL

**125.** The placenta is essential in the growth and development of a healthy fetus. It allows transport of certain things, facilitates transports of others, and is hormonally active. Which of the following statements regarding the placenta is true?

(A) High-molecular-weight substances and protein-bound substances cross readily.

(B) In the placenta, fetal blood is in lacunae that bathe maternal capillaries.

(C) Infectious organisms cannot cross the placenta from mother to fetus.

(D) The placenta fulfills some of the functions of lung, kidney, and intestine for the fetus.

(E) The placenta produces only hCG.

**126.** The pulmonary system of the fetus is one of the key facets of a newborn successfully transitioning to an air environment. Characteristics of the fetal respiratory system include which of the following?

(A) anatomic maturation is independent of amniotic fluid volume

(B) high level of surfactant by term

(C) no evidence of respiratory movement until 8 months' gestation

(D) normal maturation sufficient to support long-term extrauterine existence by the end of the fifth lunar month

(E) slow aspiration of amniotic fluid

**127.** Characteristics of the fetal digestive tract include which of the following?

(A) esophageal atresia until the seventh lunar month

(B) lack of hydrochloric acid until after delivery

(C) peristalsis starting at approximately 20 weeks' gestation

(D) production of meconium only in the eighth month of gestation

(E) swallowing of amniotic fluid by 16 weeks' gestation

**128.** A term infant is born with normal external female genitalia. Which of the following is not possible?

(A) There is androgen insensitivity.

(B) There is functional dihydrotestosterone (DHT).

(C) There is inadequate androgen production.

(D) There are no functioning gonads.

(E) There are ovaries.

**129.** Which of the following is a muscle of the external genitalia?

(A) the gluteus

(B) the sartorius

(C) the superficial transverse perineal

(D) the deep transverse perineal

(E) the levator ani

**130.** A patient develops a fever of 102°F, and a tender abdomen and uterus at 4 days postpartum. She also notices dark brown urine, and when blood is drawn the serum is red. A flat plate X-ray of the abdomen shows air in the uterus. Gram's stain of uterine curettings reveals gram-positive plump rods. On the basis of this information, which of the following is the most likely organism?

(A) *Bacteroides*

(B) *Clostridium perfringens*

(C) *Enterococcus*

(D) *Escherichia coli*

(E) *Gonococcus*

**131.** A 34-year-old patient developed an endometritis postpartum and was treated for 6 days in the hospital with bed rest, antibiotics, and fluids. She was improving when, on the eighth day, shortness of breath, anterior chest pain, and tachycardia occurred suddenly. Which of the following is the most likely diagnosis?

(A) amniotic fluid emboli

(B) Mendelson syndrome

(C) myocardial infarction

(D) pelvic abscess

(E) pulmonary embolism

**132.** A 40-year-old nulligravida female pediatrician comes to see you for irregular vaginal bleeding of 1-year duration. She has not been using birth control and had hoped to conceive. Endometrial biopsy revealed endometrial hyperplasia. She would like medical treatment and wants to know which factor is most important in determining premalignant potential. Which of the following is the best way to advise your patient?

(A) age of the patient

(B) degree of cystic atrophy

(C) persistence of bleeding

(D) thickness of endometrial hyperplasia

(E) degree of cytologic atypia

**133.** A 32-year-old woman with polycystic ovary syndrome (PCOS) has infertility of 1-year duration. Her menses occur at irregular intervals, and BBTs are monophasic. An endometrial biopsy shows endometrial hyperplasia with mild cytologic atypia. Which of the following is the most appropriate therapy?

(A) danazol

(B) medroxyprogesterone acetate

(C) OCs

(D) clomiphene citrate

(E) human menopausal gonadotropins (hMGs)

134. An 80-year-old woman who has never taken estrogen develops a pink vaginal discharge. An endometrial biopsy shows adenocarcinoma of the endometrium. Papanicolaou smear is negative. Which of the following is the most important prognostic indicator?

    (A) body habitus
    (B) level of CA-125
    (C) nutritional status
    (D) histologic type of tumor
    (E) presence of peptide hormone receptors

135. A 60-year-old woman with a 4-month history of pelvic pain, constipation, urinary urgency, and a complex adnexal mass with ascites is counseled by a gynecologic oncologist about the potential diagnosis of ovarian cancer. Which of the following is the most important principle in the treatment of ovarian cancer?

    (A) removal of all resectable disease
    (B) examination of tumor cells cultured in vitro
    (C) choice of chemotherapy
    (D) calculation of radiation dose
    (E) measurement of tumor hormone receptors

136. Which of the following is the most important prognostic indicator of survival from advanced ovarian carcinoma?

    (A) stage of disease
    (B) grade of tumor differentiation
    (C) nutritional status
    (D) body mass index
    (E) presence of sex steroid receptors

137. A 58-year-old woman is having surgery for an ovarian mass. At surgery there are external papillary excrescences. the pathologist on frozen notes psammoma bodies. Which of the following ovarian epithelial tumors is the most likely etiology of her pelvic mass?

    (A) mucinous cystadenomas
    (B) serous cystadenomas
    (C) dermoids

    (D) lutein cysts
    (E) Brenner tumors

138. A 56-year-old postmenopausal woman complains of paroxysmal flushing of the face and neck. Facial flushing is associated with colicky abdominal pain with diarrhea and shortness of breath. She has been told by her friends that she needs estrogen replacement therapy. Physical examination is normal. Pelvic examination demonstrates a 5-cm right adnexal mass. What is the most appropriate diagnostic test?

    (A) a serum FSH
    (B) a serum TSH
    (C) serum thyroid function studies
    (D) a urinary 5-hydroxyindole acetic acid
    (E) urinary catecholamines

139. A 16-year-old phenotypic girl is seen for primary amenorrhea. Karyotyping shows 46,XY. In counseling, you advise gonadectomy under which of the following circumstances?

    (A) when she is finished growing
    (B) if the gonads are not in the normal location in the pelvis
    (C) primarily because of the risk of malignancy
    (D) primarily because there is no chance of pregnancy
    (E) primarily because she will become virilized

140. A 75-year-old woman has bilateral, solid adnexal masses. Mammography is normal. GI studies show a stomach lesion suspicious for malignancy. Which of the following is the most likely diagnosis?

    (A) Pick's adenoma
    (B) Krukenberg's tumor
    (C) Brenner tumor
    (D) struma ovarii
    (E) carcinoid

141. Ovarian tumors can be derived from each of the embryologic components of the ovary. Which of the following ovarian tumors is derived from the ovarian "germinal" epithelium?

    (A) dysgerminoma
    (B) fibroma
    (C) theca cell
    (D) endometrioid
    (E) teratoma

142. Your patient asks you, "What are the advantages of mammography." Which of the following statements can you correctly tell her?

    (A) It can detect some breast cancers as early as 2 years before they would reach a palpable size.
    (B) It can detect all cancers greater than 1 cm in diameter.
    (C) It can effectively screen all women after age 30.
    (D) It is an equally effective screening technique in both premenopausal and postmenopausal women.
    (E) It can be decreased to every 3 years in women older than 70 years because their risk of breast cancer is decreased compared to the 50–70-age group.

143. An 88-year-old woman complains of itching of the nipple on her left breast over the past 2 months. On examination, you see excoriation and superficial ulceration of the nipple area. How should you counsel this patient?

    (A) She most likely has eczema of the breast and should be treated with corticosteroids.
    (B) This is a common finding in postmenopausal women. If her mammogram is negative, topical estrogen therapy or oral estrogen therapy is indicated.
    (C) Wearing gloves to bed will usually stop the scratch–itch cycle and resolve the problem. A small bandage over the area at night may also accomplish this task.

    (D) This presentation is nearly pathognomonic for breast cancer in a woman this age. A mammogram should be performed to confirm the diagnosis.
    (E) The woman may have Paget's disease of the breast. The eroded area should be biopsied.

144. A 68-year-old woman consults with you because she has discovered a single firm nodule in the upper outer quadrant of her left breast. Examination reveals a discrete nodule with no skin edema, no enlargement of lymph nodes, no retraction, no redness, and no pain. What should the immediate course of action include?

    (A) needle aspiration of the nodule
    (B) repeat examination in 2 weeks
    (C) radiation therapy
    (D) biopsy of the lesion
    (E) mastectomy

145. A 24-year-old primigravida at 36 weeks' gestation is exposed to chickenpox. She has no history of varicella. What is the most appropriate next step in the management of this patient ?

    (A) varicella vaccine within 48 hours of exposure
    (B) immediate administration of varicella zoster immune globulin (VZIG) and acyclovir
    (C) IV acyclovir and the varicella vaccine within 96 hours
    (D) immediate serologic testing for varicella, and if negative, administration of VZIG
    (E) VZIG within 96 hours

146. A 39-year-old woman presents complaining of severe, low abdominal–pelvic pain that began the day after her menses ended. She has noticed some increase in vaginal discharge. Her social history shows she and her late husband had been medical missionaries throughout their entire lives. He was her only sexual partner, and since his death 1 year ago, she has not had intercourse. Physical examination shows a temperature of 102°F. She is on the examining table on her side, doubled over, and clutching her abdomen with both arms. She has abdominal tenderness with rebound (right greater than left), cervical motion tenderness (greatest on rectal examination), and mild tenderness in the area of the right adnexa with no masses felt. Gram's stain of her cervix shows a "few WBCs"; WBC is 14,400 (normal 3,600–10,000), and an ESR of 47 mm/h (normal 0–25). A urine pregnancy test is negative. What is the next logical step in evaluation of this patient?

   (A) admit her to the hospital with presumed PID, begin parenteral antibiotics, and wait 24 to 48 hours to assess her progress
   (B) perform culdocentesis
   (C) perform a pelvic ultrasound
   (D) order a computed tomography (CT) scan of the abdomen and pelvis
   (E) take her to the operating room for diagnostic laparoscopy

**DIRECTIONS (Questions 147 through 150): The following groups of questions are preceded by a list of lettered options. For each question, select the one lettered option that is most closely associated with it. Each lettered option may be used once, multiple times, or not at all.**

**Questions 147 and 148**

   (A) bowel perforation
   (B) erosion of the urethra
   (C) foreign body granulomatous response
   (D) osteitis pubis

   (E) osteomyelitis
   (F) retropubic abscess
   (G) retropubic space hematoma
   (H) urinary tract infection (UTI)

147. A 42-year-old woman is 6 weeks' postoperative from a Marshall–Marchetti–Krantz (MMK) procedure for stress incontinence. She complains of suprapubic pain and burning with walking and standing. She is voiding fine and denies fever or vaginal discharge. On examination, she has tenderness over the pubic symphysis and limitation of abduction. WBC is 9,500. Microscopic urine evaluation shows no pyuria.

148. A 60-year-old woman had a Mersilene pubovaginal sling placed for recurrent stress incontinence after a prior MMK. She has had prior pelvic radiation for cervical cancer. For what serious complication does this procedure put her at risk?

**Questions 149 and 150**

   (A) isoimmunization
   (B) maternal alpha-thalassemia
   (C) maternal parvovirus
   (D) placenta angioma
   (E) cystic adenomatoid malformation of the fetal lung
   (F) fetal congenital heart disease
   (G) fetal nephrotic syndrome
   (H) fetal cardiac arrhythmia

149. A mother has hydramnios and positive [Sjögren's Ro (SSA) and La (SSB)] antibodies.

150. A mother had a slight rash, low-grade fever, and red cheeks for several days approximately 3 weeks ago. She is well now, but has developed a rapidly enlarging uterus at 30 weeks' gestation.

# Answers and Explanations

1. **(B)** CIN III includes severe dysplasia and CIS. It is not invasive and therefore is not cancer. If it is not treated appropriately, however, approximately 30% will progress to invasive cancer. We do not know what causes CIN III, but it is not due to bacterial infection. It is more severe than one would predict from the prior LGSIL found on her Pap smear. If her Pap smear had been an HGSIL, the Pap smear and the biopsy would be better correlated.

2. **(D)** Most medical professional liability claims represent negligence torts. Intention is not a factor in tort cases. Torts require proof of four elements of negligent action: duty, breach of duty, causation, and damage. Duty is the physician's responsibility to act in accordance with a standard of care to prevent or avoid patient injury. Breach of duty involves violation of this standard of care. Causation, or proximate cause, is the essential element of a liability claim. It links the physician's negligent act to actual damages.

3. **(E)** Pad use is protective. Predisposing factors for TSS include high-absorbency tampons (which obstruct or ulcerate the vagina), neutral vaginal pH created by vaginal blood, and high vaginal oxygen content (due to tampon insertion). In addition, the longer a tampon is left in place, the greater the risk for developing TSS. Coital frequency is not a factor.

4. **(C)** Persons with O-negative blood are called universal donors. O-type blood may have factors that can cause reactions to other factors in other blood group systems; however, they lack A or B antigens.

5. **(E)** Siblings have one chance in four of being the same human leukocyte antigen (HLA) haplotype. Parents or more distant relatives are unlikely to have both haplotypes, the same as those of the child.

6. **(D)** The principal hypothalamic locus for GnRH secretion is the arcuate nucleus. Lesions in this area cause gonadal atrophy and amenorrhea. Cell bodies for dopamine synthesis are found in the arcuate and periventricular nuclei. Separate cells in the paraventricular and supraoptic nuclei make vasopressin and oxytocin.

7. **(D)** Although the pathway from pregnenolone to aldosterone would function, there would be no cortisol production. Without cortisol negative feedback on the pituitary, adrenocorticotropic hormone (ACTH) secretion increases, causing adrenal hyperplasia in an attempt to maintain cortisol production. In the absence of sex steroid production, gonadotropin secretion also increases.

8. **(A)** The major problem in children with idiopathic precocious puberty is that increased circulating sex steroid levels induce accelerated childhood bone growth but premature epiphyseal closure. Affected individuals are taller than peers as children but short in stature as adults. A radiogram of the wrist is the easiest test to confirm changes in bone composition

induced by sex steroids. GnRH analogues have been used in children with true sexual precocity to suppress the hypothalamus and delay epiphyseal closure.

9.  **(A)** In the absence of 17-hydroxylase, circulating levels of cortisol and sex steroids are low. Without negative feedback of cortisol and sex steroids, ACTH and gonadotropin levels are elevated. The resulting increase in circulating gonadotropin levels accompanying absence of gonadal sex steroids is referred to as hypergonadotropic hypogonadism. This rare cause of congenital adrenal hyperplasia causes delayed puberty and is associated with hypertension due to accumulation of mineralocorticoids (e.g., deoxycorticosterone).

10. **(C)** Of the many follicles present at birth, only about 400 follicles ever mature and extrude on ovum. Most that start to develop become atretic. No new follicles are formed after birth. Usually, only one follicle ovulates during each cycle.

11. **(B)** Estrogen deficiency causes atrophy of estrogen-dependent tissue. Consequently, postmenopausal women commonly develop amenorrhea, vaginal stenosis, atrophic vaginal mucosa, and small labia minora. Clitoromegaly accompanies high circulating androgen levels and raises the real possibility of an androgen-producing tumor.

12. **(C)** The rotation usually occurs to the right and is thought to be due to the presence of the rectosigmoid on the left. Rotation should be determined prior to performing cesarean section. A pelvic mass on the right, such as transplanted kidney, will result in levorotation.

13. **(E)** The saliva may be related to nausea. The symptom may be helped by atropine. It will spontaneously regress after pregnancy.

14. **(C)** Although the total amount of hemoglobin increases in pregnancy, the plasma volume increases to a greater extent and the hemoglobin and hematocrit both fall. Blood volume increases by 45%, while hematocrit, in total, in-

creases by only 33%. Adequate iron supplementation will decrease this disparity.

15. **(C)** Some dependent edema is normal during pregnancy. It can be alleviated by instructing the patient to rest on her side and to wear fitted, graded, pressure elastic support hose without constricting bands. The heart, however, remains an effective pump. Decreased plasma oncotic pressure helps to exacerbate this edema. Serum sodium concentration is nearly normal in spite of sodium retention because of the increase in plasma volume.

16. **(D)** Cesarean section is indicated for a transverse lie. The incision on the uterus will depend on assessment at surgery for ease of delivery.

17. **(D)** Compensation of a lowered $P_{CO_2}$ is affected by metabolic reduction of bicarbonate. The pH change is minimal. Pulmonary function is not impaired by pregnancy. Changes are physiologically compensated.

18. **(D)** This woman may be experiencing a placental abruption. The bleeding and late decelerations signify the need for prompt delivery.

19. **(A)** With this history she has a >10% risk of venous thromboembolism durig pregnancy. Heparin therapy is indicated for this patient. Aspirin will not be sufficient and platelet inhibitors are poorly studied. Coumadin crosses the placenta and so is contraindicated in pregnancy.

20. **(D)** The exact relationship these varying compounds have in promoting lipoprotein synthesis and surfactant production is unclear, but some evidence exists supporting roles for each of the compounds listed. Perhaps some complex interaction of all of them is needed. One of the few widely used clinical techniques to promote the development of fetal lung maturity is the maternal administration of glucocorticoids. There is appreciable evidence supporting the administration of glucocorticosteroids in large amounts to the mother at certain critical times during gestation to effect an increased rate of maturation in the fetal lungs when preterm delivery is anticipated.

21. **(A)** Androgens are the only hormones relevant to the embryogenesis of the external genitalia. In the absence of androgens, female external genitalia will form. The active androgen is DHT.

22. **(A)** Obviously, some catastrophic event has occurred. Laparotomy is indicated. Oxygen should also be given but that is not the main issue.

23. **(D)** The U.S. Food and Drug Administration has established categories for medications with regard to the drug's fetal effect. For category B drugs, animal studies show no fetal risk and there are no human studies or there have been adverse effects in animals, but human studies have shown no risks. Category A has no fetal risk in human studies. In category C, there may be adverse effects in animals, but there are no available human data. Category D drugs have fetal risk, but the benefits may outweigh risks. Category X has proven significant fetal risks.

24. **(E)** The Lewis antigen is not associated with fetal hydropic disease; therefore, one should not plan termination of pregnancy, serial amniocentesis, or any invasive procedure because of this finding. On the other hand, the patient is Rh-negative and should receive a dose of 300 $\mu$g D-immunoglobulin if she is not immunized, at 28 to 32 weeks and within 3 days after delivery if the infant is proved to be Rh-positive. This is done routinely to prevent sensitization from an Rh-positive infant.

25. **(A)** The greatest advantage to CVS is that fetal cells can be obtained at an earlier stage of gestation and, because of their rapid division, obviate the need for cell culture, thereby allowing earlier results. A disadvantage is that fetuses with chromosomal abnormalities, which would spontaneously abort if one waited a slightly longer time, may be present. One can perform enzyme studies on cells after either CVS or amniocentesis, so that it in itself is not a specific benefit of the CVS. CVS is associated with a slightly increased fetal risk when compared to amniocentesis. The cell sample is good, but, because of maternal contamination, the possibility exists of fetal and maternal chromosomes being confused. CVS also requires a greater learning time for the clinician to perform it adequately.

26. **(C)** The diagonal conjugate is the distance from the pubic arch to the sacrum promontory and should be at least 11.5 cm. By subtracting approximately 1.5 cm, you will have a good approximation of the obstetric conjugate. The intertuberous distance should be approximately 8 cm. The angle of the pubic rami should be approximately from 85° to 90°. The sacrum should be hollow and deep. The midpelvis is difficult to measure clinically, and X-ray or CT examinations have been used in special situations. A thorough clinical examination of the bony pelvis allows one to predict the ease or difficulty of delivering a normal-sized infant.

27. **(A)** Ventilation and cardiac massage must all be done simultaneously in the depressed, acidotic apneic infant with a very slow or absent heartbeat. If no blood circulates, neither oxygen nor base will get to the peripheral cells, where metabolism occurs. Anything short of successful ventilation and circulation will result in a severely damaged or dead baby.

28. **(E)** All the procedures must be done, but none will be of any avail if the airway is not clear. A clear airway is the first priority in any emergency, for without availability of oxygen, the patient will die in a few minutes regardless of what else is done.

29. **(B)** Profuse, thin, acellular cervical mucus reflects high circulating estrogen levels that occur prior to ovulation. If the patient is postmenopausal, there is little to no estrogen. If she is pregnant or on birth control pills, there is a high level of progesterone, which prevents this type of mucus. If she is ovulatory, this cervical mucus pattern can be used to detect the presence of a developing ovarian follicle.

30. **(B)** When the placenta is firmly attached to the myometrium, it is a placenta accreta, if it

invades but has not penetrated the entire depth of the myometrium it is placenta increta and it is placenta percreta if it has penetrated the entire depth. These defects in placental site attachment occur most commonly after previous cesarean section or curettage or with women of high parity. They are dangerous because hemorrhage may occur antepartum, intrapartum, and/or postpartum. This is particularly true if it is in the lower uterine segment, where thin myometrium does not allow adequate compression of the enlarged, ruptured blood vessels after an attempt is made to deliver the placenta.

31. **(B)** A face presentation with mentum posterior presents a large cephalic diameter to the pelvis and does not allow extension as a normal mechanism of labor. To deliver the head, rotation to mentum anterior must occur to allow extension. Often, the rotation will be spontaneous.

32. **(D)** Cardiac arrhythmias and pulmonary edema are serious side effects of beta-adrenergic stimulation. Pulmonary edema usually occurs only with concomitant infection or corticosteroids. Plasma glucose increases and blood pressure usually decreases. Hypokalemia is seldom a major problem. Beta-mimetic agents are used to treat asthma.

33. **(B)** This patient has delivered a large infant, and without other sources of bleeding such as lacerations, the most likely cause of bleeding is uterine atony. The first best step is to add oxytocin to her IV solution. Other steps, though helpful, will be secondary.

34. **(D)** Remember the common association of genital and urinary malformations. A longitudinal vaginal septum does not usually constitute a barrier to either conception or delivery. If the uterus is deformed, implantation may be compromised.

35. **(B)** The tamponade effect of the myometrium is remarkable. Patients on heparin therapy whose blood does not clot do not bleed unusually at delivery if the uterus contracts well and no lacerations are present. Uterine atony can be a serious problem.

36. **(D)** The diagnosis that must be ruled out immediately is placenta previa. Ultrasound should be used to confirm or eliminate this as the diagnosis. Pelvic examination for the purpose of diagnosis is contraindicated without a double setup (the performance of the examination in the operating room where an emergent cesarean section can be done if bleeding occurs). The fetus is mature enough to be delivered now if a placenta previa is found since it is unlikely that the placenta will migrate out of the way at this point and the risk of a major hemorrhage persists. If no placental problem is found, the bleeding stops and mother and fetus are stable, it may be appropriate to send the patient home without delivery.

37. **(A)** The most common cause of bleeding during the hour after delivery is uterine atony, especially if a proper postpartum examination of the cervix and vaginal canal has been done to help rule out lacerations. However, the excess bleeding necessitates rapid assessment to rule out other factors. If they are ruled out and massage causes the bleeding to cease, you can maintain uterine tone and continue observation. If bleeding persists, examination under anesthesia (EUA) and D&C may be done to rule out retained secundae or uterine tears not visible from below.

38. **(B)** Nursing is contraindicated in industrialized countries with availability of good alternative sources of formula, when the mother has active CMV, chronic active hepatitis B, or HIV. If the mother has an active outbreak of varicella at delivery, she should avoid contact with the infant until the vesicles are gone, which includes breast-feeding. As long as there are no herpetic lesions on the breast, nursing is acceptable with the mother observing good hand-washing technique. The main issue with genital herpes is the mode of delivery, not breast-feeding.

39. **(A)** The plasma fibrinogen remains high for several days and as a result the ESR remains

moderately elevated as well. The hematocrit should remain stable unless there was excessive blood loss. Diuresis should occur, rather than fluid retention.

40. **(B)** The immediate care of the newborn is directed toward the same concepts as the critical care of any patient—make sure the patient is breathing and the airway is clear. Once this has been accomplished, attention must be directed to protecting the infant from the hazards of heat loss. Since the infant is naked and wet and will lose heat to the atmosphere, predisposing to metabolic problems, it should be dried and warmed. The most effective way to accomplish this end is vigorous and immediate drying of the newborn. A quick physical examination is indicated but is not an immediate priority. Hematocrit is indicated only if anemia or blood dyscrasia is suspected, and then only after the newborn has been stabilized.

41. **(C)** The infant's liver does not have adequate enzyme systems to conjugate the bilirubin load. Mild jaundice often occurs because unconjugated bilirubin is poorly excreted. It can be photoabsorbed with great therapeutic results by light, even simple sunlight. This is associated more with breast-feeding than the use of bottle-feeding. Carotene production and meconium have no bearing on the development of jaundice.

42. **(B)** A cephalhematoma lies beneath the periosteum in the subperiosteal space and, therefore, is limited by the midline periosteal attachment to the skull. Subdural hemorrhage, subarachnoid hemorrhage, and tentorial tears result in bleeding directly into the CNS.

43. **(C)** Facial paralysis may occur after either spontaneous (one-third of cases) or forceps delivery (two-thirds of cases) by pressure at the stylomastoid foramen. It is most often transient and rapidly clears within a few days after delivery.

44. **(E)** Renal agenesis (Potter syndrome) occurs about 1 in 4,000 births. It is more frequent in male infants. Prenatally, a low amniotic fluid volume is seen (because there is no urine made). The constellation of findings described in the problem are found in addition to the lack of kidneys. One-third of infants with this syndrome are stillborn; the others die within 48 hours of life. A diaphragmatic hernia does not present with the other anomalies but will have respiratory difficulty and difficulty ventilating. Pyloric stenosis is usually an isolated event without other anomalies and may be associated with excessive amniotic fluid volume. Postmaturity will also not have the anomalies noted or the difficulty ventilating the fetus.

45. **(E)** *Unexplained infertility* is a term used to define couples who have completed their entire infertility workup with no clear etiology for their infertility problem. In this case, although the hysterosalpingogram demonstrated unilateral proximal obstruction, the diagnostic laparoscopy demonstrated patent tubes bilaterally. It is important to note that the laparoscopy is necessary for the workup to exclude endometriosis or pelvic adhesions. The semen analysis is normal with excellent concentration, motility, and morphology. Luteal-phase deficiency is unlikely given the normal-length luteal phase and serum progesterone level (>10 ng/mL).

46. **(A)** Autosomal trisomy is the most common chromosomal abnormality associated with first-trimester spontaneous abortion. X monosomy is the next most common chromosomal abnormality. Triploidy commonly accompanies hydropic placental degeneration. Tetraploidy and sex-chromosome polysomy are rare causes of first-trimester spontaneous abortion.

47. **(C)** Clomiphene citrate is typically utilized as a first-line agent in the treatment of anovulation in patients. The course of therapy usually involves clomiphene citrate for 5 days, with ovulation usually occurring in 7 days after the last tablet has been ingested. It is quite successful, causing ovulation in 75% to 80% of all patients with a multiple pregnancy rate of 7%. There is no increased risk of congenital anomalies in clomiphene citrate-induced pregnancies.

Severe ovarian hyperstimulation syndrome occurs rarely in patients treated with clomiphene citrate.

48. **(A)** The presence of ovarian hyperandrogenism (HA), insulin resistance (IR), and hyperpigmentation of the neck, axillae, and skin folds [acanthosis nigricans (AN)] constitutes the HAIR-AN syndrome, a variant of PCOS. Normal values of serum DHEAS and 17-hydroxy-progesterone exclude a primary adrenal disorder (CAH) or a neoplastic process. The treatment of hirsutism under these conditions depends on the desires of the patient. Women with PCOS-induced hirsutism who do not wish to conceive should receive OCs to suppress gonadotropin secretion and ovarian androgen production thereby decreasing hirsuitism progression. The estrogen component of the OC also stimulates hepatic SHBG synthesis. As SHBG-bound testosterone (T) levels increase, the amount of biologically active T in the circulation decreases. The progestin component of the OC opposes estrogen-induced endometrial stimulation. GnRH analogues also have been used for treatment of PCOS-related hirsutism, but the risk of bone demineralization and the complaints of menopausal side effects (e.g., hot flashes and vaginal dryness) limit the usefulness of this therapy unless it is combined with exogenous hormones. Antiandrogens block T action by competing with T for its skin receptors but may also inhibit steroidogenic enzymes, causing menstrual irregularity. Antiandrogens are contraindicated during pregnancy because they may enter the fetal circulation and antagonize T action during sexual differentiation. For these reasons, antiandrogens are usually combined with OCs for treatment of hirsutism. Anovulatory women with PCOS who wish to conceive should receive ovulation-inducing agents (e.g., clomiphene citrate).

49. **(A)** Secondary amenorrhea refers to absence of menses for 6 months or a duration of three of the previous menstrual cycle lengths. Although the distinction between primary and secondary amenorrhea tends to identify groups of individuals with different disorders (e.g., abnormal gonadal development occurs in 30% to 40% of women with primary amenorrhea but occurs less frequently in women with secondary amenorrhea), the diagnostic approach to primary and secondary amenorrhea is similar. After obtaining a history regarding sexual activity, contraception, use of medication associated with amenorrhea, stress, exercise, weight change, and instrumentation of the uterus (e.g., induced abortion), a serum hCG level should be obtained to exclude pregnancy. Serum prolactin and TSH should also be measured because abnormalities of prolactin secretion and thyroid function disrupt ovulation. The next step is to determine whether menstruation occurs 2 to 7 days after progesterone administration (progesterone challenge). The ability of progesterone to induce menstruation (positive response) requires a circulating $E_2$ value of about 40 pg/mL and an endometrium responsive to estrogen. Individuals with a positive response to progesterone challenge have a functional hypothalamic–pituitary–gonadal axis and do not have an anatomic abnormality of the hypothalamus or pituitary.

50. **(E)** The IUCD string may retract into the cervical canal so that it is not palpable. It may also become displaced because of pregnancy, malposition, expulsion, and perforation. The latter complication accompanies about 1:1,000 IUCD insertions and occurs more frequently with insertions performed postpartum when uterine involution is incomplete. The IUCD string can often be found by gently probing the cervical canal with a Q-tip or cytobrush. If cervical probing is unsuccessful, further studies, including colposcopy with an endocervical speculum, pelvic ultrasound, abdominal radiography, or hysteroscopy may be necessary.

51. **(A)** The most common side effect associated with OC use is breakthrough bleeding. It usually occurs during the first one or two cycles and resolves spontaneously. Another common problem is amenorrhea. Persistent breakthrough bleeding and amenorrhea commonly reflect an atrophic endometrium and may be corrected by using a pill with a higher estrogen or lower progestin content. Other side

effects include nausea, fluid retention (and perhaps weight gain), mood change, headache, breast tenderness (mastalgia), and a brownish discoloration of the face, particularly the forehead and cheeks (chloasma). Nausea usually not only remits spontaneously but also may decrease by taking pills with food or at bedtime. Generally, these side effects are minimal with "low-dose pills." OCs decrease PG levels in menstrual fluid and lessen dysmenorrhea.

52. **(E)** Excessive tubal destruction during female sterilization can create a small cornual fistula between the uterine and peritoneal cavities. This complication occurs most commonly when the tube is fulgurated near its uterine insertion rather than at its midportion. Spermatozoa migrating through the fistula can enter the fimbriated end of the tube. If fertilization occurs, 50% of the resulting pregnancies are ectopic. The remaining intrauterine pregnancies probably result from spontaneous tubal recannulation, failure of mechanical devices, and incomplete tissue damage by electrocoagulation. Although pelvic pain and menstrual abnormalities after tubal ligation have been called the "post–tubal ligation syndrome," there is no evidence that female sterilization increases the risk of dysmenorrhea, anovulation, irregular bleeding, or ovarian cyst formation.

53. **(E)** Second-trimester pregnancy termination may be accomplished by either surgical evacuation of the uterus or induction of labor. D&E is a surgical procedure in which the cervix is dilated and the intrauterine contents are removed with forceps and blunt curet. Unlike the evacuation of the uterus employed with early (first-trimester) terminations, evacuating the contents of a pregnancy at 25 weeks is associated with a much increased risk of perforation, sepsis, and retained products (incomplete removal). Labor may be induced by parenteral, vaginal, or intra-amniotic administration of PGs. IV oxytocin administration is less effective in inducing labor, although it is frequently used in conjunction with PG therapy.

54. **(E)** This is a description of lichen sclerosis, a common problem in postmenopausal women. It has been shown to exhibit increased metabolic activity. It must be followed closely and biopsied if other abnormal areas appear. Experience using the topical corticosteroid clobetasol propionate ointment has shown improved results over previously recommended testosterone and progesterone ointment. About 25% of patients with lichen sclerosis will have associated areas of squamous cell hyperplasia and up to 5% will be associated with intraepithelial neoplasia. Lichen sclerosis should not be confused with the changes found in atrophic (postmenopausal) vulvitis. In atrophic vulvitis, the tissues are thinned and shiny but lack the whitish coloration found in lichen sclerosis.

55. **(E)** Endometrial carcinoma must be ruled out in a postmenopausal woman who bleeds from the vagina, even if the bleeding is of short duration. Once a woman of this age has gone for 12 consecutive months without menstrual bleeding, she is considered menopausal. An office biopsy or curettage is recommended. However, if the woman refuses a sampling, a transvaginal sonogram may be a reasonable alternative since she is at low risk for endometrial cancer (she is not obese, was on OCs until age 42, is not hypertensive, and is recently menopausal; she also bled after a progesterone withdrawal). An endometrial stripe of $\leq 5$ mm on ultrasound is very unlikely to be associated with a premalignant or malignant process.

56. **(E)** The PG synthetase inhibitors [nonsteroidal anti-inflammatory drugs (NSAIDs)] decrease the formation of Prostaglandin F2 (PGF2)-alpha in the endometrium. They have side effects similar to aspirin but are very effective. Most dysmenorrhea can be treated successfully with these medications.

57. **(B)** The usage of combined estrogen and progesterone eliminates hormonal cycling and gradually produces atrophy of the ectopic endometrial glands. This atrophy is the desired treatment effect. Antiestrogens, gonadotropin analogues, and androgens will produce similar suppressive results.

**58. (B)** Luteectomy (removal of the corpus luteum of pregnancy) before 42 days will result in spontaneous miscarriage with a dramatic drop in progesterone and estradiol levels. However, after 7 weeks, loss of pregnancy does not occur because of the ability of the placental unit to produce progesterone. The normal biphasic shift of the luteal-phase BBT remains elevated during pregnancy. It is thought that this persistent shift is mediated via progesterone and interleukins (IL-1).

**59. (D)** Endometriosis affects 10% to 20% of reproductive-age women and is the most common reason for hospitalization. The classic symptoms are increasingly severe dysmenorrhea, pelvic pain, and infertility. It is diagnosed by direct visualization and biopsy. Ectopic endometrial glands surrounded by endometrial stroma should be seen. It can be treated either by surgical extirpation or by hormonal suppression of the ectopic endometrial glands.

**60. (B)** The Burch operation has a quoted success rate of 85% to 95%. The risk of ureteral injury is 0.1% to 1.5%. The risk of permanent urinary retention is fortunately rare, but altered voiding habits are not uncommon (slower stream of urine), as immediate postoperative urinary retention is reported to occur 16% to 25% of the time following a Burch procedure. The risk of later enterocele and/or rectocele is 15% to 20%.

**61. (A)** She has detrusor hyperreflexia with impaired contractility probably due to a neurologic etiology and/or a diabetic neuropathy. Most patients with good hand dexterity can easily master CISC with few risks. Long-term continuous drainage with a Foley has a much higher complication rate with infection, stones, contracted bladder, discomfort, and urethral dilation. While both medications might help the leakage, they both can worsen the voiding dysfunction. Once CISC is mastered, medications can be added if needed.

**62. (B)** Forty percent of abdominal masses in children under the age of 2 years are renal in origin. An ectopic pelvic kidney occurs in up to 15% of girls without a uterus or vagina. The pelvic kidney may be palpable abdominally or rectally.

**63. (A)** A functional ovarian cyst is the most common pelvic mass in menstruating reproductive-age women. It is usually nontender, mobile, and less than 8 cm in diameter. A unilocular smooth ovarian cyst without internal excrescences is usually a functional cyst. Functional ovarian cysts commonly regress spontaneously over 1 to 2 months and also may be suppressed with OCs. With a history of thrombophlebitis when taking OCs, observation is the safest for this patient. OCs for the purpose of cyst suppression are generally not recommended for cysts greater than 8 cm because the chance of neoplasia is too great.

**64. (D)** A painful adnexal mass in an amenorrheic, reproductive-age woman is suspicious of an ectopic pregnancy (implantation of an embryo outside the uterine cavity). One to two percent of all pregnancies are ectopically located, most of which occur in the fallopian tube (tubal pregnancy) as a consequence of chronic salpingitis. Hemorrhage at the implantation site causes a painful adnexal mass due to tubal distention. A serum pregnancy test should be performed in all reproductive-age women with pelvic pain, amenorrhea, and irregular vaginal bleeding. Sonography may be helpful in determining the location of the pregnancy, but knowing if the pregnancy test is positive and the level of hCG will greatly influence the interpretation of the examination.

**65. (B)** The incidence of multifetal pregnancies has risen dramatically with increased use of agents for ovulation induction and transfer of multiple embryos during IVF. Generally, the number of fetuses is inversely related to pregnancy duration and birth weight. This patient has a grand multi-fetal pregnancy, defined as four or more embryos. She has a significant risk of developing pregnancy complications (including preterm delivery and pregnancy-induced hypertension) leading to low-birth-weight infants and high perinatal mortality. Although this case presents several ethical dilemmas, the patient should be offered selective termination, a technique in which the number of fetuses is reduced. It is commonly performed by ultrasound-directed transcervical injection of potassium chloride into the fetal thoracic cavity.

66. **(A)** Any solid tumor of the vulva in a woman of this age should be biopsied without delay. It will most often be benign. An excision biopsy may be curative, and most important, you will find any cancer present.

67. **(C)** Cellular atypia extending less than the full thickness of the squamous cervical epithelium justifies the diagnosis of dysplasia, in this case, probably a moderate dysplasia. More recent terms for classifying the degrees of atypia are CIN grades I, II, and III; the grades depend largely on the distance the atypical cells extend through the epithelium.

68. **(B)** The criteria for staging of carcinoma of the cervix should be memorized (see Table 27–1). Once performed, the clinical stage remains the same, even if subsequent events prove that the tumor was either more or less extensive than thought at the time of the initial staging. Staging is mainly by clinical examination and the few tests used for staging are readily available.

69. **(B)** Such cysts, though rare, can cause technical difficulties during examination, during intercourse, or during tampon insertion. The cysts, also known as Gartner duct cysts, are invariably benign and need to be removed only when they cause problems for the patient.

70. **(C)** Endometrial biopsy allows a histologic evaluation of the endometrial lining in a patient who has several risk factors for endometrial cancer, including age, obesity, and unopposed estrogen replacement therapy (ERT). The sampling done by the biopsy must be complete. Transvaginal sonography is playing an increasing role in evaluating postmenopausal bleeding. An endometrial stripe thickness of less than 5 mm indicates a very small chance of endometrial cancer. However, no tissue is obtained for diagnosis.

**TABLE 27–1.   International Classification of Cancer of the Cervix (FIGO, 1994)**

| Stage | Description |
| --- | --- |
| **Preinvasive carcinoma** | |
| Stage 0 | Carcinoma in situ, intraepithelial carcinoma. |
| **Invasive carcinoma** | |
| Stage I | Strictly confined to the cervix. Extension to corpus should be disregarded. |
| IA | Preclinical carcinomas of the cervix (those diagnosed only by microscopy). |
| IA1 | Measured microscopic stromal invasion no greater than 3-mm deep and 7-mm wide. |
| IA2 | Microscopic lesions larger than IA1. The upper limit of the measurement should not show a depth of invasion of >5 mm from the base of the epithelium, either surface of glandular, and the horizontal spread must not exceed 7 mm. |
| IB | Lesions confined to the cervix of greater dimensions than stage IA2 lesions, whether seen clinically or not. |
| Stage II | Carcinoma extends beyond the cervix but has not extended onto the pelvic wall. The carcinoma involves the vagina, but not the lower third. |
| IIA | No obvious parametrial involvement. |
| IIB | Obvious parametrial involvement. |
| Stage III | Carcinoma has extended onto the pelvic wall. On rectal examination, there is no cancer-free space between the tumor and the pelvic wall. The tumor involves the lower third of the vagina. All cases with hydronephrosis or nonfunctioning kidney unless known to be due to another cause. |
| IIIA | No extension onto the pelvic wall, but involvement of the lower third of vagina. |
| IIIB | Extension onto the pelvic wall and/or hydronephrosis or nonfunctioning kidney due to tumor. |
| Stage IV | Carcinoma extended beyond the true pelvis or clinically involving the mucosa of the bladder or rectum. |
| IVA | Spread of growth to adjacent organs (i.e., rectum or bladder with positive biopsy from these organs). |
| IVB | Spread of growth to distant organs. |

71. **(C)** Sarcomas can occur at any age but are most common after age 40. Most women with uterine sarcoma experience symptoms of short-term duration, including abdominal pain (from a rapidly enlarging uterus), vaginal discharge, and/or vaginal bleeding. Based on similar patterns of disease spread, staging of uterine sarcoma uses the same system as that for endometrial carcinoma. Sarcomas tend to disseminate systemically by hematogenous spread. Therefore, they are often diagnosed at an advanced stage and associated with a poor prognosis (25% overall 5-year survival rate). The tumor may also extend by lymphatic channels and contiguous spread. Distant metastases

commonly occur in the liver, abdomen, brain, and lung.

72. **(C)** Ovarian cancer usually spreads along the peritoneal surfaces of pelvic and abdominal viscera, including the undersurface of the diaphragm. Sites of metastases from ovarian carcinoma, in decreasing order of frequency, are peritoneum (85%), omentum (70%), contralateral ovary (70%), liver (35%), lung (25%), uterus (20%), vagina (15%), and bone (15%). Malnutrition and death usually occur when malignancy invades beyond pelvic structures and spreads along the peritoneal serosa and surface of the bowel, leading to intestinal obstruction. Lymphatic dissemination, particularly to para-aortic nodes, also occurs. Hematogenous metastases and spread of disease to liver and lungs are less common.

73. **(D)** Pseudomyxoma peritonei refers to massive intra-abdominal accumulation of gelatinous material from rupture of mucinous tumors or appendiceal mucoceles. The material is histologically benign but can cause intestinal obstruction. Mucinous cystadenomas are often large tumors (up to 15–30 cm in diameter) and are associated with a lower rate of malignancy (15%) than serous cystadenomas.

74. **(B)** In primary dysmenorrhea, there is no apparent lesion associated with the pain. In secondary dysmenorrhea, there is, and it might include processes within the uterus, within the uterine wall, or external to the uterus (Table 27–2). While hysterectomy would be definitive, the best therapy for secondary dysmenorrhea is always directed toward the underlying cause. In this case, the most appropriate alternative of those given would be OC therapy based on the ability of these agents to produce a thin, atrophic endometrium, even in ectopic endometrial implants. Testosterone in high enough dosage will stop ovulation but causes hirsutism and acne, and its use is generally avoided. Many patients will be helped by one of many PG inhibitors during episodes of dysmenorrhea, but again, OCs are more effective by preventing the cause of the pain.

**TABLE 27–2.  Possible Causes of Secondary Dysmenorrhea**

| Uterine Causes | Extrauterine Causes |
|---|---|
| Adenomyosis | Endometriosis |
| Cervical stenosis and cervical lesions | Inflammation and scarring (adhesions) |
| Congenital abnormalities (outflow obstructions, uterine anomalies) | Nongynecologic causes: Musculoskeletal, gastrointestinal, urinary |
| Infection (chronic endometritis) | "Pelvic congestive syndrome" (debated) |
| Intrauterine contraceptive devices (IUDs) | Psychogenic (rare) |
| Myomas (generally intracavitary or intramural) | Tumors: myomas, benign or malignant tumors of ovary, bowel, or bladder |
| Polyps | |

Reproduced, with permission, from Smith RP. *Gynecology in Primary Care*. Baltimore, MD: Williams & Wilkins, 1996.

75. **(A)** The differential diagnosis for this patient must include ectopic pregnancy and bleeding into a corpus luteum cyst. Transvaginal ultrasonography will provide the best imaging of both the uterine contents (if any) and the adnexa. This superiority over transabdominal ultrasonography is both by proximity and by the higher frequency sound waves allowed by this proximity. Since the resolution of ultrasonographic images is a function of the frequency of the sound used, higher frequency results in better resolution. Higher frequency sound waves do not travel as far in the body, so transabdominal ultrasonography generally uses lower frequencies, resulting in lower resolution. While all of the imaging techniques listed would probably yield diagnostically useful information, the use of ionizing radiation should be avoided when possible in early pregnancy. Magnetic resonance imaging does not have this problem, but its higher cost and limited availability suggest other alternative would be better.

76. **(C)** Stromal hyperthecosis is a benign ovarian disorder in which nests of luteinized stromal cells are present within the gonadal stroma. Circulating androgen levels may be markedly elevated, mimicking those accompanying an ovarian tumor. Virilization occurs gradually over several years, and gross ovarian morphology is similar to that of polycystic ovaries.

77. **(C)** A single, firm nodule is statistically more worrisome than multiple nodules, and cancer

is most common in the upper outer quadrant. Any firm lump in a postmenopausal woman's breast must be biopsied, aspirated, or shown to be a smooth unilocular cyst on ultrasound regardless of the mammographic findings. However, a mammogram should be done both to evaluate the lump and to rule out other suspicious areas in both breasts.

78. **(C)** Bladder and bowel are the greatest concerns in the radiation treatment of cervical cancer. The dosage to kill tumor is very close to the dosage that will seriously harm these organs. Small bowel is generally far enough from the field so that it survives. Pelvic muscles are very radioresistant. Radiation seldom induces infection.

79. **(C)** Influenza vaccine is a multivalent agent in most cases, given subcutaneous (SQ) or IM, usually in the fall (at the beginning of the flu season). It is an annual vaccination for those at risk of serious complications and also for medical care personnel. Because she is in a high-risk occupation, she should take it in spite of her age.

80. **(E)** No amount of imaging can replace direct observation when there is concern about the possibility of uterine rupture during pregnancy. This is an obstetric emergency and the infant needs to be delivered emergently to avoid compromise.

81. **(E)** Although these changes could represent an anxiety- or stress-related disorder, those are diagnoses of exclusion. Women are at increased risk for thyroid dysfunction, including hyperthyroidism. Even without a clinical goiter, this patient may be hyperthyroid. A very low TSH and an elevated thyroxine (T4) will make the diagnosis. A thyroid scan may become part of the workup but is not the initial screening test. If the thyroid workup is negative, an evaluation for mitral valve prolapse with a good cardiac examination or echocardiogram, or even an evaluation for dysautonomia, if postural blood pressure changes are present, may be warranted.

82. **(C)** The rectus sheath serves to both support and control the rectus muscles. The posterior rectus fascia (sheath) ends at the arcuate line (also called the semicircular line, linea semicircularis, line of Douglas) midway between the umbilicus and pubic symphysis. The rectus muscles are attached mainly to the anterior rectus sheath.

83. **(B)** The occipitomental diameter is about 13.5 cm. A brow presentation tries to force the greatest diameter of the head through the pelvis. The greatest circumference is the occipitofrontal (see Figure 27–1).

84. **(D)** Ether also produces great uterine relaxation but is seldom used in modern obstetric

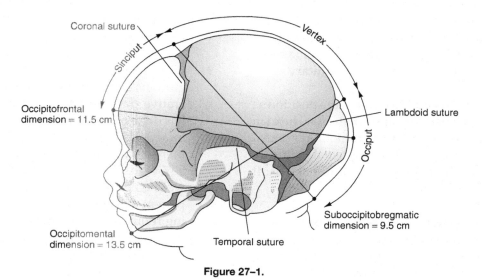

**Figure 27–1.**

units. The regional techniques may decrease uterine contractions but will not result in the profound uterine relaxation caused by halothane. Halothane should be used only when profound uterine relaxation is desired. Atony is seldom desired unless a fetus is "trapped." Often the use of nitroglycerin can get a similar effect for a shorter duration.

85. **(C)** The ovary has hormonally active stroma and follicles. The germ cells are also stored here prior to ovulation. These are the two primary functions of the ovaries. The ovary can vary normally in size from the postmenopausal patient, measuring 1 cm × 1 cm × 0.5 to 4 cm × 3 cm × 2 cm in the reproductive-age patient with multicystic ovaries. The ovary lies in the ovarian fossa of the true pelvis, overlying the iliac vessels. It is attached by a mesentery (mesovarium) to the posterior broad ligament and to the pelvic side-wall by a fold of peritoneum called the infundibulopelvic or suspensory ligament and is normally freely mobile.

86. **(C)** All women with galactorrhea and amenorrhea should be questioned regarding the use of birth control and lactotropic medication. Reproductive-aged women should be considered pregnant until proven otherwise, by measuring urinary or serum hCG. In the absence of pregnancy, evaluation of galactorrhea also includes determination of serum prolactin, TSH, and thyroid function studies. A serum creatinine with blood urea nitrogen (BUN) and chest radiogram also may be indicated if renal or pulmonary disease is suspected. The presence of hyperprolactinemia requires radiologic assessment of the hypothalamus and pituitary.

87. **(A)** A common error is to refer to the position as the lie. A transverse position of the fetal head in labor carries a far different connotation than a transverse lie in labor. The lie is usually directly in line with the maternal longitudinal axis. It may also be oblique or transverse.

88. **(B)** Group B streptococcus is a pathogen carried in the maternal vagina. When pathologic, it may be associated with an overwhelming sepsis in the first 5 days of life, most commonly

in the first 24 hours of life. Mortality can be as high as 10% in term babies and 66% in preterm babies.

89. **(B)** TB was the leading cause of death in the United States in the early 1900s. It has a higher incidence in southeast Asian and Native American populations. Skin tests should be performed routinely during pregnancy in high-risk populations. Only patients with abnormal skin tests or strongly suggestive histories or symptoms (and a negative skin test) should be followed up with chest X-ray. Multidrug therapy can and should be used in pregnancy, with the exception of streptomycin because of its ototoxicity in the fetus. In general, if found and treated in pregnancy, TB has no adverse effect on mother or child.

90. **(C)** The greatest concern here is that the patient may have hepatitis (hepatitis A, B, C, Delta, or non-A, non-B). The patient is at risk for hepatitis B because of her occupation (handling of blood products). The differential diagnosis should not include preeclampsia because her blood pressure is normal, and the symptoms she has are strongly suggestive of a viral syndrome. Since there is no effective treatment for most causes of hepatitis, the most important task is to establish a diagnosis (measuring liver enzymes) and determine, as well as possible, the cause from the serum markers used for hepatitis screening (after screening elevated liver enzymes). Although fatty liver is a possibility, it is a rare complication of pregnancy and unlikely in this setting.

91. **(C)** Passage of a large amount of serosanguinous fluid through the wound on postoperative days 5 to 8 indicates that this wound has dehisced (deep fascial layers are no longer intact). Rather than the fascia just separating, there is more likely a tear of the fascia. About 50% of the time, the wound is also infected. The wound must be explored, and in most cases the patient will have to be taken back to the operating room, debrided, and closed again with internal or external retention sutures. Since this is a serious complication, it must be actively ruled out immediately. Although a delay in the

spontaneous drainage of a hematoma or urinary injury is possible, it is unlikely.

92. **(C)** Sarcoma botryoides (embryonal rhabdomyosarcoma) is a malignant tumor that can involve the vagina, uterus, bladder, and urethra of young girls. It usually begins on the anterior vagina near the cervix and grows to fill the vagina. Eventually, patients experience vaginal discharge and bleeding associated with passage of grape-like lesions. The tumor may also appear as a grape-like mass prolapsing through the vaginal introitus. The combination of surgery, chemotherapy, and radiation therapy offers effective treatment for children with localized disease.

93. **(C)** The history of painless, early labors, five consecutive times, combined with the findings of effacement and dilation make incompetent cervical os the best bet. The history does not make one think of true labor with uterine contractions, although that is a possibility. A mechanical weakness of the cervix is more likely.

94. **(D)** Meticulous repair by layers (i.e., the mucosa, fascia, anal sphincter, perineal muscles, and vaginal mucosa) with interposition of fascia between the rectum and the vagina will yield the best results. If a laceration involves the rectal mucosa, it may be called a fourth-degree laceration.

95. **(A)** Four milligrams of folic acid taken preconceptually will decrease the risk of recurrence of an open neural tube defect by about 50%.

96. **(E)** Shoulder dystocia is a problem of disproportion of fetal shoulders and maternal pelvis. It occurs after the fetal head is delivered. Fundal pressure and increased maternal pushing simply push the shoulders into the symphysis and is contraindicated. The Ritgen maneuver is used for delivery of the head. Correct maneuvers to aid delivery of a baby with shoulder dystocia include McRobert's (flexion of the maternal thighs and knees), and Wood's screw—rotating the fetal shoulders to disimpact the anterior shoulder from behind the symphysis.

97. **(C)** The fetus needs maternal thyroid in the first trimester; it does not make its own thyroid until about 12 weeks. Maternal needs increase by up to 50% in the first trimester. Since she cannot make her own thyroid hormone, she should increase her dose.

98. **(A)** The vacuum extractor is applied to the fetal scalp. The most common complications involve traumatic injury to the scalp, including tentorial tears, cephalhematomas, and subgaleal hemorrhage. The last are the most severe and may be life threatening. Retinal hemorrhages occur up to 30% of the time. Facial lacerations are very uncommon, and rib fractures are not associated with vacuum extraction.

99. **(D)** The clinical utilization of prolactin measurements should be reserved for situations in which the potential causes of hyperprolactinemia may be suspected. These include galactorrhea, experienced by a woman with significant hyperprolactinemia. The amenorrhea/oligomenorrhea is induced by direct effects of prolactin on inhibiting GnRH secretion from the hypothalamus and gonadotropin secretion from the pituitary gland. If radiographic evidence of an enlarged sella turcica is seen, a pituitary adenoma must be suspected. Pituitary adenomas that elevate prolactin secretion are either prolactinomas (prolactin-secreting adenomas) or nonsecretory adenomas, which increase prolactin via a mass effect inhibiting dopamine secretion to the prolactin-secreting cells. Prolactin is always elevated in normal pregnancy.

100. **(A)** Uterine contractions normally cease for a short time immediately after delivery and then continue whether or not the placenta has separated. These uterine contractions are instrumental in causing placental separation by cleavage through the decidual plane of attachment. Traction does not aid in normal placental separation. The lack of change from discoid to globular should raise question of undiagnosed twins.

101. **(A)** Conditions of inappropriate prolactin secretion cause nongestational lactation, referred

to as galactorrhea. The most common cause is a prolactin-secreting pituitary adenoma (prolactinoma). Although one-quarter of the general population harbors a pituitary adenoma (most of which are biologically inert), about one-half of patients with symptomatic hyperprolactinemia have radiologic evidence of a pituitary adenoma. Prolactinomas cause an elevation in circulating prolactin levels. A concomitant suppression of pulsatile GnRH secretion results in amenorrhea. Prolonged estrogen deficiency under these conditions increases the risk of osteoporosis since estrogen plays a role in inhibiting bone reabsorption. Primary hypothyroidism accounts for about 3% to 5% of patients with symptomatic hyperprolactinemia. The compensatory increase in thyrotropin-releasing hormone (TRH) stimulates prolactin release, causing galactorrhea and/or amenorrhea. These symptoms may be the only manifestation of hypothyroidism. Other less common conditions associated with hyperprolactinemia include the following:

- Hypothalamic tumors (e.g., craniopharyngioma), via interruption of dopamine release
- *Medication*: Exogenous estrogen (OCs), dopaminergic antagonists (phenothiazines, tricyclic antidepressants, reserpine, alpha-methyldopa), opiate peptide derivatives (meperidine), histamine (H2-receptor) antagonists (cimetidine), and serotonergic agonists (amphetamines)
- Areolar neural stimulation (prolonged suckling, herpes zoster, chest surgery)
- Renal failure, via reduced metabolic clearance of prolactin
- Ectopic prolactin secretion (bronchogenic carcinoma, hypernephroma)

102. **(C)** Newer formulations attempt to minimize the effects of dry mouth, urinary hesitancy, blurred vision, and confusion. Constipation and abdominal cramping are the most common side effects for all medication in this class. These side effects often will prevent the patient from being compliant with the medication.

103. **(B)** Necrotizing fasciitis is a life-threatening surgical emergency. Prompt aggressive debridement must be performed to remove the necrotic tissue involving the subcutaneous tissue and fascia. The initial presentation may be consistent with cellulitis, but the patient generally appears toxic with signs of sepsis. Surgical explorations are required to rule out necrotizing fasciitis in such suspicious cases. Broad-spectrum antibiotics are necessary for treatment. Patients with diabetes, malnutrition, obesity, and poor tissue perfusion are more susceptible.

104. **(B)** U.S. Preventive Services Task Force (USP-STF) has the following recommendations:

- Mammography every 2 years for women age 50 and older (2009).
- Pap smear at least every 3 years (American Cancer Society and American College of Ob-Gyn (ACOG). They recommend starting Pap smears at age 21 irrespective of the initiation of coitus and every 1–2 years until 30. Less frequent screening is appropriate then in women who are low risk and have had three consecutive normal results).
- *Diabetes screening*: Data are insufficient to recommend formal screening. Testing should be based on risks, patient symptoms, and signs.
- Serum creatinine should be based on risk, symptoms, and signs.
- *Lipids*: Routinely (every 5 years) starting in women aged 45; [American Heart Association follows the recommendation from the National Cholesterol Education Program's (NCEP) expert panel—check lipids at least every 5 years in women starting at age 20].

105. **(D)** If androgens are not present, female genitalia will be formed, regardless of any of the other conditions being met. If the embryonal or fetal organs have an insensitivity to androgen (testicular feminization), female genitalia will form. In the presence of androgens (some forms of congenital adrenal hyperplasia), in spite of a 46,XX chromosomal makeup, male genitalia form.

106. **(E)** The due date is primarily determined by a certain LMP in a woman who has regular monthly menses and has not recently stopped

a hormonal form of contraception or is not currently breast-feeding. Typically a confirmatory ultrasound is done to verify dating and evaluate anatomy or possibly location of the pregnancy. If the earliest ultrasound dating is consistent with the LMP dating (within error range of the ultrasound) then LMP dating is used. In this case, the patient had an ultrasound that was a 8 weeks which is accurate to within less than 1 week. For this reason, ultrasound dating would take priority. Subsequent ultrasound do *not* change dating but demonstrate that the patient is making a large for gestational age infant that appears further along than it is. The key message is: establish dating based on the initial ultrasound and do not change it.

107. **(E)** In a secondary arrest of labor, the problem may be in the attitude of the fetal head, the mismatch of the pelvic shapes and dimensions, or the strength of contractions. After adequate labor has been ensured with oxytocin, a cesarean section is indicated. A vacuum-assisted delivery is not indicated when the patient is neither fully dilated nor completely engaged and ideally +1 or +2 station or better.

108. **(B)** Intrapartum fetal heart rate monitoring is routinely used to assess fetal well-being in labor. A rate below 100 or above 160 bpm is generally regarded as evidence of distress. The association of thick meconium with abnormal heart rate is even more predictive of distress. Therefore, rapid intervention is imperative. Supplemental oxygen can be helpful, as can maternal position change to potentially alleviate cord compression.

109. **(B)** Once delivery is accomplished, most patients show marked improvement within 48 hours. Magnesium sulfate may be used for seizure prevention. Antihypertensive medication also helps prevent complications. Only delivery is a cure.

110. **(C)** Other signs of valvular disease are a harsh, loud systolic murmur, and evidence of true cardiac enlargement. As pregnancy causes some change in cardiac contour and sounds, one must be careful that the changes noticed are not physiologic only. A diastolic murmur is always abnormal. Echocardiography can detect early abnormalities.

111. **(B)** Anemia occurs as a late manifestation of folic acid deficiency. If iron is also low, the megaloblastic character of the folate deficiency may be masked.

112. **(C)** The combination of proteinuria, hypoalbuminemia, and hyperlipidemia characterizes the nephrotic syndrome, which may be due to many causes. Generally, women with nephrosis who do not have renal insufficiency or hypertension have a successful pregnancy; however, if either of these appear, prognosis becomes increasingly poor.

113. **(C)** All of the STDs listed occur in pregnancy and should be thought of in high-risk women. Herpes, HIV, and human papillomavirus are three viral conditions that are also common in pregnancy. With maternal chlamydia, there is an increased incidence of conjunctivitis and pneumonia in the newborn, and there might be late postpartum endometritis in the mother. Chancroid is a rare disease in the United States, although it is becoming more common. The causative agent is *Haemophilus ducreyi*, which causes painful, soft, genital ulcers and is associated with painful inguinal nodes.

114. **(C)** Long-acting thyroid stimulators can cross the placenta and affect the fetus for some time after delivery. The fetus may require symptomatic therapy or even antithyroid medication.

115. **(B)** This tumor probably arises from the stromal theca cells, which become luteinized, large, and eosinophilic. Hilar cells are probably homologues of the testicular Leydig cells and may resemble hyperplastic theca lutein cells. Luteoma should regress following delivery.

116. **(D)** Urine output is extremely important, as this is the only route of excretion of $MgSO_4$, which causes marked muscle and CNS depression in overdose and can be counteracted by calcium. The distress is related to overdose,

and is not an allergic or idiopathic reaction. Respiratory arrest is perhaps the most dangerous side effect. The compound, however, has a wide margin of safety.

117. **(E)** Factor V Leiden is an abnormal Factor V that cannot bind with protein C and thus cannot be inhibited. The easiest test is an activated protein C resistance; Factor V levels will not detect this allele. The treatment is controversial but if needed it should be heparin and not baby aspirin or Coumadin. Coumadin is contraindicated in pregnancy except in the setting of mechanical heart valves.

118. **(A)** Arachidonic acid is found in several tissues, including fetal membranes and decidua. The liberation of intracellular arachidonic acid is followed by enzymatic oxidation via cyclooxygenase to form PGs.

119. **(E)** The response of circulating gonadotropins to exogenous GnRH differentiates children with true sexual precocity (exhibiting an adult-pattern rise) from those with pseudoprecocious puberty (exhibiting an attenuated, prepubertal rise). Pseudoprecocious puberty, as evidenced in this patient, is responsible for 20% to 30% of sexual precocity and does not lead to fertility. It can be due to estrogen-secreting neoplasms of the adrenal glands and ovary (e.g., gonadoblastoma, teratoma, and granulosa cell tumor) benign ovarian follicular cysts, and sex steroid-containing creams and medications. Although its mechanism is unclear, hypothyroidism is also associated with pseudoprecocious puberty and regress with thyroid hormone replacement.

120. **(B)** Serum beta-globulins increase in pregnancy, including corticosteroid-binding globulin and thyroid-binding globulin. Triglyceride levels rise two- to threefold. The elevation in free cortisol seen after the first trimester is related in part to an increase in corticotropin-releasing hormone (CRH) during pregnancy. Because of increased renal loss, serum iodide levels fall. Serum-ionized calcium levels are unchanged during pregnancy, and PTH levels remain in the low-normal range. While antibody-mediated immunity is enhanced in pregnancy, the levels of immunoglobulins A, G, and M decrease.

121. **(C)** Increased levels of erythropoietin are found, which apparently stimulate increased RBC production. Reticulocyte count is slightly elevated. However, there is a greater increase in plasma, so the hematocrit tends to drop slightly. Adequate iron supplementation will attenuate this drop. In a typical pregnancy, this increase can be the equivalent of 2 units of packed red blood cells (PRBCs).

122. **(D)** Progesterone affects both the respiratory center and the smooth muscles of the bronchi. The smooth muscles generally are relaxed by progesterone, leading to decreased GI motility and ureteral dilation, as well as bronchodilation. Tidal volume, minute volume, and oxygen uptake, all increase (see Figure 27–2).

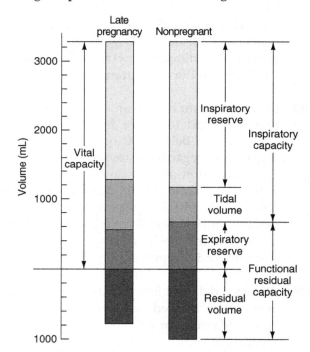

**Figure 27–2.** Lung volumes in pregnancy. (Reproduced, with permission, from DeCherney AH, Nathan L. *Current Obstetric and Gynecologic Diagnosis and Treatment,* 9th ed. New York: McGraw-Hill, 2003.)

123. **(D)** In the supine position, the compression of the inferior vena cava in late pregnancy markedly diminishes venous return, stroke volume, and cardiac output. Symptoms of

supine hypotension include dizziness, light-headedness, nausea, and even syncope. The lateral recumbent position increases cardiac output 10% to 30% over the supine position.

124. **(B)** Blood volume increases 40% to 45% in pregnancy, but plasma volume increases by 50%, whereas erythrocyte production increases by only 30%. Because of the greater increase in plasma, a physiologic anemia of pregnancy occurs and hematocrit reaches a nadir at 30 to 34 weeks' gestation. The fifth percentile of hemoglobin concentration for normal iron-supplemented women at 32 weeks' gestation is 11.0 g/dL. The Centers for Disease Control and Prevention defined *anemia* as less than 11 g/dL in the first and third trimesters and less than 10.5 g/dL in the second trimester. The woman in question has likely depleted her iron stores. All other laboratory values presented are normal for pregnancy. This woman's symptoms are those of heartburn (pyrosis), common in pregnancy, caused by reflux of gastric contents into the lower esophagus. The physical findings are normal.

125. **(D)** The fetal blood is totally contained in the fetal vascular bed and the maternal blood is in lacunae. Small amounts of fetal and maternal blood do cross the placental barrier, but they do not mix freely. Spirochetes (e.g., *Treponema pallidum*) can cross the placenta and have been known to do so. The placenta is a respiratory and excretory organ for the fetus and is capable of producing several hormones, including hCG and human placental lactogen (HPL).

126. **(B)** Surfactant, which decreases surface tension of the alveoli, is not present in high amounts until near term. Fetal breathing of amniotic fluid is present early on in pregnancy and may be an indicator of fetal well-being. Amniotic fluid is the medium allowing for prebirth lung expansion. In fact, preterm rupture of membranes at an early gestational age (<24 weeks) with resultant oligohydramnios interferes with the normal breathing process and hence pulmonary development. If severely affected, the fetus can have pulmonary hypoplasia with increased risk of neonatal death.

127. **(E)** The fetus has peristalsis by 11 weeks' gestation and swallows amniotic fluid from 16 weeks onward. Esophageal atresia should not be present since the consequent inability to effectively swallow will cause the development of hydramnios. Gastric acid and meconium continue to be produced from early on, although an extremely preterm infant may have transient deficiencies of digestive enzymes.

128. **(B)** Functional androgens with active androgen receptors are required for the phenotypic male development. In the presence of inactive androgens (androgen insensitivity syndrome), no gonads (gonadal dysgenesis), inadequate androgen production, or normally functioning ovaries, the infant phenotype will be female even though the chromosomes may be 46,XY.

129. **(C)** The muscles of the external genitalia are the ischiocavernosus, bulbocavernosus, superficial transverse perineal, and external anal sphincter. The paired bulbocavernosus muscles surround the distal vagina and vestibule on each side. The muscle originates on the perineal body and inserts into the fibrous tissue dorsal to the clitoris. It surrounds the crura of the clitoris and with the ischiocavernosus muscle contributes to the voluntary urethral sphincter, but it is not a sphincter. The ischiocavernosus muscle takes origin from the ischial tuberosity and inferior ischial ramus and inserts under the pubic symphysis on each side. Each clitoral crura is covered by the ipsilateral ischiocavernosus muscle. Contraction of these muscles allows arterial blood to flow into the body of the clitoris but inhibits venous outflow, thereby maintaining clitoral erection.

The superficial transverse perineal muscle is a muscle of the external genitalia and arises from the ischial tuberosity and inferior ischial ramus. It inserts into the central tendon between the posterior vagina and the anterior rectum, referred to as the perineal body. The perineal body serves as a central connection for all the superficial muscles of the external genitalia and also for the muscles of the anus and anal canal. The deep transverse perineal, the levators, and the gluteus muscles are deep to the

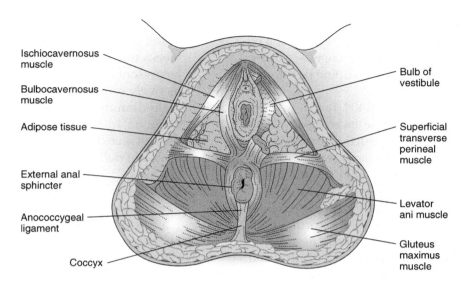

Ischiocavernosus muscle

Bulbocavernosus muscle

Adipose tissue

External anal sphincter

Anococcygeal ligament

Coccyx

Bulb of vestibule

Superficial transverse perineal muscle

Levator ani muscle

Gluteus maximus muscle

**Figure 27–3.** Inferior pelvic musculature. (Reproduced, with permission, from DeCherney AH, Nathan L. *Current Obstetric and Gynecologic Diagnosis and Treatment*, 9th ed. New York: McGraw-Hill, 2003.)

external genitalia. The sartorius is a muscle of the thigh (see Figure 27–3).

130. **(B)** *C. perfringens* is a club-shaped, gram-positive rod that produces a potent lecithinase toxin causing intravascular hemolysis. Other enzymes cause hydrolysis of glycogen, releasing hydrogen, and causing gas gangrene. *Bacteroides* and *Clostridium* are both anaerobes, and only *Clostridium* and *Enterococcus* are gram-positive.

131. **(E)** Chest pain, tachycardia, and dyspnea of sudden onset, up to 10 days postpartum, must be regarded as resulting from a pulmonary embolus until proven otherwise. Immediate tests to confirm the diagnosis should be done. Amniotic fluid emboli will occur in the immediate peripartum period. Pelvic abscess would present as pelvic pain and fever and typically more around 5 days. Myocardial infarction is a young woman without preexisting heart disease is uncommon.

132. **(E)** Patient age and degree of cytologic atypia are important factors in management planning of endometrial hyperplasia. Recent evidence suggests that the degree of cytologic atypia is the most important determinant of premalignant potential. One study found that 18%

of women with endometrial hyperplasia developed endometrial carcinoma within 1 to 30 years of initial diagnosis. In women of childbearing age desiring fertility, endometrial hyperplasia with or without cytologic atypia may be treated with progestins (e.g., OCs, medroxyprogesterone acetate, and megestrol acetate). An endometrial biopsy should be repeated in 3 to 6 months. If repeat endometrial sampling shows normal endometrium, progestins may be continued or the patient may be observed without hormone therapy for evidence of ovulation. Anovulatory patients interested in childbearing should be treated with ovulatory agents. Persistent symptomatology despite adequate therapy requires hysteroscopy combined with D&C to confirm adequacy of endometrial sampling and to identify coexisting uterine pathology. Perimenopausal women may be treated by progestins or hysterectomy, depending on severity of hyperplasia, desire for sterilization, or persistence of symptoms. Patients with moderate-to-severe atypical hyperplasia should consider hysterectomy. Individuals with lesser disease may receive progestin therapy but require hysterectomy if symptoms persist to eliminate the possibility of concomitant endometrial carcinoma or discover ovarian estrogen-producing tumors. Unless they are poor surgical candidates, most postmenopausal women with endometrial hyperplasia should consider hysterectomy with bilateral salpingo-oophorectomy, since uterine or ovarian disease may coexist.

133. **(B)** This patient with PCOS is anovulatory, as confirmed by the absence of a biphasic shift in BBTs. Acyclic estrogen production unopposed by progesterone stimulates endometrial proliferation, increasing the risk of developing endometrial hyperplasia and carcinoma. In patients desiring to preserve fertility, high-dose protesting such as 10-20 mg of MPA is appropriate. A biopsy should be repeated in 3 to 6 months. If the biopsy is then normal, she may need ovulation induction. The method of choice for this patient with PCOS is clomiphene citrate. Intramuscular administration of hMGs is expensive and inconvenient and requires close monitoring.

134. **(D)** Important prognostic indicators of survival from endometrial carcinoma include (1) histologic tumor type, (2) grade of tumor differentiation, (3) lymphatic/hematogenous spread, and (4) stage of disease at the time of detection. The histologic types papillary serous and clear cell confer the highest risk of poor prognosis. They are biologically more aggressive tumors. They have a higher propensity for lymphovascular invasion, and intraperitoneal as well as extra-abdominal spread. Stage of disease is inversely correlated with 5-year survival rate (stage I, 86%; stage II, 66%; stage III, 44%; stage IV, 16%). In stage I disease, depth of myometrial invasion by tumor is an important prognostic factor. Tumor penetration beyond the middle half of the myometrium adversely affects survival and relapse rates. Malignant cells in peritoneal washings are found in 12% to 15% of women with early disease by clinical assessment and reduce the chance for survival. Other tumor indicators of poor prognosis are size (>2 cm), absence of sex steroid receptors, and DNA ploidy. Many of these prognostic indicators are interrelated and occur together. Five-year survival rates range from 95% (in women with well-differentiated tumors that do not invade the myometrium) to 20% (in patients with poorly differentiated tumors that invade deeply into

the myometrium). CA-125 may be of value only in the case of advanced disease for follow-up of these patients.

135. **(A)** Exploratory laparotomy with complete surgical cytoreduction is the most important aspect of ovarian carcinoma management because it establishes the diagnosis, serves as effective therapy, and determines the extent of disease for planning of adjunctive therapy. Most patients will need adjuvant chemotherapy as determined by final stage and histologic type. Radiation plays no significant role in ovarian cancer management.

136. **(A)** Important prognostic indicators of survival from ovarian carcinoma include stage of the disease, age of the patient, and amount of residual tumor after surgery. The stage of ovarian malignancy is inversely correlated with the 5-year survival rate. Poorly differentiated (high-grade) tumors are commonly diagnosed in advanced stages, while well-differentiated (low-grade) tumors tend to be diagnosed in earlier stages. Grade is not incorporated into the FIGO classification of ovarian cancer. Grade is a useful prognostic indicator in early-stage cancer, but this has not been proven in advanced stages. Older women are more likely than younger women to have advanced stage, poorly differentiated tumors. Moreover, women over age 50 have a worse prognosis than younger women after correction for tumor stage and grade. Individuals with residual tumor masses less than 2 to 3 cm in size after surgery have a longer length of survival than those with larger amounts of disease.

137. **(B)** Serous tumors, whether benign or malignant, tend to form calcific "sand-like" concretions, called psammoma bodies (from the Greek word *psammos*, meaning sand). Serous tumors may have papillations, or excrescences, on their external or internal surfaces. Excrescences do not prove malignancy, so one should wait for histologic examination before deciding further surgical management. Serous cystadenomas have a malignancy rate of 30%.

**138. (D)** Highly specialized teratomas include carcinoid and struma ovarii. Primary ovarian carcinoid originates from GI or respiratory epithelium within a teratoma. It is diagnosed by finding an elevation in the amount of urinary 5-hydroxyindoleacetic acid. One-third of cases produce the carcinoid syndrome (paroxysmal flushing of the face and neck, colicky abdominal pain with diarrhea, and asthma-like respiratory distress). Although the tumor is usually benign and treated by simple excision, malignant transformation is possible.

**139. (C)** Gonadectomy is indicated at the time the abnormality is detected because of the risk of malignancy. These patients can develop gonadoblastoma or malignant germ cell tumors (primarily dysgerminoma). Gonadectomy is indicated regardless of the location of the gonad. These abnormal gonads are almost always useless for fertility and many will become virilized, but the primary reason for removal is the cancer risk.

**140. (B)** One type of metastatic ovarian tumor is Krukenberg's tumor. It is characterized histologically by nests of mucin-filled cells with a "signet ring" appearance in a cellular stroma. Krukenberg's tumors form large, bilateral masses, containing gelatinous necrosis and hemorrhage. They usually arise in the GI tract, primarily the stomach. The next most frequent primary site of origin is the large intestine. These tumors occasionally arise from the breast and other mucus-producing organs, such as the appendix and urinary bladder.

**141. (D)** There are three predominant histologic types of ovarian tissue. They are the serosa (germinal epithelium), germ cells, and stromal cells, which are divided into undifferentiated stroma and specialized stroma. Neoplasms may be derived from each of these histologic types. Other neoplasms may be metastatic to the ovary. Dysgerminoma and teratomas are derived from the germ cells, not from the germinal epithelium. Fibromas are derived from the stroma and granulosa thecal cell tumors from the specialized stroma. Germinal epithelium is a misnomer. It does not give rise to

germ cells or tumors derived from germ cells. Epithelial tumors of the ovary (serous, mucinous, and endometrioid) derive from it. There may also be mixed forms of tumor, but they are rare.

**142. (A)** Many breast cancers may take 8 to 10 years to reach a palpable size. Mammograms may detect them several years before they become palpable. On the other hand, many breast cancers can be palpated that are not seen on mammograms. The clinical examination and mammography are complementary. While there are differences of opinion regarding when mammogram screening should begin and how often it should be performed in premenopausal women, there is agreement that all post-menopausal women 50 and older should have mammographic screening every 1 year (ACOG and ACS) or 2 years (USPTF). ACOG now recommends that women should be offered a screening mammography at age 40 and then every 1-2 years. There are groups of high-risk patients such as those shown to be at genetic risk, who should begin screening in their thirties. Mammographic lesions are more difficult to detect in young women that lesions in postmenopausal women because the density of the young women's breast tissue is greater. Their breast parenchyma has not yet been replaced by less dense fat. Women over 50 should have regular mammograms. Screening should not be stopped at age 70. Unlike many other cancers the longer a woman lives the more likely she is to get breast cancer.

**143. (E)** Paget's carcinoma of the breast is uncommon. It classically presents as itching and an erosion. Biopsy of the erosion makes the diagnosis. There may be no palpable mass, and the mammogram is unlikely to help in making the diagnosis. There are two learning points here: (1) Breast pruritus is an uncommon complaint and (2) a physical finding suggestive of tissue destruction merits biopsy.

**144. (D)** Any breast nodule in a postmenopausal woman should be biopsied immediately. Aspiration may be indicated for cystic masses during the menstrual years but has no place in this age group. Therapy, of course, is dependent on the pathology. If you do not perform radical breast surgery, immediate referral for biopsy and further care is indicated.

145. **(D)** Primary infection with the varicella-zoster virus causes chickenpox, which has an attack rate of 90% in seronegative individuals. Fortunately, over three-quarters of adults are immune from prior symptomatic or asymptomatic infection. Therefore, the best course of action is to determine whether this patient is immune. If so, nothing more need be done. If not, then administration of VZIG within 96 hours of exposure is recommended to attenuate varicella infection. The varicella vaccine, a live, attenuated vaccine, is not recommended for pregnant women and would not be effective in preventing infection after exposure has already occurred. Finally, IV acyclovir is recommended for the treatment of varicella pneumonia, which has been found to lower the mortality rate in pregnancy from 35% to 15%.

146. **(E)** While this woman meets the standard criteria for PID on the basis of clinical criteria, her history is disparate with this diagnosis. Admitting and treating for a disease she is unlikely to have "in order to see how things go" is poor medicine. Culdocentesis has generally fallen out of favor, because if you find pus, it will not tell where the pus comes from. Pelvic ultrasound or CT may reveal an ovarian mass or appendicitis; however, she is displaying signs of an acute abdomen and thus waiting for these tests would only delay necessary surgery for evaluation and management. Diagnostic laparoscopy should be used in cases in which the diagnosis is unclear. In this case, it was appendicitis.

147. **(D)** Osteitis pubis occurs 2.5% of the time following MMK. It probably occurs because of suture placement in the periosteum covering the pubic rami. The condition can be incapacitating. ESR is elevated. The treatment is bed rest, pain medications, and anti-inflammatory agents. The condition is self-limiting, although it can last for months.

148. **(B)** Pubovaginal slings can be performed with autologous or synthetic, inorganic materials. Autologous materials have less risk of infection and subsequent poor healing. Given her prior radiation and increased risk of poor healing, Mersilene was probably not a good choice, and urethral erosion is a serious risk.

149. **(H)** Women who are positive for Ro (SSA) and La (SSB) often have infants with heart blocks, which can lead to hydrops. These antibodies, or systemic lupus erythematosus (SLE) antibodies, can cross the placenta and cause fibrosis and inflammation of the fetal cardiac conducting system.

150. **(C)** Parvovirus ($B_{19}$) infection of the mother is often mild and causes few symptoms, one of which is a red face—the slapped-cheek sign—along with low-grade fever, mild arthritis, and a faint rash on the trunk and extremities. The fetus may have a transient aplastic crisis with anemia and high-output congestive heart failure. It is diagnosed by testing for maternal immunoglobulin M (IgM) and immunoglobulin G (IgG) antibodies to parvovirus.

# References

Agency for Health Care Policy and Research. *Clinical Handbook of Preventive Services.* 2nd ed. Washington, DC: US Department of Health and Human Services, 1998.

Beckman CRB, Ling F, Smith RP, Barzansky BM, Herbert WN, Laube DW. *Obstetrics and Gynecology.* 5th ed. Baltimore, MD: Williams & Wilkins, 2006.

Carr BR, Blackwell RE, Azziz R. *Essential Reproductive Medicine.* New York: McGraw-Hill, 2005.

Copeland LJ, Jarrell JF. *Textbook of Gynecology.* 2nd ed. Philadelphia, PA: WB Saunders, 2000.

Cunningham FG, Leveno KJ, Bloom S, Gilstrap LC, Hauth JC, Wenstrom KD. *Williams Obstetrics.* 22nd ed. New York: McGraw-Hill, 2005.

DeCherney AH, Nathan L. *Current Obstetric and Gynecologic Diagnosis and Treatment.* 10th ed. New York: McGraw-Hill, 2007.

Greenspan FS, Strewlar GJ. *Basic and Clinical Endocrinology.* 6th ed. New York: McGraw-Hill, 2001.

Lemcke DP, Pattison J, Marshall LA, Cowley DS. *Current Care of Women, Diagnosis and Treatment.* New York: McGraw-Hill, 2004.

Ling FW, Duff P. *Gynecology: Principles for Practice.* New York: McGraw-Hill Medical Publishing Division, 2001.

# Index

Note: Page numbers followed by an "*f*" denote figures and those followed by a "*t*" denote tables respectively.

Lightning Source UK Ltd.
Milton Keynes UK
UKOW05f0727270717

306141UK00009B/55/P